Rachael Prendergast

PROFESSIONAL ISSUES IN SPEECH-LANGUAGE PATHOLOGY AND AUDIOLOGY: A TEXTBOOK

Professional Issues In Speech-Language Pathology and Audiology: A Textbook

Edited by

ROSEMARY LUBINSKI, Ed.D.

CAROL FRATTALI, Ph.D.

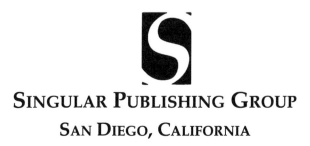

SINGULAR PUBLISHING GROUP

SAN DIEGO, CALIFORNIA

Published by Singular Publishing Group, Inc.
4284 41st Street
San Diego, California 92105-1197
©1994 by Singular Publishing Group, Inc.

Typeset in 10/12 Palatino by So Cal Graphics
Printed in the United States of America by BookCrafters

Library of Congress Cataloging-in Publication Data

Professional issues in speech-language pathology and audiology: a textbook/edited by
  Rosemary Lubinski, Carol Frattali.
      p.   cm.
    Includes bibliographical references and index.
    ISBN 1-56593-171-8
    1. Speech therapy—Practice.   2. Audiology—Practice.   I. Lubinski, Rosemary.
  II. Frattali, Carol.
    [DNLM: 1. Speech-Language Pathology.   2. Audiology.   3. Professional Practice.
    WM 475 P9635 1994]
  RC428.5.P755 1994
  616.85′5—dc20
  DNLM/DLC
  for Library of Congress   93-44521
                                                                          CIP

■ CONTENTS ■

SECTION I. OVERVIEW OF THE PROFESSIONS

SECTION II. EMPLOYMENT OPPORTUNITIES AND ISSUES

■ CONTRIBUTORS ■

Dolores Battle, Ph.D.
Associate Professor
Dept. of Communication Disorders
State University College at Buffalo
Buffalo, New York

Marlene Bevan, Ph.D.
Audiologist, Private Practice
Audicare Hearing Center
Traverse City, Michigan

Bonnie A. Curl, M.S.
Information Manager
Health Services Division
American Speech-Language-Hearing
   Association
Rockville, Maryland

Carol Frattali, Ph.D.
Director, Health Services Division
American Speech-Language-Hearing
   Association
Rockville, Maryland

Therese Goldsmith, M.S.
Assistant Director
Speech-Language Pathology Service
National Rehabilitation Hospital
Washington, D.C.

Hortensia Kayser, Ph.D.
Postdoctoral Fellow
Center for Neurogenic Communication
   Disorders
University of Arizona
Tucson, Arizona

Rebecca Kooper, J.D.
Educational Audiologist
Nassau BOCES
Program for the Hearing Impaired
Long Beach, New York

Angela Loavenbruck, Ed.D.
Audiologist, Private Practice
New City, New York

Rosemary Lubinski, Ed.D.
Associate Professor
Dept. of Communicative Disorders
   and Sciences
Clinical Associate Professor
Dept. of Otolaryngology
University of Buffalo, SUNY
Amherst, New York

Jane R. Madell, Ph.D.
Director of Communicative Disorders
Long Island Medical College
Associate Professor of Otolaryngology
SUNY Health Sciences Center
Brooklyn, New York

M. Gay Masters, Ph.D.
Clinical Assistant Professor
Dept. of Communicative Disorders and Sciences
University of Buffalo, SUNY
Amherst, New York

Nancy J. Minghetti, M.A.
Deputy Executive Director
American Speech-Language-Hearing Foundation
Rockville, Maryland

Judith B. Montgomery, Ph.D.
Assistant Professor of Special Education
Chapman University
Orange, California

Paul Rao, Ph. D.
Director, Speech-Language Pathology Service
National Rehabilitation Hospital
Washington, D.C.

Judith A. Rassi, M.A.
Director of Clinical Education
Associate Professor
Vanderbilt University
School of Medicine
Division of Hearing and Speech Sciences
Nashville, Tennessee

Charlena M. Seymour, Ph.D.
Professor
Department of Communication Disorders
University of Massachusetts
Amherst, Massachusetts

Cynthia M. Shewan, Ph.D.
Senior Vice President of Research, Analysis
  and Development
American Physical Therapy Association
Alexandria, Virginia

Becky Sutherland Cornett, Ph.D.
Director, Speech Pathology Dept.
The Ohio State University Hospitals
Columbus, Ohio

Peggy S. Williams, Ph.D.
Deputy Executive Director
American Speech-Language-Hearing
  Association
Rockville, Maryland

Margo E. Wilson, Ph.D.
Speech-Language Pathologist,
Private Practice
Scottsdale, Arizona

■ FOREWORD ■

I am very pleased to have been asked to write a Foreword for *Professional Issues in Speech-Language Pathology and Audiology: A Textbook.* I occasionally teach the University of Arizona's departmental graduate proseminar in this area, and have longed for just such a text. For a wide range of professional issues affecting practitioners (and future practitioners) of Speech-Language Pathology and Audiology, there has been no place where these materials are gathered together. What I particularly appreciate about this textbook is that the materials are gathered together in a well-organized, current, and principled way.

This compilation has had the advantage of being organized by two individuals with unmatched experience in recognizing the importance of grounding students not only in the discipline and its scientific underpinnings, but in the professional context of prac-

tice. Rosemary Lubinski and Carol Frattali represent the discipline with experience in the most critical of professional issues. Their breadth of understanding permitted them to choose a group of uniquely qualified authors for this book's broad coverage of issues relevant to both Audiology and Speech-Language Pathology.

This is a textbook, to be sure, but it has two broader functions as well. The first is as a reference book. Most practitioners would do well to have a copy handy for referral. But it also serves a unique spot in the history of the professions. Because it deals so directly with issues that affect the practice in this time of great change and upheaval, and because it so clearly tells its readers how to seek more help and to stay current, a future historian of the professions will likely value it as much as we do today.

Audrey L. Holland, Ph.D.
University of Arizona

■ PREFACE ■

Three words capture the essence of the professions of audiology and speech-language pathology: caring, diversity, and change. We come with a need to assist others in their ability to communicate and do this through clinical service, research, administration, and teaching. We come from many cultural and geographical backgrounds, take an array of course work ranging from basic sciences to clinical disorders and blend these with supervised clinical experiences involving a variety of clients and in a variety of settings. We are truly an integrated science in that we have bases in anatomy and physiology, neurology, psychology and behavioral studies, linguistics, electronics, education, and physics, as well as traditional courses in hearing, speech, and language disorders. We are also professions that are technology-driven—from our use of alternative and assistive communication devices and systems to instrumental diagnostic procedures and automated management information systems. We are challenged by the diversity and complexity of our clients' problems, by the need to translate clinical research into functional outcomes for our clients, and by the need for continuing education to stay abreast of developments in the field. But this is just the beginning.

Our professional lives lie within a much broader context that reflects a spectrum of national issues and trends. To remain competitive and viable in today's society, audiologists and speech-language pathologists must also be aware of issues affecting our professional service. Individually and collectively, these issues affect our service delivery and include the cultural and epidemiological makeup of our country, political and economic climates, and health care, education, and social priorities. Today's clinician must look beyond the clinic door to the changing social, economic, and political arena to clearly understand who we are, whom we serve, what we do, and how we do it.

This text, *Professional Issues in Speech-Language Pathology and Audiology: A Textbook,* arose from the need to introduce readers to the scope of professional issues facing clinicians today and expected in the future. The text presents a scope of current and critical issues that are shaping our professional lives. The text also challenges the reader to go beyond the written word through debate and discussion.

The text is divided into six sections. Section I, Overview of the Professions, introduces you to our discipline of human communication sciences and disorders and the professions of speech-language pathology and audiology. This section includes issues related to professional education, certification and licensure, standards, ethics, and the professions in other countries. Section II focuses on Employment Opportunities and Issues. Topics here include epidemiological issues that help us understand who our clients are and who we are as professionals. It also includes a discussion of ways to prepare for employment and an introduction to the changing populations we serve and the diversity of clinical settings. Sections III and IV feature federal legislation and service delivery issues in health care and school settings. Section V concentrates on topics that promote a high quality of care. These topics include the policy and procedural manual, quality improvement, marketing, infection prevention, and professional liability. Section VI, the last section of the book, highlights some of the most current professional issues facing us: multiculturalism, supervision, functional assessment, autonomy, burnout, and the professional doctorate.

Each chapter begins with a section entitled Scope of Chapter in which the major topics of the chapter are introduced. This is followed by the body of the chapter in which the topic is discussed in detail. Each chapter concludes with a Summary, Discussion Questions, References, and Resources (if appropriate). We hope that you will consider additional discussion questions that arise as you read the text.

The authors of the chapters—audiologists and speech-language pathologists—were selected from several perspectives. Each person has a particular interest in the topic discussed. The authors are practitioners, administrators, and/or academicians. All have served the professions of audiology and speech-language pathology at the national, state, and local levels. All contributors have devoted their work to improving our professional practices.

The professions of speech-language pathology and audiology have a rich although relatively short history. Maturity will develop partly as a result of insightful and critical discussion of professional issues among colleagues both within and outside the discipline. This process allows our roots to go deeper and our professions to branch out meaningfully to meet the needs of a changing society.

■ ACKNOWLEDGMENTS ■

The editors of this book would like to offer sincere appreciation to each of the chapter authors for their contributions to this text. We thank you for your willingness to participate and to generously share your expertise and time.

The following chapter authors wish to acknowledge assistance they received in preparation of their manuscripts:

Carol Frattali: would like to thank the following individuals from the American Speech-Language-Hearing Association National Office staff for their assistance, direction, or review and comments on various chapters throughout the book: Amie Amiot, Zenobia Bagli; Evelyn Cherow; Constance Lynch; Susan Karr; Mark Kander; Vickie King; Roger Kingsley; Janet McCarty; Mary Beth Nowinski; Sarah Slater; Maureen Thompson; and Cheryl Wohl. I would like to extend special gratitude to Steven White for his careful review and substantive comments on Chapter 14, Health Care Legislation: Implications for Financing and Service Delivery.

Rosemary Lubinski: would like to thank the following persons for their assistance in preparing or reviewing her chapters: Joan Arvedson, Terri Cinotti, Jack Katz, Janet Mahar, Rose Nager, and Richard Welland.

Nancy Minghetti: would like to thank Judith Cooper, James Gelatt, Leslie Olswang, Brad Stach, and Lisa Tolino for sharing insights and thoughtful comments during preparation of this chapter.

Cynthia M.Shewan: would like to thank Sarah Slater for her expert help with the tables and figures in her chapters. Thanks are also given to the American Speech-Language-Hearing Association for facilitating this work and generously providing me with access to the data used in the chapters.

■ DEDICATION ■

To our parents, the memory of Leo and Agnes Lubinski, and August and Rita Frattali
for a lifetime of unselfish love and steadfast support.

CHAPTER 1

Overview of the Professions: Beginning the Dialogue

■ ROSEMARY LUBINSKI, Ed.D. ■
■ CAROL FRATTALI, Ph.D. ■

SCOPE OF CHAPTER

"Talking is what keeps me alive." This quote from an 80-year-old nursing facility resident illustrates in its simple elegance how vital communication is to our existence. Our ability to communicate involves reception of auditory, visual, and other sensory information; integration of this information; conceptual and motor formulation of a reply; and some combination of oral, written, or nonverbal expression of thoughts. A breakdown somewhere in this chain creates difficulty for communication partners to successfully engage in this important human process. When such breakdowns occur, a natural reaction by communication partners is to seek assistance in developing the needed communication skills, in repairing the difficulties, or in facilitating interaction through any means possible. The professions of speech-language pathology and audiology are uniquely devoted to meeting these needs.

The professions of speech-language pathology and audiology are relatively new within the broad scope of helping professions— although the need to communicate and the natural inclination to help when communication difficulties occur have been eternal. When you decided to enter one of these professions you had some internal recognition or real-life experience that inspired you to pledge your professional life to helping others communicate. Providing this assistance is governed not only by your recognition of the value of communication, your cognitive and interpersonal skills and internal needs, but also by a vast and dynamic array of societal and professional issues. As a speech-language pathologist or audiologist you will need to develop and refine your knowledge base about normal communication development and communication disorders, *and* you will need to be aware of and conversant in the many issues that directly, powerfully, and continually influence where, how, and with whom you practice your profession.

This chapter will raise your consciousness and open a dialogue about issues that will influence your professional life. Provision of high quality services emanates from practitioners who are knowledgeable about the amalgam of ever-changing societal, political, and economic factors that influence these services. After reading this chapter, and indeed this text, you may say "I just wanted to help people communicate." Yet, for practicing clinicians, you are likely to say, "but the authors forgot to mention X issue and Y issue."

Today, professional issues affecting our service delivery stem both from trends external to our professions and from internal dynamics. External trends reflect long-term, global societal changes. Two such changes include technology breakthroughs and concern for our national economy. The rapid technological advances of the last 10 to 20 years influence our everyday and professional lives in countless, but often unrecognized, ways. The high-risk infant who may not have survived years ago may become the preschooler with language-learning problems. New client populations (e.g., individuals with AIDS, multicultural populations, those receiving cochlear implants) require that our professions develop the expertise necessary to provide effective and efficient services. Further, changes in our national economy influence funding sources and thus determine who will receive services, by whom, for how long, and with what expected outcomes.

Regardless of the source or immediacy of an issue, viable professions must constantly face, analyze, and prepare to meet issues that are both current and looming. Academic and clinical preparation is not enough. Speech-language pathologists and audiologists who are in the vanguard of service delivery must recognize the broad scope of matters that determine our professional practice and shape our future. Professionals must be prepared to articulate, justify, and implement alternatives that place us on the cutting edge. Unless our professions assume responsibility for tackling these issues, we will be in defensive, reactive positions rather than in control of our professional destinies.

This chapter introduces a range of current issues affecting our professional practice and sets the framework for the remainder of the book. The issues are addressed broadly. The text is designed to stimulate your thinking and dialogue with yourself and others to explore the issues influencing your professional practice.

MODEL OF PROFESSIONAL ISSUES

The model of professional issues presented here is a theoretical construct of the variety of issues affecting our service delivery as speech-language pathologists and audiologists. This is only *one* model, and undoubtedly others could be constructed and factors added, eliminated, or described differently. This model is based on systems theory, as the individual components are not as important as their relationship with each other in forming a dynamic whole. Although factors are divided into those emanating from external and from internal forces, this division is somewhat artificial. Our professions simultaneously react to and initiate new ideas; our work reciprocally enhances and is enhanced by interaction with other disciplines and the larger society. Further, our professions may be influenced differentially by these issues as will individual practitioners in various settings and with diverse clientele.

EXTERNAL ISSUES

In a 1991 guest editorial in *Asha* magazine, D. C. Spriestersbach (1991) reminds us that "We are part of the planet, you know!" In this article, Spriestersbach identifies eight current issues he believes influence our individual and professional lives. These include: the (a) increasing world population; (b) changes in world health needs; (c) growing alienation of the underclass; (d) increasing population of minorities in the United States; (e) national fiscal situation; (f) technological factors influencing national productivity; (g) tension between the needs of the larger society and those of the individual; and (h) demands to change health care delivery and financing in the United States. These factors are merged with others to define the issues affecting all aspects of our society as well as our professional service delivery. A brief discussion of each issue follows to stimulate your thinking and discussion.

Changing Demographics and Diversity of Clinical Populations

As will be mentioned in several chapters in this text, the population of the United States is not only increasing but is changing. At least two of these demographic changes have important implications for speech-language pathologists and audiologists: the aging of America and the growing cultural diversity within the population. In 1990, individuals over the age of 65 constituted more than 12% of the U.S. population. This population continues to grow rapidly and may approach 22% of the population by 2040, with the largest increases among those beyond 85 years of age (*Statistical Abstracts of the United States, 1992*). Such precipitous growth among the older population will create demand for services from both speech-language pathologists and audiologists. Among this population the increasing prevalence of presbycusis, dysphagia, and neurological disorders such as stroke and dementia will intensify this demand.

Similarly, the continuing increase in the number of minorities in the United States challenges our professions to provide appropriate services to these diverse populations. In the period 1980 to 1990, the percentage of increase among African Americans was 13.2%; 37.9% among American Indians, Eskimos, or Aleuts; 107.8 % among Asian or Pacific Islanders; and 53% among those of Hispanic origin (*Statistical Abstracts of the United States*, 1992). What we have not seen, however, is significant growth in the number of speech pathologists and audiologists who are from minority backgrounds. Only about

4.5% of our practioners are from such backgrounds (Keough, 1990). (See Chapter 9 by Shewan on characteristics of members of the American Speech-Language-Hearing Association [ASHA], Chapter 22 by Kayser on multiculturalism, and Chapter 12 by Lubinski and Masters on special populations and settings for more in-depth discussions.)

Increasing Number of High-Risk and Clinically Complex Populations

The clients we serve are also presenting with more complex needs: from the premature babies of substance abusing mothers and elderly nursing facility residents with a multitude of physical, sensory, and psychological problems to adolescent head trauma survivors who must return to school and persons who are multiply and severely disabled whose communication can be tapped with assistive communication devices. Today we serve clients with AIDS, dementia, dysphagia, and cochlear implants. The problems that each of these population groups and their families present are far more involved than that of the traditional client with a frontal lisp. (See Chapter 12 by Lubinski and Masters on special populations and Chapter 21 by Lubinski on infection prevention.)

Changing Societal Conceptions of Disability

Historically, Americans have had an approach–avoidance attitude toward those with disabilities, including those with communication problems. On the one hand, Americans tend to be compassionate and altruistic and pride themselves for a spirit of equality. On the other hand, many of these same persons feel a certain physical and psychological aversion to individuals with disabilities. This uneasiness may stem from prejudicial and stereotypic images of those with disabilities largely created by media, inadequate opportunities for interaction with these individuals, discriminatory and exclusionary laws, and the unfortunate and often permanent labels given to those with disabilities by service providers (Spiegel, Simon, & Fiorito, 1981). Henderson and Bryan (1984) state that, "even the most liberal of individuals do not treat all people the same" (p. 31).

These conflicting attitudes translate into social action and, hence, laws such as the Americans with Disabilities Act—considered to be the most important civil rights legislation for individuals with disabilities. Nevertheless, it is not axiomatic in our society, particularly in times of cost containment, that every individual with a disability will receive needed services for an unlimited amount of time at the expense of third-party payers. There appears to be a rapidly growing mandate that services must be clearly justified, have relevance to a person's everyday life, and be for a predetermined length of time. Society will pay only for so much assessment and intervention and that amount has to be perceived as functionally useful to integrating the individual into the mainstream of home, school, work, and community. Erikson (1981) stated that all human service professionals must be required to define "what is helpful?" (Chapter 24 by Frattali on functional assessment addresses the critical need for changes in our assessment process.)

Ongoing Health Care Reform

Dramatic changes lie ahead for how health care in this country will be financed and delivered. The health care system is encountering a complete philosophic shift from a "more is better" to a "more with less" approach. The current system is one of many contradictions. We spend more on health care than any other industrialized nation, yet 37 million Americans are without care (Schieber & Poullier, 1991). We are reputed to have the best health care in the world, yet we have one of the highest infant mortality rates among industrialized countries (Lewit & Monheit, 1992). We have the most advanced life saving technologies, yet these advances are creating ethical dilemmas (Callahan, 1990). For example,

Americans are living longer but with increasingly complex and chronic medical problems diminishing quality of life. Are the burgeoning costs associated with managing these medical problems worth the extension of life if the individual is devoid of self-sufficiency, vocational or avocation abilities, and meaningful social relationships?

Current reform proposals carry common themes that will substantially alter our traditional service delivery models. These proposals consistently focus on cost controls, prevention, meaningful patient outcomes, equal access, professional collaboration, and practitioner accountability. Our services will be judged by their "value"—that is, the provision of services using the most cost-effective means. Practitioner credentials will be deemphasized and practitioner competence as measured by results emphasized. Thus, health care reforms will open the door to greater overlap of service provision by professionals from other fields. Coordination of care and professional collaboration will be requisite. You may be required to develop or follow critical paths—coordinated maps that chart the flow of clinical care for a specific diagnosis by all practitioners involved in providing that care. You may also find it in your best interest to form interdisciplinary alliances with other professionals and to package your services within a broader context, such as stroke rehabilitation or hearing health care, to successfully negotiate contracts with managed care plans. And most definitely, you will be required to quantify your practice. In other words, you will need to develop plans of treatment using accepted standards of care or clinical guidelines (that are ideally derived from available efficacy studies) and document the effectiveness of treatment using reliable and valid outcome measures (including functional outcome measures and measures of patients' judgments of treatment). (See Chapters 19 and 24 by Frattali on functional assessment and quality improvement.)

Health care reform will shatter some perceived models of service delivery. The traditional one-on-one approach to client care provided by a certified speech-language pathologist or audiologist may be just one of several service delivery options. The use of support personnel under the supervision of qualified professionals, a perhaps more cost-effective means of service delivery, will become more widespread, as will interdisciplinary team models of service, computer-assisted treatment, and increased family participation in treatment. More than ever, we will be challenged to be flexible and innovative in providing services to those with communication disorders who are entitled to be treated. In fact, the degree to which we can be flexible and innovative will dictate our ability to compete effectively in a reformed health care system.

Growing Emphasis on Outcome
Measurement and Quality Improvement

As long as we have rendered clinical care, we have been asked to provide objective evidence of the outcome of our services. We have been queried by hospital-based directors of rehabilitation programs, third-party payers, physicians, and local or state education officials, among others who have a stake in service delivery. As early as the 1960s, we were asked to translate such information into functional terms or terms relevant to a client's everyday life skills. Thirty years later, we have made little progress in the development and universal use of reliable and valid instruments for measuring functional outcomes. The consequences today, in the absence of data derived from the use of outcome measures, may be a loss of competitive position and, thus, jobs in the education and health care systems.

Practitioners must be able to answer the question, "Does clinical intervention make a difference?" This question, asked by policy makers on a national scale, has prompted the creation of federal agencies, restructuring of accreditation agency standards, and funding of national demonstration projects to underscore the importance of outcome evaluation and its relationship to improved quality of care. The Federal Agency for Health Care

Policy and Research within the U.S. Public Health Service was created, in part, to promote improvements in clinical practice and patient outcomes through more appropriate and effective health care services (Agency for Health Care Policy and Research, 1990). Its Center for Medical Effectiveness Research supports extramural research on treatment effectiveness and client outcomes. Research conducted under this program addresses the following questions: Do clients benefit? What treatments work best? Are resources well spent? The Joint Commission on Accreditation of Healthcare Organizations (JCAHO), a private, nonprofit agency that accredits a range of health care programs, is nearing completion of its ambitious "Agenda for Change." The Agenda for Change includes the development of clinical indicators and the restructuring of accreditation standards from ones that evaluate the capability to perform to ones that evaluate actually performance (Joint Commission on Accreditation of Healthcare Organizations, 1987). Finally, the National Demonstration Project on Quality Improvement in Health Care (Berwick, Godfrey, & Roessner, 1990), hosted by the Harvard Community Health Plan, was a 1-year project designed to answer this question: Can the tools of modern quality improvement with which other industries have achieved breakthroughs in performance (or outcomes) help in health care as well? Twenty-one health care organizations participated in this national endeavor and conducted a series of pilot team projects. The project documented some early successes in the ability to use measures of quality from the manufacturing industry and apply them to the human services industry.

Quality improvement is becoming more science than art—more objective measurement than subjective judgment. It often involves the use of statistical tools and a sound methodology that borrows from the works of Deming (1986) and Juran (1988), two statisticians who made important contributions to improving the quality in the manufacturing industry. To build on the knowledge base pertaining to clinical outcomes, professionals must now be versed and skilled in quality improvement methods. These methods should be integrated into routine professional practice, rather than regarded as an activity external to professional activities—another profound change for today's professionals.

Burgeoning Technological Advances

In the early years of the professions, the use of technology played a relatively small role in clinical care. Audiometric screening and evaluation procedures were perhaps the most technological of procedures conducted by speech-language pathologists and audiologists, respectively. With advances in technology came digital hearing aids, more instrumental diagnostic procedures, and computerized augmentative and alternative communication devices and systems. Today, technology plays a large and vital role in the course of clinical care. You need just consider national practice guidelines, developed recently by the ASHA Ad Hoc Committee on Advances in Clinical Practice (ASHA, 1992), to appreciate the breadth of technology applied currently in the field:

■ Balance function assessment (involves the use of computerized electronystagmography and ocular motor tests, rotational tests of the vestibularocular reflex, and dynamic posturography)
■ Electrical stimulation for cochlear implant selection and rehabilitation (entails the application of electrical current to the audiovestibular nerve to assess its integrity, monitor functional status of electrodes during surgery, or determine parameters for cochlear implant operation)
■ Evaluation and treatment for tracheoesophageal fistulization/puncture (TEF) (involves the ability to interpret videoaudiographic findings, and fitting a TEF prosthesis)
■ Instrumental diagnostic procedures for swallowing (includes the use of videofluorography, ultrasonography, scintigraphy, fiberoptic endoscopic examination of swallowing, electromyography, and manometry)

■ Neurophysiologic intraoperative monitoring (involves electrophysiologic measurement and interpretation of myogenic and neural responses to intraoperative events or modality-specific, controlled stimulation during the course of surgery)
■ Vocal tract visualization and imaging (includes the use of endoscopy).

As clinicians, you must stay abreast of advances in the field. Technological, as well as scientific advances, carry an inherent mandate to upgrade skills to maintain clinical competencies. Clinicians performing such procedures must also be aware of state licensure restrictions on scope of practice, informed consent issues, infection prevention, safety, professional liability, and the need for emergency protocols.

Increasing Litigation

In today's world, malpractice suits are at an all-time high. To date, however, this trend is not evident for the professions of audiology and speech-language pathology. Lawsuits, however, are not unusual in the field. ASHA members, with their multiple professional responsibilities, often are exposed to the risk of a lawsuit or penalty (ASHA, 1990a). The following are just a sampling of claims that have been paid under the Albert H. Wohlers and Company plan (the professional liability plan that is offered by ASHA):

■ $101,430—An ASHA member was accused of leaving hearing aid impression material in the ear of a client.
■ $97,037—An ASHA member allegedly failed to properly test an infant for hearing loss.
■ $53,724—A 2-year-old child swallowed the battery of a hearing aid that had been prescribed by an ASHA member.

Today, it is inconceivable to practice your profession without liability coverage. You must be aware of the potential risks associated with working in your profession. As the professions continue to engage in invasive or technologically complex procedures that carry an element of risk, and as society becomes more aware of these associated risks, practitioners must take individual responsibility for their own potential exposure to liability. (See Chapter 13 by Kooper on liability for further discussion of this topic.)

Education Reform

In 1983, a landmark report titled "A Nation at Risk" was released (Boyer, 1983). According to the ASHA Ad Hoc Committee on Changes in Educational Policies and Practices (ASHA, in progress), the report, warning of a rising tide of mediocrity, spawned a decade of educational reform initiatives aimed at regaining a competitive edge globally in the academic preparation of American students. Consequently, a multipronged approach involving national, state, and local governments; school boards; corporate businesses; and citizen groups is redesigning the educational system in this country. These educational reform initiatives converged in the development of national educational goals, which later were recast in the Goals 2000: Educate America Act of 1993. The proposed federal legislation was introduced by U.S. Secretary of Education Richard Riley in April 1993. These goals address school readiness, school completion, competence in core subjects, upgraded math and science skills, adult literacy and job performance, and a positive and safe school climate.

The changing cultural fabric of the nation, which now reflects a rich multiculturally diverse population, adds yet another dimension to the challenges facing school-based speech-language pathologists (ASHA, 1993b). Thus, a large segment of professionals are practicing while facing impending and far-reaching change in their work sites.

The work of speech-language pathologists and audiologists will figure prominently in education reform for several reasons: Communication is considered the foundation of learning, the national education goals are based on the premise that students have effective communication skills, and the rights of students with disabilities must be protected (ASHA, in progress). Germane to the rights of individuals with disabilities is access to technology to allow effective communication (e.g., assistive listening devices, augmentative and alternative communication systems). As technology advances, however, speech-language pathologists and audiologists are faced with dilemmas created largely by shrinking budgets. Thus, you will be challenged to do more with less, find alternative cost-efficient ways to deliver effective services consistent with national education goals, and become more accountable for student outcomes. Your success will depend largely on the partnerships formed with other practitioners, administrators, parents, payers, and policy makers.

The future in education is already sketched lightly in blueprint. Your services will become totally integrated into the regular classroom curriculum. Services will be provided predominantly in collaboration with regular and special education teachers. Support personnel will play a more prominent role. Emphasis will be placed on application of speech and language skills to learning and daily life. The speech-language pathologist and audiologist will provide services both inside and outside the classroom. In short, our professions must be poised to enter a new era of practice in school settings to more aggressively and effectively meet the increasingly diverse needs of students and gain a competitive edge in education worldwide.

INTERNAL ISSUES

Our professions of audiology and speech-language pathology are dynamic. To remain viable, introspection is necessary. This can be accomplished through involvement with professional organizations, readings of a broader scope of literature, dialogue, and a willingness to appreciate the commonalities and differences of our professions. More discussion with related professions such as medicine, dentistry, nursing, physical therapy, occupational therapy, clinical psychology, social work, and education could facilitate our own introspection. Finally, more discussion with the consumers of our services will sharpen our vision.

Three internal issues are identified here. Each generates numerous related issues that may be powerful agents for change in our professions.

Expanding Scopes of Practice

During the past 20 years, client populations, work settings, and assessment and treatment methods employed have changed dramatically. Twenty years ago few speech-language pathologists were versed in discourse analysis, facilitated communication, instrumental analysis of respiratory and laryngeal function, assessment of and intervention in cognitive disorders, or provision of augmentative and alternative communication device systems. Similarly, audiologists now offer an expanded scope of assessment and rehabilitative services requiring more expertise in the peripheral and central auditory systems, vestibular functions, and electrophysiological measurements. Who would have predicted 20 years ago that many audiologists would be dispensing hearing aids, performing balance function assessment and intraoperative monitoring, and providing clinical management for those with cochlear implants and assistive listening devices. (See Appendix 1A for ASHA's 1990 definition of Scope of Practice in Speech-Language Pathology and Audiology.)

Many professional issues spawn from our expanding scopes of practice including those related to educational preparation within the professions, specialty certification, and fragmentation and fractionation of the discipline.

EDUCATIONAL PREPARATION. A major issue facing both professions is determining the basic and continuing education necessary to prepare professionals to meet the ever-expanding scopes of practice. Consumers and payers demand that professionals provide state-of-the-art, efficacious, and efficient services. More than 25 years ago, our professions recognized that such expertise could not be gained at the undergraduate level and the master's degree became the recognized entry-level degree in most settings. Today's discussion focuses on the continually expanding knowledge base necessary to provide services, the sufficiency of the masters' degree as the entry level degree, and the need for specialty certification within the professions. Audiologists and speech-language pathologists will be debating the need for a professional or clinical doctorate as the entry level in years to come. Also of issue is the viability of support personnel to supplement the professional services of audiologists and speech-language pathologists. The expanding scopes of practice also have direct implications for what will be taught in the academic setting, the type and amount of practice necessary to develop clinical skills, and the relationship between research and clinical practice. (See Chapter 3 by Battle on professional education and Chapter 29 by Loavenbruck on the professional doctorate in audiology.)

SPECIALTY CERTIFICATION. A related issue growing from our expanding scopes of practice relates to specialty certification. Increasingly, practitioners are struggling to be expert in many areas of human communication sciences and disorders, particularly at the entry level. For example, the hospital-based speech-language pathologist may, in one day, assess or treat persons with a laryngectomy, aphasia, phonological and voice disorders related to progressive neurological disease, cognitive/communicative problems secondary to head trauma, and dysphagia. Both speech-language pathologists and audiologists find that the mix of clients and their complex needs necessitate sophisticated skills that cannot be acquired easily at the master's degree level. Will needs be served more effectively by increasing the requirements of the master's degree, by mandating the doctoral level as the entry, or by encouraging specialty certification whereby a professional may specialize in one or more communication areas? Will such specialty certification enhance our services or confuse the public regarding who we are and what we do? (See Chapter 5 by Madell on professional standards and Chapter 3 by Battle on professional education for more discussion of this topic.)

FRACTIONATION AND FRAGMENTATION. The growth of our professions through the years resembles a puzzle. At first there were a few pieces that appeared to fit logically and easily together. But as our client populations became more diverse and our service delivery more specialized and complex, so did our professions. As the number of puzzle pieces have increased, their fit seems less exact. Cooper (1993) recently warned of the fractionation of our disciplines with Kent (1989–90) earlier alerting us to a similar fragmentation between clinical service and clinical science in communicative disorders. This issue forces us to study our identity as professions and to answer such questions as: What are our goals, our commonalities, our differences? Are the issues that bind us stronger than those that separate us? How does our education prepare us to meet the challenges of new client populations and technological advances? How do our professional associations meet the needs of a diverse membership? How does our identity ultimately affect our service delivery and our effectiveness to our clientele? At the heart of these professional issues is need for continuing redefinition of the discipline of human communication sciences and disorders.

Need for Efficacy Research

A second major internal force influencing our professions is the need for clinical research to demonstrate the efficacy and efficiency of our services to ourselves, our clients, their families, and others. This need stems both from our own long recognition that efficacy research is necessary and from pressure from consumers and insurers to demonstrate that what we do makes a real difference in the everyday lives of our clients that would not have been realized without professional intervention. Efficacy research must also focus on numerous

other issues including determining: (a) what clinical approach(es) best achieve desired clinical outcomes for specific types and severity of disorders; (b) the cost effectiveness of various treatment approaches even when resulting in favorable clinical outcomes; (c) the effectiveness of alternative approaches to therapy, such as enhancing the physical and social environment of our clients to result in more fulfilling communicative opportunities for our clients even when specific communication skills remain impaired; (d) what characteristics of our clients and their environments optimize clinical progress, (e) what research methods best evaluate our clinical effectiveness; and finally, (f) how can practicing clinicians participate in designing and implementing efficacy studies.

Of imminent necessity is our need for new tools to measure functional outcomes among a variety of client types. Functional assessment measures are needed that focus on specific client populations and on significant individuals, such as family members and caregivers. Academic programs need to focus coursework and practica on functional assessment, and our research funding agencies and journals need to include more research on this topic. The repercussions of not developing functional assessment measures and conducting efficacy research are loss of client referral, loss of income for professionals, and negative perceptions about the value of our professional services by policy or decision makers.

For those of you interested in treatment research in communication disorders, ASHA has organized one of its Special Interest Groups and national conferences on this topic. For more reading on efficacy research see the January, 1993, issue of *Asha*, Chapter 25 by Minghetti on research needs and grant seeking, and Chapter 24 by Frattali on functional assessment .

Establishing Professional Autonomy

A rite of passage of any profession is to establish autonomy. Autonomy, as defined by a profession's scope and standards for practice, code of ethics, and the ability to police itself through licensure, certification and accreditation, often is a long and arduous process attained slowly in incremental steps during the course of the profession's development. In view of the above interpretation, the professions of speech-language pathology and audiology would be considered autonomous. The professions have a defined scope of practice (ASHA, 1990b) and a Code of Ethics (ASHA, 1993a). Their standards of practice are defined by the Preferred Practice Patterns (ASHA, 1993c) and numerous practice guidelines. Most professionals hold a Certificate of Clinical Competence awarded by ASHA and are licensed in the 43 states that issue licensure for speech-language pathology and/or audiology. Finally, many professionals have been graduated from academic programs accredited by ASHA's Educational Standards Board, and the clinical programs in which they work are voluntarily accredited by ASHA's Professional Services Board.

We have navigated our rite to autonomous practice. Or have we? Professional autonomy is not immune to forces external to the professions. These forces include federal and state regulations, third party requirements, and national accreditation agency standards— many emanating from health care and education reforms. Autonomy also is misinterpreted by many professionals as suggesting independence in the traditional sense. Given the technological, social, and political complexities of the health care and education systems nationwide, autonomy proceeds naturally from a state of independence to interdependence. Today, no one professional can afford to work in isolation from other professionals whose practice is integrally related to ours as a part of client care. Thus, we must learn to function as team members. Our knowledge must extend beyond the boundaries of our own discipline to that of other disciplines. Finally, we must learn the art of collaboration and compromise. Today, professionals must all sit on the same side of the fence, must rise above territorial concerns, and feel comfortable with their autonomy as defined by degrees of interdependence.

SUMMARY

The most critical professional issue on the horizon is the impending change in national health care funding. Never before in our history has it been so imperative that federal legislators and other health care policy makers understand the nature and value of our professions. Our services need to be considered fundamental, rather than optional, in the basic package of health care. Regardless of the health care program receiving final approval, our professions must be prepared to unambiguously define our goals and methods, to present evidence that unquestionably justifies inclusion in health care programs, and to develop better tools for measuring clinician productivity and client outcomes. Achievement of these goals requires a concerted effort and a sustained commitment on the part of all professionals.

Numerous other issues loom on the horizon in addition to health care reform. Educational reforms such as outcome-based education, individual education plans, cooperative learning, and inclusion programs necessitate continued redefinition of our roles as speech-language pathologists and audiologists in school settings. Our expanding scopes of practice in both audiology and speech-language pathology require that our code of ethics keep pace with these changes and that our academic and clinical programs review curricula to ensure that graduates are ready to meet an increasing diversity of clients and inevitable technological changes. Similarly, our professional organizations, through educational programs and literature, must keep us informed of the challenges to and advances in our professions and provide forums for continued public debate. The dialogue begins with you.

DISCUSSION QUESTIONS

1. What factors influenced your decision to enter the profession of audiology or speech-language pathology?

2. What new clinical populations do you perceive on the horizon? What are their needs? How will you prepare to meet these needs?
3. What similarities do you perceive between the changes in national health care reform and educational reform?
4. How do you think technology will continue to influence our delivery of clinical services?
5. In 10 years, do you expect the professions of audiology and speech-language pathology to be more or less united? Why?
6. How would the introduction of specialty certification affect service delivery in our professions?

REFERENCES

Agency for Health Care Policy and Research. (1990). Medical treatment effectiveness research. *AHCPR Program Note*. Rockville, MD: U.S. Department of Health and Human Services.

American Speech-Language-Hearing Association. (1990a). Professional liability insurance available. *Asha, 32*, 9–10.

American Speech-Language-Hearing Association. (1990b). Scope of practice, speech-language pathology and audiology. *Asha, 32*(Suppl. 2), 1–2.

American Speech-Language-Hearing Association, Ad Hoc Committee on Advances in Clinical Practice. (1992). Position statements and guidelines. *Asha, 34*(Suppl. 7), 9–37.

American Speech-Language-Hearing Association. (1993a) Code of ethics. *Asha, 35*, 17–18.

American Speech-Language-Hearing Association. (1993b). *Demographic profile of the ASHA membership*. Rockville, MD: Author.

American Speech-Language-Hearing Association. (1993c). Preferred practice patterns for the professions of speech-language pathology and audiology. *Asha, 35*(Suppl. 11), 1–97.

American Speech-Language-Hearing Association, Ad Hoc Committee on Changes in Educational Policies and Practices. (in progress). *Technical report to the Executive Board*. Rockville, MD: Author.

Berwick, D., Godfrey, A. B., & Roessner, J. (1990). *Curing health care: New strategies for quality improvement*. San Francisco: Jossey-Bass.

Boyer, E. (1983). *A nation at risk*. Princeton, NJ: Carnegie Foundation for Education.

Callahan, C. (1990). *What kind of life: The limits of medical progress*. NY: Simon & Schuster.

Cooper, E. (1993). The fractionation of our discipline. *Asha, 35*, 51–54.

Deming, W. E. (1986). *Out of the crisis*. Cambridge: Massachusetts Institute of Technology, Center for Advanced Engineering Study.

Erikson, K. (1981). *Human services today*. Reston, VA: Reston Publishing.

Henderson, G., & Bryan, W. (1984). *Psychosocial aspects of disability*. Springfield, IL: Charles C. Thomas.

Joint Commission on Accreditation of Healthcare Organizations (JCAHO). (1987). *Agenda for change*. Oakbrook Terrace, IL: Author.

Juran, J. M. (1988). *Juran on planning for quality*. New York: The Free Press.

Kent, R. (1989–90). Fragmentation of clinical service and clinical science in communicative disorders. *National Student Speech Language Hearing Association Journal, 17*, 4–16.

Keough, K. (1990). Emerging issues for the professions in the 1990s. *Asha, 32*, 55–58.

Lewit, E. M., & Monheit, A. C. (1992). Expenditures on health care for children and pregnant women. *The future of children*. (pp. 95–114). Rockville, MD: Agency for Health Care Policy and Research.

Schieber, G., & Poullier, J. (1991). International health spending: Issues and trends. *Health Affairs, 10*, 106–115.

Spiegel, A., Simon, P., & Fiorito, E. (1981). *Rehabilitating people with disabilities into the mainstream of society*. Park Ridge, IL: Noyes Medical Publications.

Spriestersbach, D. C. (1991). We are part of the planet, you know!, *Asha, 33*, 34–35.

Statistical Abstract of the United States. (1992). Washington, DC: Department of Commerce.

APPENDIX 1A: Scope of Practice, Speech-Language Pathology and Audiology

The following document, prepared by the American Speech-Language-Hearing Association (ASHA) Committee on Interprofessional Relationships, was adopted as an official statement by the ASHA Legislative Council (LC 6–89) in November 1989. Current and past members of the committee responsible for the development of the document include Crystal S. Cooper, 1988–1990 chair; John L. Peterson, 1988 chair; Rachel E. Stark, 1986–87 chair; Brenda L. B. Adamovich; Katherine G. Butler; Janina K. Casper; Becky S. Cornett; Ted A.

Culler; Frank De Ruyter; Elaine S. Dunn; Anita S. Halper; Anne E. Seltz; Rosalind R. Scudder; Barbara Shadden; and Brenda Y. Terrell. Michelle M. Ferketic, 1988–89 ex officio; Lynette R. Goldberg, 1989–90 ex officio; Carol Kamara, 1986–87 ex officio; Patricia G. Larkins, 1988 ex officio. Ann L. Carey, current vice president for professional and governmental affairs, and Nancy Becker, vice president for professional and governmental affairs, were monitoring vice presidents.

PREAMBLE

The purpose of this statement is to define the scope of practice of speech-language pathology and audiology in order to: (1) inform members of ASHA and certificate holders of the activities for which certification in the appropriate area is required in accordance with the ASHA Code of Ethics; and (2) educate health-care and education professionals, consumers, and members of the general public of the services offered by speech-language pathologists and audiologists as qualified providers.

The scope of practice defined here, and the areas specifically set forth, are part of an effort to establish the broad range of services offered within the profession. It is recognized, however, that levels of experience, skill and proficiency with respect to the activities identified within the scope of practice will vary among the individual providers. Similarly, it is recognized that related fields and professions may have knowledge, skills and experience which may be applied to some areas within the scope of practice. By defining the scope of practice of speech-language pathologists and audiologists, there is no intention to exclude members of other professions or related fields from rendering services in common practice areas for which they are competent by virtue of their respective disciplines.

Nothing in the scope of practice statement is intended to affect the licensure laws of the various states or the implementation or interpretation of such laws.

Finally, it is recognized that speech-language pathology and audiology are dynamic and continuously developing practice areas. In setting forth some specific areas as included within the scope of practice, there is no intention that the list be exhaustive or that other, new, or emerging areas be pre-

cluded from being considered as within the scope of practice.

STATEMENT

Speech-language pathologists and audiologists hold either the master's or doctoral degree, the Certificate of Clinical Competence of the American Speech-Language-Hearing Association, and state license where applicable. These professionals identify, assess, and provide treatment for individuals of all ages with communication disorders. They manage and supervise programs and services related to human communication and its disorders. Speech-language pathologists and audiologists counsel individuals with disorders of communication, their families, caregivers and other service providers relative to the disability present and its management. They provide consultation and make referrals. Facilitating the development and maintenance of human communication is the common goal of speech-language pathologists and audiologists.

The practice of speech-language pathology includes:
■ screening, identifying, assessing and interpreting, diagnosing, rehabilitating, and preventing disorders of speech (e.g., articulation, fluency, voice) and language (ASHA, 1983, 1989);
■ screening, identifying, assessing and interpreting, diagnosing, and rehabilitating disorders of oral-pharngeal function (e.g., dysphagia) and related disorders;
■ screening, identifying, assessing and interpreting, diagnosing, and rehabilitating cognitive/communication disorders;
■ assessing, selecting and developing augmentative and alternative communication systems and providing training in their use;
■ providing aural rehabilitation and related counseling services to hearing impaired individuals and their families;
■ enhancing speech-language proficiency and communication effectiveness (e.g., accent reduction); and
■ screening of hearing and other factors for the purpose of speech-language evaluation and/or the initial identification of individuals with other communication disorders.

The practice of audiology includes:

- facilitating the conservation of auditory system function; developing and implementing environmental and occupational hearing conservation programs;
- screening, identifying, assessing and interpreting, diagnosing, preventing, and rehabilitating peripheral and central auditory system dysfunctions;
- providing and interpreting behavioral and (electro) physiological measurements of auditory and vestibular functions;
- selecting, fitting and dispensing of amplification, assistive listening and alerting devices and other systems (e.g., implantable devices) and providing training in their use;
- providing aural rehabilitation and related counseling services to hearing impaired individuals and their families; and
- screening, of speech-language and other factors affecting communication function for the purposes of an audiologic evaluation and/or initial identification of individuals with other communication disorders.

REFERENCES

American Speech-Language-Hearing Association. (1987a). Ad Hoc Committee on Dysphagia report. *Asha, 29*(4), 57–58.

American Speech-Language-Hearing Association. (1987b). The role of speech-language pathologists in the habilitation and rehabilitation of cognitively impaired individuals: A report of the Subcommittee on Language and Cognition. *Asha, 29*(6), 53–55.

American Speech-Language-Hearing Association. (1983). Definition of language, *Asha, 25*(6), 44.

American Speech-Language-Hearing Association. (1988). The role of speech-language pathologists in the identification, diagnosis, and treatment of individuals with cognitive-communication impairments. *Asha, 30*(3), 79.

American Speech-Language-Hearing Association. (1989). Standards for the certificates of clinical competence. *Asha, 31*(3), 70–71.

■ CHAPTER 2 ■

Professional Organizations

■ PEGGY S. WILLIAMS, Ph.D. ■

SCOPE OF CHAPTER

This chapter defines and identifies the parameters of professional organizations and reviews rationales for affiliation by individuals and related groups. The intent is to answer the questions: What is a professional organization and why should you get involved? To work effectively in your career requires more than just the knowledge of speech, language, hearing, and related disorders and the remediation of those disorders. An understanding of how a profession is represented to the world at large and how one can participate in making decisions for the benefit of all the individuals in a profession and thus improve the standing for oneself and/or the consumer requires an understanding of how the governance of the profession takes place. What is the governance? How is it structured? How do I get involved? These are all questions one must answer when entering a profession.

STANDARD FEATURES OF PROFESSIONAL ORGANIZATIONS

Professional organizations, also called associations, share a number of common features: (a) they have a definable scope (local, state, national, international); (b) their members are persons from a specific, recognized area such as a degreed profession; (c) they are financially identified as nonprofit; (d) there are recognized membership requirements; and (e) there is an identifiable governing structure and process. National activities include the services of membership development, educational programs, publications, interface with federal and state governments, public information and relations, finance, and administration. These activities are usually handled by departmental units within the organization. That is, individuals can call the organization and ask for the membership unit for questions about membership issues.

Other types of associations, such as trade (usually representing for-profit groups), educational, civic, consumer, and religious associations, are prevalent in society. All, like the professional organization, focus on a common topic. Their memberships may also consist of individuals, but are more likely to be agencies, companies, or other group-type affiliates.

The governing structure of a nonprofit organization has an identified body of individuals who direct the affairs of the overall organization. They are elected by the membership and operate according to a set of bylaws. The elected leadership usually includes a president, president-elect, past president, and a number of vice presidents who oversee various areas of the organization's activities, such as standards, practice, governmental affairs, academic affairs, public information, finance and administration, planning, quality improvement, membership, and so forth. These individuals, or officers, usually appoint a number of committees to assist in their work. The bylaws represent a set of agreed-on goals, objectives, and guidelines for operation of the organization—a governing plan and structure.

Typical activities conducted by a professional association are educational and scientific meetings, scholarly publications, input into and monitoring of educational standards for the profession, the provision of public information, governmental lobbying, development of public and private position statements on aspects of the profession, and involvement and cooperative projects with other related organizations. In most cases, there are state chapters, or recognized state organizations, that coordinate work on behalf of the profession and work with the national association. The state affiliates aim at furthering the mission of the national organization and increasing the strength of the national goals.

Income for the operation of a national professional organization is primarily from membership dues and secondarily from such sources as publications and products, trade exhibits and meetings, mailing list sales, grants and contracts, and fees for specific services. Revenue may also be generated from investments, property sales or rentals, and service contracts (e.g., bank credit cards, insurance programs). This income is fed into:

- Membership activities, services, projects (television, articles, special events);
- Publications (journals, magazines, brochures);
- Educational programs (workshops, conferences teleconferences);
- Educational materials (books, audio and video tapes);
- Lobbying (written and oral input and responses to laws and regulations);
- Continuing education programs (ensuring quality programs offered in the field, maintaining a registry service for members);
- Membership and career development (supporting a call-in telephone line for member—use Actionline 800 service);
- Recruiting new members for the association and prospective students for universities;
- Helping students choose careers and helping members be aware of career opportunities within the profession;
- Ensuring and maintaining quality education (setting standards and monitoring, certifying new members);
- Ethics administration (establishing and monitoring ethical conduct of individuals in the profession);
- Supporting the operations of an office staff to handle business operations (in national and some state organizations staff handle many logistics of the above-named operations along with managing the financial and administrative operations).

Most organizations have some form of a long-range strategic plan that sets a direction and provides a focus for day-to-day management. The plan contains a mission statement, or statement of purpose, and identifies outcomes expected from plan objectives. That is, the plan outlines what the organization's goals are and the results expected from the implementation of activities to meet the goals. The plan also indicates the cost to the organization for the successful completion of the objectives and therefore helps the association decide what it can or cannot do on the basis of what it can afford.

ASHA: A NATIONAL PROFESSIONAL ORGANIZATION

The American Speech-Language-Hearing Association (ASHA) currently exists as the primary national association for the professions of audiology and speech-language pathology. ASHA was founded in 1925 by a group of 22 individuals in the profession who thought that gathering and forming a national organization could give visibility to the professions, help members know and learn from one another, and provide educational opportunities beyond their formal education. The association has grown from 22 interested professionals at inception to more than 75,000 members, affiliates, and nonmember certificate holders from around the world who still join for the same reasons identified in 1925. Most reside in the continental United States.

At this writing, of the approximately 68,000 certified members and affiliates, 84% are certified speech-language pathologists; 14% are certified audiologists; 2% hold dual certification; 90% are female; 10% are male; 94% are Caucasian; 74% provide clinical services; and the median age is 37 years. (See Chapter 9 by Shewan for more details on characteristics of ASHA membership.)

The association has changed in both scope and size since 1925. It has achieved national and international recognition and offers a broad range of membership services and activities, such as an annual convention that draws more than 10,000 people, a large publications program that produces numerous scholarly journals and publications, and many educational events to support life-long learning. Also, a student association has been added (National Student Speech Language Hearing Association), a consumer affiliate organization (National Association for Hearing

and Speech Action), and a foundation (American Speech-Language-Hearing Foundation).

PURPOSES

The purposes of the Association as stated in the bylaws (ASHA, 1993b) are:

The purposes of this Association shall be: (1) To encourage basic scientific study of the processes of individual human communication with special reference to speech, language, and hearing; (2) To promote appropriate academic and clinical preparation of individuals entering the discipline of human communication sciences and disorders and promote the maintenance of current knowledge and skills of those within the discipline; (3) To promote investigation and prevention of disorders of human communication; (4) To foster improvement of clinical services and procedures concerning such disorders; (5) To stimulate exchange of information among persons and organizations thus engaged and to disseminate such information; (6) To advocate the rights and interests of persons with communication disorders; and (7) To promote the individual and collective professional interests of the members of the Association. (p. 11) (article II, 2.1)

In all cases, you can look to the ASHA bylaws when seeking current and specific answers to questions about the association's purpose, membership, governance, standards, publications, stance on discrimination, honors, recognition of other organizations, special interest divisions, parliamentary authority, and amendments. These eleven areas define the purpose, nature, and scope of the organization.

GOVERNANCE

The governance structure of ASHA is addressed in detail in article IV of the bylaws. In general, the legislative council (LC) constitutes the overall policy making body of the association, and the executive board (EB) constitutes the management body. A visual display of the structure is presented in Figure 2–1.

The LC establishes the policies of the Association and as such represents the intention of

Association Governance Structure

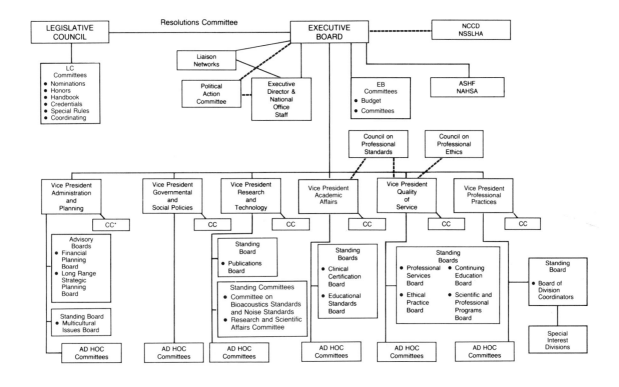

*Coordinating Committee

Figure 2–1. Association governance structure. (Reprinted from *Asha*, 35, p. 41. Copyright 1993 by American Speech-Language-Hearing Association, by permission.)

the entire ASHA membership. The LC is made up of ASHA members who are elected by and from the general membership through state balloting. That is, LC members of ASHA are elected by their fellow ASHA members who live in the same state. Numbers of Councilors vary per state based on the number of ASHA members in the state—one councilor is elected for every 150 members in the state. The District of Columbia is included as a state, and members whose mailing addresses are outside the United States choose Councilors from among themselves or vote with the state from which they are long-term based.

The executive board (EB), made up of individuals elected by and from the membership

at-large, is considered the legally responsible management body. This means that its members supervise, control, and direct the affairs of the association, implementing all objectives and activities in compliance with the programs and policies set forth by the bylaws and the LC. The EB disburses funds within the policies, including the annual budget, approved by the LC. The actions of the EB are monitored by the LC and are formally reported to the LC each year.

The intention of the structure described above is to ensure that the membership of the association has access to decision making and has a voice in setting policy, primarily via the LC. The membership also elects the members of the management body (EB) that then administers the day-to-day operations of the association in compliance with approved policies. The LC and the EB, in combination, not only have mutually supportive though separate roles, but also provide a mechanism for a balance of legislative power.

To accomplish the work set forth by the LC, the EB may establish different types of governance working groups to assist with the work. Such groups are identified as ad hoc committees, task forces, networks, and working groups. These bodies may also recommend, for LC approval, the establishment of standing committees and boards to handle long-range, ongoing work such as monitoring the accreditation of clinical and educational programs. These latter bodies allow members to participate directly in the governance process, to learn about how the governance process works, and to contribute to the association. Members who wish to serve on these groups submit a committee pool form (printed annually in the March reference issue of *Asha*). Members who submit committee pool forms remain in the committee pool for 3 years from the date the form is received at the national office.

NATIONAL OFFICE

In addition to the governance structure, the association maintains a national headquarters based in Rockville, MD. The 170 members of the national office staff work in seven departments: executive, multicultural affairs, professional practices, professional affairs, governmental affairs, public information, and business management (see Figure 2–2). The staff carry out the day-to-day implementation of activities, programs, policies, and procedures of the Association under the guidance of the members of the EB. The executive director serves as the chief administrative officer of the association and is a nonvoting member of the EB.

The goal of activities of the association, on a daily basis, is to accomplish the purposes, implement select objectives, and monitor long-term operations. Activities may vary from year to year within these three areas.

Also, there are ongoing publications such as *Asha, Language, Speech, and Hearing Services in the Schools, American Journal of Audiology, American Journal of Speech-Language Pathology,* and the *Journal of Speech and Hearing Research,* as well as an annual convention—all are intended to keep the members and affiliates informed and involved.

As mentioned earlier, the long-range plan (LRP) for an organization provides focus and sets the direction for action. ASHA's 1994–1999, long-range plan contains a vision, mission, eight guiding principles, and seven critical issues with intended outcomes to guide the association in the next few years. The LRP is made available to members each year in the March *Asha* reference issue.

To apply the information in this section to the individual member, such as yourself, a case study is presented to illustrate how the association works.

CASE STUDY: NATIONAL ORGANIZATION

Many individuals become disenchanted and frustrated with an organization after repeatedly voicing an objection or expressing a need with no result. This situation usually develops when individuals do not know how to translate their need or request into an action to bring about the desired result. Understanding how the system is organized and designed to work aids the individual in knowing how to enter and make an impact. An example of how to translate a need into action and the desired result follows.

One member of ASHA noted that there were areas of clinical practice of speech-language pathologists and audiologists in their day-to-day management of clients with certain types of communication disorders that had few guiding principles. The individual became acutely aware of this as a member of a state licensing board. The licensing board was faced with making decisions about the practice of the professions in the state and

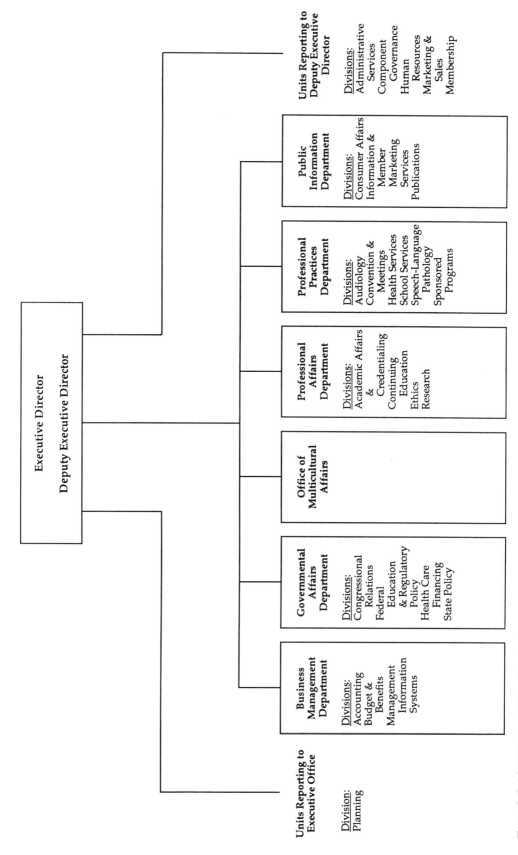

Figure 2–2. ASHA National Office Organization.

needed some consensus directions from national associations (i.e., the members of the professions nationally).

The member contacted an officer of the ASHA executive board who, by title of office, best represented the area of the member's concern—the vice president for clinical affairs. (The member could also have contacted the state legislative councilor for similar assistance.) The vice president explained that the issue needed to be formulated into a clear statement of need (or needs) and a request for action. This is defined as a "charge" (specific request of what needed to be done) for a resolution (request for action to either the EB or LC).

The vice president assisted the member in developing the resolution and it was submitted to the EB at its next meeting. The WHEREAS statements stated the problem; the RESOLVED statements stated the actions desired and a time line for completion. The resolution presented below was passed by the EB, and an ad hoc committee of ASHA members was appointed to address the concern. The committee was named the Ad Hoc Committee on Extended Practice Issues.

WHEREAS, speech-language pathologists and audiologists are becoming increasingly involved in potentially high risk invasive procedures (e.g., evoked potential measurement, [ABR], nasal endoscopy, tracheoesophageal puncture), and

WHEREAS, there is increasing need for clarification of the speech-language pathologists's and audiologists's role in the delivery of these procedures, and

WHEREAS, there is a need to define appropriate training protocols, and

WHEREAS, there is a need to clarify insurance coverage for such procedures; therefore

EB 115–88. RESOLVED, That the Executive Board of the American Speech-Language-Hearing Association appoints an Ad Hoc Committee on Extended Practice Issues to be comprised of not more than seven people including both speech-language pathologists and audiologists; and further

RESOLVED, That this Committee is charged with studying the extent to which: (1) procedures (e.g., evoked potential measurement, (ABR), nasal endoscopy, tracheoesophageal puncture) are being utilized by speech-language pathologists and audiologists; (2) the role of the speech-language pathologist and audiologist in conducting these procedures is clearly specified; (3) educational preparation is being provided; (4) reimbursement is being provided for these procedures; and (5) these procedures have an impact on professional liability insurance; and further

RESOLVED, That a report be prepared which will include background information including the extent to which these procedures are used by speech-language pathologists and audiologists and recommendations regarding the action(s) the Association should undertake in addressing the practice, education/training and third-party reimbursement issues identified; and further

Resolved, That the report of the Ad Hoc Committee on Extended Practice Issues be presented to the Executive Board at its May 1989 meeting.
[Approved (7–0)]
Origin: Vice President for Clinical Affairs (ASHA, 1988, p.11)

The ad hoc committee developed a preliminary report to the EB, asking for approval to circulate the report to other groups in the governance structure to obtain further input and refinement. The EB approved the action. The resolution, with EB action, is:

EB 120–89. RESOLVED, That the Executive Board receive the preliminary report of the Ad Hoc Committee on Extended Practice Issues; and further

RESOLVED That the recommendations indicated in the Executive Summary of the Preliminary Report of the Ad Hoc Committee on Extended Practice Issues be referred for study and comments by appropriate committees, boards, councils, and National Office staff.
[Approval (8–0)]
Origin: Ad Hoc Committee on Extended Practice Issues (ASHA, 1989, p.36)

After input was obtained and the report completed, the ad hoc committee then submitted a new request to the EB. It was determined that the topic needed to be broken down into several position statements and guidelines for different practice areas. The EB approved this request and reconstituted the ad hoc committee to do the work.

EB 131–89. RESOLVED, That a reconstituted Ad Hoc Committee on Extended Practice Issues be appointed and charged with the responsibility for drafting position statements and guidelines for delivery of service for each of the extended practices identified in the report where no positions or guidelines already exist; and further

RESOLVED, That the Ad Hoc Committee on Extended Practice Issues consist of no more than nine (9) members representing the designated extended practices; and further

RESOLVED, That the Ad Hoc Committee on Extended Practice Issues prepare the position statements and guidelines for Executive Board action no later than August, 1990.
[Approved (7–0)]
Origin: Ad Hoc Committee on Extended Practice Issues (ASHA, 1989, p. 42)

After a few months of work, the ad hoc committee requested, and obtained, a name change to the Ad Hoc Committee on Advances in Clinical Practice because "extended practices" incorrectly implied that these procedures were beyond the boundaries of current clinical practice.

The ad hoc committee then completed its work and presented for approval the position statements and guidelines in 1991. The EB approved the work and forwarded it to the LC for final approval (recall that only the LC can approve association policies, positions, and guidelines).

The LC reviewed and approved the documents at its November 1991 meeting, and the results were published for member use in the March 1992 *Asha* supplement (ASHA, 1992). The documents then became part of the *Asha Desk Reference* (ASHA, 1993a) for long-term retrieval as an approved document of the association.

Thus, one member's need and subsequent effort were translated into effective action and benefited the full membership. The process took 3 years.

The length of time required for such work is often seen as a stumbling block to initiating action, but was necessary in this case to ensure a democratic process. However, emergency issues, or those affected by external time lines, can be targeted to move faster. In those cases, a task force, instead of an ad hoc committee or board, is usually formed.

You, as a member, can always access the governance structure by learning to formulate your concerns into a resolution format and asking your state legislative councilor, or an EB member, to take it forward to an EB or LC meeting. You may get current copies of resolution forms from your legislative councilor or directly from the national office by contacting the administrative assistant to the executive board. LC, EB, and national office staff are available to assist you in working effectively in the process, including the development of resolutions. The process of developing ASHA policies is shown in Figure 2–3.

Contributions such as the one described above enhance your growth as a professional and a leader and also benefit the professions at large. This "50–50" principle (50% work contributions and 50% leadership training) offers members the opportunity to gain personally, as well as contribute professionally. What better reasons to get involved?

STATE AND LOCAL PROFESSIONAL ORGANIZATIONS

Organizations in audiology and speech-language pathology formed at the state and local levels generally share the same or markedly similar purposes to the national organization. These local organizations also develop bylaws and implement a governing structure. For new members entering the profession, the state and local organizations are key places to begin professional involvement. After joining the organizations, you can become acquainted with the officers and volunteer to become a

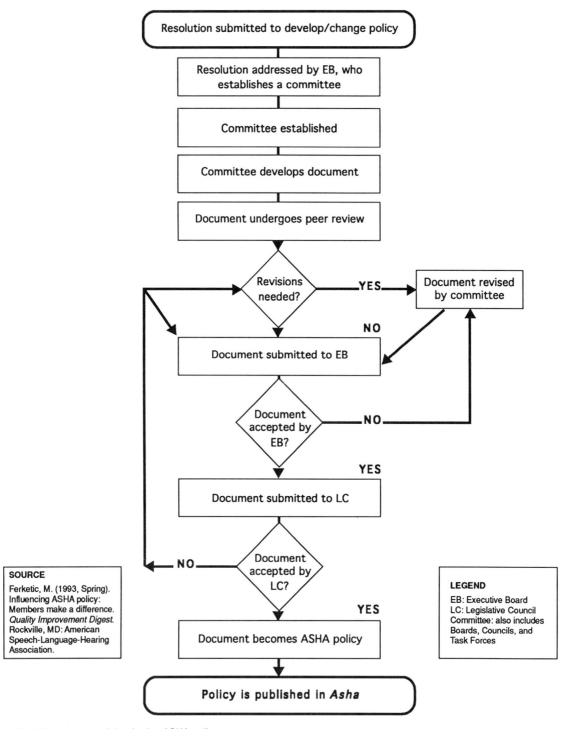

Figure 2–3. The process of developing ASHA policy.

The flowchart contains the following elements:

- Resolution submitted to develop/change policy
- Resolution addressed by EB, who establishes a committee
- Committee established
- Committee develops document
- Document undergoes peer review
- Revisions needed? — YES → Document revised by committee
- NO
- Document submitted to EB
- Document accepted by EB? — NO → (back to Document revised by committee)
- YES
- Document submitted to LC
- Document accepted by LC? — NO → (back to Document submitted to EB)
- YES
- Document becomes ASHA policy
- Policy is published in *Asha*

SOURCE
Ferketic, M. (1993, Spring). Influencing ASHA policy: Members make a difference. *Quality Improvement Digest*. Rockville, MD: American Speech-Language-Hearing Association.

LEGEND
EB: Executive Board
LC: Legislative Council
Committee: also includes Boards, Councils, and Task Forces

member of a committee. After gaining some experience, you should seek to chair a committee and then try for an elected office. Learning the local and state organization structures assists in the development of leadership skills and builds a strong future national leader.

State associations representing audiologists and speech-language pathologists, by their own choice, are not part of the ASHA governing structure nor do they represent national chapters as is the case for many other national organizations. However, ASHA has a formal recognition process to recognize states that have similar membership requirements to the national organization. Also, there is a strong working relationship between the national and state organizations, along with a joint committee of the national and the state organizations that promotes communication and mutual support between the groups.

Local organizations are less formally recognized and may exist as a group of audiologists and speech-language pathologists who live in the same city or in a regional area of a number of small towns. Individuals need to ask colleagues in their local area about such groups and how to affiliate, as these groups provide a good opportunity to network and learn about governance practices.

State and local groups advocate for recognition by state and local governments, conduct public recognition projects, monitor state licensure requirements—including continuing education, champion ethical practice standards, monitor education and health laws and regulations, seek consumer recognition and involvement, conduct educational meetings, develop and disseminate newsletters, and set up networks for communication. Many national objectives are furthered by state and local assistance and vice versa. For example, the national organization spends both time and money in assisting states with the development of licensure laws and other laws and regulations influencing the practice of audiology and speech-language pathology within the states.

STUDENT ASSOCIATION

Available for students in speech-language pathology and audiology is the National Student Speech Language Hearing Association (NSSLHA). The organization has chapters at many universities and is an excellent means of becoming involved in a governance activity before entering the profession. The NSSLHA has elected offices and an annual meeting. If your university does not have a chapter, think about organizing one. The NSSLHA has its own staff, housed at the ASHA headquarters. They can be reached by calling ASHA.

INTERNATIONAL PROFESSIONAL ORGANIZATIONS

Often, audiologists and speech-language pathologists wish to become active internationally, offering papers at meetings and serving on governing boards. A number of organizations exist that may be directly or indirectly related to the professions. Examples are the International Society of Audiology, the International Association of Logopedics and Phoniatrics, the International Academy for Research in Learning Disabilities, and the International Affairs Association. Most international organizations meet annually in various countries. Two of the organizations are described below. (See Chapter 7 by Wilson for more discussion of international associations.)

The International Association of Logopedics and Phoniatrics (IALP) is concerned with communication and its disorders. IALP is composed of organizations similar to ASHA and individuals whose major interests lie in the field of communication and communication disorders.

The International Society of Audiology (ISA) aims to facilitate the knowledge, protection, and rehabilitation of human hearing, including the effects of pharmacological and surgical measures, but excluding matters relating to the applications of these measures. It coordinates and disseminates information, particularly through courses, regular international congresses, published proceedings of these congresses, and other communications in the field of audiology.

RELATED PROFESSIONAL ORGANIZATIONS

Approximately 30 related professional organizations meet in conjunction with the ASHA annual convention, as well as conduct many separate meetings and conferences. Example groups are the Academy of Dispensing Audiologists, Air Force Audiology Association, American Academy of Audiology, American Academy of Private Practice in Speech-Language Pathology and Audiology, American Auditory Society, Computer Users in Speech and Hearing, Council of Supervisors in Speech-Language Pathology and Audiology, National Black Association for Speech, Language and Hearing, Public School Caucus, and the Society of Hospital Directors of Communicative Disorders Programs.

These organizations focus on specific issues and areas of interest, allowing a forum for networking with individuals with similar interests. All have governance structures and provide opportunities for professional growth and contribution through committee and office-holding opportunities, as well as fellowship and education.

There is a relatively close working relationship between these groups and with ASHA and other organizations, as the memberships share the same populations. Occasionally, coalitions are formed or mutual working groups and joint committees work together to form a unified position. In other cases, there *are* differing opinions and directions taken as change naturally occurs in the progress and growth of the professions.

SUMMARY

Affiliation with a professional association that represents the profession you enter strength-

ens both you and the organization. You have the opportunity—and the obligation—to contribute to your profession through service and leadership and in return grow in personal abilities. The organization benefits from your ideas and the impetus in combination with others' and helps the profession survive and accomplish needed changes. As part of your professional growth, you should consider membership as soon as eligible and work at all levels—local, state, national, international, and related areas of interest. The rewards are certain to be mutually beneficial.

DISCUSSION QUESTIONS

1. Describe the activities of associations that are national in scope.
2. What are the purposes of the American Speech-Language-Hearing Association (ASHA)?
3. Describe the role of each of the following ASHA governance groups: legislative council, executive board, committees/boards/task forces, and national office staff.
4. Using an issue of professional concern to you, describe how you would use ASHA's governance system to get that concern addressed.
5. Describe the 50–50 principle in relationship to professional organization member volunteers.
6. How does professional organization membership benefit the individual member? The association itself? The professions?

REFERENCES

American Speech-Language-Hearing Association. (1992). *Asha, 34*(March, Suppl. 7), 9–40.

American Speech-Language-Hearing Association. (1993). *ASHA desk reference—guidelines, position statements, and relevant papers.* (pp. II-14A, II-28A, II-28E; II-28J; II-32A; II-74B; II-122A). Rockville, MD: Author.

American Speech-Language-Hearing Association. (1988, August). Executive board meeting minutes, p. 11.

American Speech-Language-Hearing Association. (1989, August). Executive board meeting minutes, pp. 36, 42.

American Speech-Language-Hearing Association. (1993). *Membership directory* (p.11) [Bylaws]. Rockville, MD: Author.

RESOURCES

American Speech-Language-Hearing Association
10801 Rockville Pike
Rockville, MD 20852
(301) 897-5700
FAX (301) 571-0457

State Associations:
See the annual March reference issue of *Asha* for current addresses.

■ CHAPTER 3 ■

Professional Education

■ DOLORES BATTLE, Ph.D. ■

SCOPE OF CHAPTER

Speech-language pathologists and audiologists must have appropriate knowledge and skills to ensure that quality services are provided to the public. The preparation for a career in speech-language pathology or audiology is a lifelong commitment. Preparation begins at the undergraduate or preprofessional level and continues through to the master's degree. The doctoral degree, which represents the highest achievement in the field, is awarded for advanced study in communication sciences and disorders. This chapter provides you with information on the goals and objectives, admission requirements, curricula, and degree requirements for undergraduate and graduate education in communicative sciences and disorders. It also provides you with information on continuing education for the continued competence to practice the professions.

UNDERGRADUATE PREPROFESSIONAL EDUCATION

Undergraduate preprofessional education in communicative sciences and disorders is the foundation of the educational continuum. There are 282 college and university programs in the United States that provide undergraduate education in communication sciences and disorders. Of these, 68 provide only the baccalaureate degree, 164 provide the bachelor's and master's degrees, and 50 provide the bachelor's, master's, and doctoral degrees. Six programs provide only the master's and doctoral degrees, 8 provide only the master's degree, and 2 provide only the doctoral degree (ASHA, 1994a). In the 1990–91 academic year there were 15,227 undergraduate students in the discipline. Approximately 3,826 bachelor's degree were awarded in 1989–90. This was a 16.7% increase in the number of bachelor's degrees granted over the past 10 years. (Creaghead, Bernthal, & Gilbert, 1991)

Historically, programs that provide only the bachelor's degree have been referred to as terminal bachelor's degree programs because additional education was not necessary for independent practice. More recently, the goals of the undergraduate education in speech-language pathology and audiology provide introductory-level education in the discipline and prepare students for graduate study in the discipline. Preprofessional programs do not prepare students for independent professional practice. For this reason the undergraduate programs are considered to be *preprofessional* programs.

Undergraduate education in speech-language pathology and audiology is usually provided within the context of the traditional liberal arts and sciences program. Thirty-five percent of the undergraduate programs are located in colleges of arts and sciences; 19% are located in colleges of education; 23% are in allied health. The remaining programs are located in schools of communication, professional studies, behavioral studies, or human sciences. Sixty percent of communication sciences and disorders departments exist as independent departments and 40% exist as programs within departments of education, special education, or communication (Creaghead et al., 1991). Students wishing to obtain undergraduate preparation in communicative sciences and disorders usually major in communication sciences and disorders, speech-language pathology, or related areas such as linguistics, communication, education, or special education.

PREPROFESSIONAL CURRICULUM

Students completing the undergraduate major in communicative sciences and disorders must demonstrate skill in: (a) oral and written communication, technological literacy, computational skills, and scientific reasoning; (b) the ability to think critically and solve problems; (c) understanding of cultural diversity; (d) understanding of human development across the life span; and (e) the ability to analyze, synthesize, and apply information (ASHA, 1990). The American Speech-Language-Hearing Association (ASHA) standards for the Certificates of Clinical Competence (CCC) (ASHA, 1990) reflect the need for a liberal education. The requirements include 12 semester hours in physical or biological sciences and mathematics and 6 semester hours in behavioral or social sciences. In addition,

effective January 1, 1995 some coursework must include, where appropriate, human development across the life span and coursework in cultural diversity (ASHA, 1994a). These requirements are often completed as part of the liberal arts education requirements for the bachelor's degree.

The major curriculum for undergraduate programs in communication sciences and disorders varies although 50% of those who belong to the National Academy of Pre-professional Programs feel that there should be some standardization (Terrizzi, 1988). This group has recommended a model curriculum for preprofessional programs. The curriculum includes coursework in basic human communication, the nature of communication disorders, and an introduction to the principles of assessment and treatment. Although specific coursework is defined by the institution granting the degree, academic coursework usually includes a minimum of 30 semester credits in:

1. Human anatomy and physiology, specifically systems involved in communicative functions;
2. Articulatory and acoustic phonetics, including transcription skills and appropriate experiences in auditory discrimination;
3. Physics of sound and the use of instrumentation essential to the measurement of sound;
4. Normal development of speech and language;
5. Diversity of normal communication behaviors and developmental patterns found in the multicultural society;
6. Nature and prevention of speech and language disorders and delays;
7. Principles commonly used by professionals in the assessment of communication differences, disorders, and delays;
8. Nature and prevention of hearing loss;
9. Measurement of auditory sensitivity;
10. Principles commonly used by professions in the re/habilitation of persons with hearing impairment.

The clinical education component of pre-professional education provides students with the basic principles of assessment and treatment of communication differences, delays, and disorders. This usually includes a minimum of 25 hours of observation of assessment and treatment with a variety of cases. Although many programs do not include clinical practicum in the undergraduate program, others include up to 100 hours of supervised clinical practice as a part of the undergraduate program. Undergraduate clinical practicum is usually obtained in an on-campus clinic but may also include an off-campus school-based practicum. All undergraduate clinical observation and practicum must be supervised by a person holding the ASHA CCC if the student intends to use the experiences as part of the requirements for the CCC.

ADMISSION

Applicants for admission to undergraduate programs in communication sciences and disorders must provide evidence of a strong secondary school preparation including courses in laboratory science, computational mathematics, and preferably a language other than English. Many programs require a satisfactory score on the Scholastic Aptitude Test or a similar standardized test used to predict success in college. In addition, applicants who have had experience in human services through volunteer work or employment are preferred.

ACCREDITATION

The Educational Standards Board (ESB) of ASHA accredits graduate programs in speech-language pathology and audiology. Accredited programs meet standards established by the ASHA Council on Professional Standards. The ESB does not accredit undergraduate or preprofessional programs. In institutions where there are both bachelor's and accredited master's-level programs, the standards for accreditation of educational programs apply to both programs. This is particularly important for clinical education standards, because several of the standards

for clinical certification may be met at the undergraduate level.

Information on undergraduate preprofessional programs is available from the National Academy of Preprofessional Programs in Communication Sciences and Disorders. (See the Resource section at the end of this chapter for further information.)

MASTER'S DEGREE IN SPEECH-LANGUAGE PATHOLOGY AND AUDIOLOGY

The master's degree is the minimal degree required for practice of the professions of speech-language pathology and audiology. It is required for the CCC and for state licensure.

The first master's degrees in speech-language pathology and audiology were awarded in the 1920s. Today there are 222 master's degree programs in communicative disorders and sciences in the United States. Ninety-nine of these programs offer the degree in speech-language pathology only; two offer the master's degree in audiology only; and 121 offer the master's degree in both speech-language pathology and audiology (ASHA, 1994a). In 1990–91, there were 10,146 students enrolled in master's level programs in communicative sciences and disorders. Of these, 8,747 were in speech-language pathology programs, 1,352 were in audiology programs, and 47 were in programs for speech and hearing science (Creaghead et al., 1991).

The major objective of master's level education in communication sciences and disorders is to prepare students for professional careers in speech-language pathology or audiology. Most master's degree programs prepare students for independent practice in the profession of speech-language pathology or audiology. Others prepare students for careers in speech and hearing science.

ADMISSION

Admission to master's programs in communication sciences and disorders usually requires a strong undergraduate record of liberal arts and sciences, in addition to preprofessional coursework. Students who have not completed a preprofessional curriculum as undergraduates usually must successfully complete 18–30 semester hours of preprofessional coursework before acceptance into a master's program. They may be classified as nondegree students, make-up students, premajor students, or conditional graduate students while they are completing needed requirements.

Although there is some variation in the admission requirements, programs usually require applicants for admission to master's degree programs to submit:

- Scores on the verbal, mathematical, and/or analytic sections of the Graduate Record Examination (GRE);
- Transcript or record of successful completion of a bachelor's degree;
- Letters of recommendation from persons knowledgeable about the student's ability to be successful in graduate study;
- A written personal statement that expresses the applicant's interest in the profession and the individual's career objectives;
- A personal interview is usually optional, but is highly recommended.

CURRICULUM

The curriculum of a specific master's degree program often reflects the interests and strengths of the individual members of the institution's faculty. The curriculum is usually designed to allow students to complete requirements for the CCC, state licensure, and, where appropriate, the certificate to practice the profession in educational settings. Master's programs usually require 4 semesters of postbaccalaureate study, if the undergraduate major was in the discipline and 7–8 semesters of study, if the undergraduate program was not in the discipline. The number of graduate credits in the discipline required for a degree ranges from 36 to 65. The average number of semester credits required for graduation is 48 semester credits postbachelor's degree for students with the

undergraduate major and 62 semester credits for students without the undergraduate major.

Master's degree programs have the following three major requirements for completion of the degree: (a) academic coursework; (b) clinical practicum, and (c) a culminating activity, such as a comprehensive examination, research project, or thesis.

Academic Coursework

The academic coursework of a master's program builds on the foundation of liberal arts, basic sciences, and human communication processes introduced in a preprofessional program. Academic coursework is not merely an extension of the preprofessional coursework, but rather represents development of the knowledge base of the profession and its application to clinical practice and research.

Although each program is different, coursework in speech-language pathology generally includes emphasis on specific disorders, such as neuropathologies, voice disorders, craniofacial anomalies, language disorders, articulatory and phonatory disorders, dysfluency, augmentative and alternative communication, diagnostic principles and procedures, and the related areas of dysphagia and cognitive disorders. In addition, coursework often includes advanced study in acoustics or neuroscience, statistics, and research methods.

Coursework in audiology generally includes anatomy and physiology of the hearing mechanism, amplification, hearing conservation, counseling, amplification, diseases and disorders of the auditory mechanism, and aural rehabilitation. As in the speech-language pathology curriculum, the audiology curriculum usually includes advanced study in acoustics or neuroscience, statistics, and research methods.

Clinical Practicum

Clinical practice at the master's level usually follows the standards for the CCC. Master's candidates must obtain a minimum of 250 supervised clinical practicum hours. Although the exact nature of the clinical practicum experiences varies with the educational program, most require at least one semester of full-time clinical practicum in a hospital, clinic, or rehabilitation facility in addition to extensive study in an on-campus clinic. See Chapter 5 on clinical certification by Madell.

Comprehensive Examination

Master's degrees require a culminating activity designed to show that a student has acquired an appropriate knowledge base of the discipline and can use that knowledge in an integrated manner to solve clinical problems. Comprehensive examinations are designed for this purpose. The tests are usually designed by the faculty of the master's program to reflect the knowledge a given program expects of each student completing the degree at that institution. Comprehensive examinations usually require that the student integrate information obtained from a variety of academic courses and clinical experiences. They are usually written; however, they may be oral or a combination of types.

According to the *Guide to Graduate Education in Speech-Language Pathology and Audiology* (American Speech-Language-Hearing Association, 1991a), a comprehensive examination is required by nearly 50% of the graduate programs, and is optional in approximately 10% of the programs. In several programs, a comprehensive examination is required if the student does not complete a thesis. In others, if a comprehensive examination is selected in lieu of a thesis, additional academic coursework must be taken to complete the degree. Some programs require students to obtain a passing score on the National Examination in Speech-Language Pathology or Audiology (NESPA) in lieu of a comprehensive examination.

Thesis or Master's Project

The thesis is an original, independent research project completed under the direction of a faculty member. It is designed to provide a student with the opportunity to apply principles of scientific research to a question or hypothesis in the discipline and to produce a written scholarly document.

The thesis is developed with the guidance of a faculty member in consultation with a committee of faculty scholars. The thesis requires that the student develop and test a hypothesis using scientific method of inquiry. Often the student must present or defend the thesis before the committee or other members of the academic community.

A thesis is required for completion of degree requirements in only seven master's degree programs. It is optional in nearly all others. There has been a decline in the number of master's graduates completing theses during the past 10 years. In 1981–92 24.9% of master's graduates completed theses; however, in 1989–90 only 19.3% of master's graduates completed theses (Creaghead et al., 1991).

A master's project is an independent project developed by the student with the guidance of a faculty member. The master's project may be a research project, a case study, a literature review, or similar activity which requires the student to integrate knowledge obtained in the program in an original manner. The master's project usually does not involve a committee of scholars or an oral defense.

Many doctoral programs require that students complete a thesis or predissertation research work before work on a dissertation. Students who are contemplating doctoral study are usually encouraged to complete a master's thesis rather than a master's project.

ACCREDITATION AND CERTIFICATION

Standard I of The Standards for the Certificates of Clinical Competence, effective January 1, 1993, states:

Applicants for either certificate must have a master's or doctoral degree. Effective January 1, 1994, all graduate coursework and graduate clinical practicum required in the professional area for which the certificate is sought must have been *initiated and completed* at an institution whose program was accredited by the Educational Standards Board of the American Speech-Language-Hearing Association in the area for which the certificate is sought. (ASHA, 1993b, p. 76)

Nearly all graduate programs in speech-language pathology and audiology are accredited by ESB. Because the accreditation status of a program can change, students must be certain that their chosen master's degree program is accredited when they begin and complete their graduate professional coursework and graduate clinical practicum. Information on how to obtain the accreditation status of a program is provided at the end of this chapter.

DOCTORAL EDUCATION IN SPEECH-LANGUAGE PATHOLOGY AND AUDIOLOGY

The first doctoral degree with an emphasis in speech-language pathology or audiology was awarded to Sara M. Stinchfield at the University of Wisconsin in 1921 (Neidecker & Blosser, 1993). At the present time there are 58 programs in the United States that offer the doctoral degree in communication sciences and disorders. Fifty doctoral programs are in institutions that offer the bachelor's, master's, and doctoral degrees; 6 offer both the master's and doctoral degrees; and 2 offer only the doctoral degree. Nine programs offer the doctoral degree in speech-language pathology only; 2 offer the degree in audiology only; 44 in both speech-language pathology; and 3 in communication sciences (ASHA, 1994a). One-hundred-twenty-seven doctoral degrees in communication sciences and disorders were awarded in 1989–90 (Creaghead et al., 1991).

The fundamental purpose of a doctoral degree in communicative sciences and disorders sciences is demonstrated achievement in three broad areas.

1. Mastery of the essential theory and knowledge in the field in which the degree is awarded;
2. Achievement of pertinent research or scholarship skills relevant to the field;
3. Dissertation or scholarly work that is an original contribution to the knowledge in the field. (Council of Graduate Schools in the United States, 1977)

DOCTORAL PROGRAMS IN COMMUNICATION SCIENCES AND DISORDERS

Doctoral programs require 2–3 years of study beyond the master's degree, or 3–4 years beyond the bachelor's degree without an intervening master's degree. All doctoral degrees require critical, basic elements.

Curriculum

The curriculum of doctoral programs is individualized with flexibility to allow individuals to prepare as researchers, university teachers, administrators, or clinicians.

The doctoral curriculum is usually based on a strong foundation of liberal arts and sciences and requires of students a common knowledge base in the discipline of communication sciences and disorders as prerequisite. The specific curriculum at each university builds on the strength of the faculty at the institution. The curriculum must ensure that students become familiar with the scientific and professional knowledge base related to their particular area of study. If the program is designed to prepare the graduate for clinical service, there must be available a sufficient base of clinical programs providing a high quality of clinical services above that expected of persons entering the profession. Laboratories must provide sufficient equipment to conduct the desired research.

If the doctorate is designed to prepare the student for clinical practice, the program must incorporate and exceed state and national minimal standards for certification and licensure.

Residency

Doctoral degree programs must allow sufficient time for the completion of the degree requirements, but not permit a time frame so long or so short as to impair the educational experience. Most doctoral degree programs require a minimum of 3 years and a maximum of 7 years for completion. For at least 1 year of the doctoral program, the doctoral student must be engaged in full-time study. The period of full-time study is called the residency.

Faculty

Doctoral faculty should demonstrate competency for scholarly and professional work in the relevant discipline. Doctoral faculty usually hold the doctoral degree and have a record of postdoctoral scholarship and research. The quality of the faculty is essential to assure students proper guidance in the completion of their research projects. The primary professional commitment of the core faculty and administration of a doctoral program must be to the sponsoring institution rather than to private practice or employment elsewhere.

Access

Doctoral programs must ensure students sufficient access, either individually or in small groups, to qualified faculty and to adequate laboratory facilities. This assures that students can pursue most of their program under the scrutiny of qualified faculty. For this reason, doctoral programs usually limit the number of enrolled students. There was an average of three doctoral students in each of the 59 doctoral programs in the United States in 1990–91 (Creaghead et al., 1991).

Preliminary and Comprehensive Examinations

Most doctoral programs require preliminary examinations taken early in the doctoral program to assess student knowledge. An appropriate course of study is then planned based on the knowledge that the student is able to demonstrate. At or near the end of the program, comprehensive final examinations are conducted by recognized scholars in the discipline to verify that the doctoral student has obtained the cognitive substrata of the discipline. The examinations usually require demonstration of knowledge and the ability to integrate knowledge within the entire discipline. Examinations may be written, oral, or

both, depending on the institution. Doctoral students must successfully complete comprehensive examinations before being admitted to candidacy for a degree and before being given permission to work on a dissertation.

Dissertation

Doctoral programs require a scholarly written project based on independent research or clinical study. Students usually must develop and defend their proposal for an independent research project that demonstrates their understanding of pertinent research skills. They must develop an original hypothesis and a plan to test the hypothesis using the methods of science. Development of the hypothesis and plan is usually accomplished with the guidance of a faculty advisor and committee of scholars from fields related to the particular project. The doctoral candidate must defend the proposal before members of the committee to demonstrate an understanding of the research methods necessary for completion of the project.

After collection and analysis of the research data, the doctoral candidate must prepare the written document. The document is reviewed by members of the dissertation committee, and an outside reader scholar must attest to the accuracy and rigor of the completed project.

Oral Defense

Doctoral programs require that a candidate defend the final dissertation or scholarly work before acknowledged scholars in the field. The oral defense before the committee of scholars and other members of the research community allows the doctoral candidate to demonstrate mastery of research skills and scholarship (Harris, Troutt, & Andrews, 1980).

TYPES OF DOCTORAL DEGREES

There are three types of doctoral degrees awarded in the United States—the research doctorate, the clinical doctorate and the professional doctorate.

The Research Doctorate

The research doctorate is the mark of the highest achievement in a field. It is awarded in recognition of preparation for creative scholarship and research, often in association with a career in teaching at a university or college or with work in a research laboratory. The most commonly awarded doctorates for study in communicative sciences and disorders are the Doctor of Philosophy (Ph.D.) and the Doctor of Education (Ed.D.) The Doctor of Philosophy, originally awarded in 1861, is a degree which is granted for study in nearly all fields of pure and applied learning. The Doctor of Education is awarded for study in areas traditionally related to education. At least two programs offer other types of doctoral degrees. Boston University offers a Doctor of Science (Sc.D.) in communication disorders and Adelphi University offers a Doctor of Arts (D.A.) in communicative disorders.

The Clinical Doctorate

The clinical doctorate is an adaptation of the research doctorate. Like the research doctorate, the clinical doctorate is a mark of highest achievement in a field. While the objective of the research doctorate is to prepare students for careers in research and scholarship, the objective of the clinical doctorate is to prepare students for clinical practice. The clinical doctorate is not intended to replace the research doctorate. Rather, it refers to a clinical track taken by those who wish to practice a profession as a direct service provider to the public or other professions. Preparation in research and the completion of a research project are usually required, but granting the degree is not contingent on research as the cornerstone of the degree. The Ph.D. is awarded to persons completing requirements for the clinical doctorate (ASHA, 1991b; The Council of Graduate Programs in the United States, 1969).

The Professional Doctorate

The Council of Graduate Schools in the United States (1971) has defined the professional doctorate as "the highest university award given in a particular field in recognition of completion of academic preparation for professional practice" (p. 1). The most common professional doctorates are Doctor of Medicine (M.D.), Doctor of Dental Service (D.D.S.), Juris Doctor (J.D.), Doctor of Psychology (Psy.D.), and Doctor of Pharmacy (Pharm. D.). The major objective of the professional doctorate is to produce professionals who are competent to provide a wide array of services associated with professional practice. While research doctorates such as the Ph.D. and Ed.D. place emphasis on research and scholarship, professional doctorates place emphasis on clinical practice.

The Doctor of Audiology (Au.D.)

The Doctor of Audiology is a postbaccalaureate professional degree primarily designed to prepare audiologists who are competent to perform the wide array of diagnostic, remedial, and other services associated with the current practice of audiology. The Au.D. places major emphasis on clinical training with students expected to engage in a variety of full-time clinical assignments. At this time, the Au.D. is offered only by Baylor University Medical Center. The specific curricula for the degree is specified by the degree-granting institution (see Chapter 28 by Loavenbruck).

ACCREDITATION AND CERTIFICATION

Standard I. The Standards for the CCCs states that graduate coursework and graduate clinical practicum required in the professional area for which the certificate is sought must have been initiated and completed at an institution whose program was accredited by the Educational Standards Board of ASHA (ASHA, 1993b). Until recently, only master's degree programs could be accredited. In

1993, a mechanism was established to allow the accreditation of graduate programs, including doctoral programs. This will allow students who complete doctoral degrees without an intervening master's degree to obtain clinical certification. This will also allow new models of education, such as the professional doctorate, to develop with the assurance that graduates will be eligible for clinical certification.

POST-DOCTORAL STUDY

Post-doctoral study in communicative sciences and disorders is specialized study undertaken by an individual after the completion of a doctoral degree. Postdoctoral study is usually for 1 to 3 years of advanced study in a specialized area of research or clinical study. The site of the study depends on the nature of the post-doctoral study. Study may be at a doctoral degree-granting-institution, a research laboratory, or a research clinic or hospital. Specific projects are usually funded by the federal government, foundations, or private agencies. Specific information about postdoctoral study can be obtained from the ASHA Research Division.

FINANCIAL ASSISTANCE

The process of obtaining an education for a career in speech-language pathology or audiology requires many years of study. Many students require financial assistance to support their course of study. Financial aid is available for students to support graduate study in the discipline. In 1990–91, 37.1% of the master's degree students and 79.6% of the doctoral level students received financial support (Creaghead et al., 1991). Although many sources of financial aid are based on financial need, graduate financial assistance is usually based on merit and the ability of the student to fulfill the requirements of the particular aid program.

Financial aid may take the form of scholarships or grants, fellowships, assistantships, teaching assistantships, traineeships, or loans. Financial aid may be awarded by a university, private agency, or state or federal government. Fellowships, scholarships, and grants are awarded to the student based on particular requirements set by the awarding agency. Such aid does not need to be repaid, nor is work required. Several scholarships are available from the American Speech-Language-Hearing Foundation.

Patricia Roberts Harris Fellowships are available from the United States Department of Education for minority students who are underrepresented in certain professional fields and who meet academic and financial need requirements. The awards are made by the institution that has been granted the fellowship program. Students should contact the United States Department of Education Patricia Roberts Harris Fellowship Program for information about programs that have received Patricia Roberts Harris Fellowships.

Assistantships for graduate students are funded by the university or by grants to the university from external sources. The United States Department of Education Office of Special Education and Rehabilitation Services provides a number of graduate assistantships through the Personnel Preparation Grants program. Personnel Preparation programs are intended to train personnel for areas of specific need. Awards are made to individual programs to complete a project designed to improve the quality of service to disabled children and youth.

Teaching assistantships which are usually awarded to doctoral students require the student to teach or assist faculty in teaching undergraduate or graduate courses. Research assistantships require a student to assist faculty in an ongoing research project. Student assistants usually receive a tuition remission or waiver and a living stipend in exchange for several hours of work each week.

Traineeships are awarded to students to allow special training for a particular population. For example, the Veteran's Administration provides traineeships to prepare students for careers in the Veteran's Administration programs.

Students who require financial assistance for graduate study should contact the program that they wish to attend. Because the application dates for several programs are usually early in the spring, students should apply for financial aid when they apply for admission to the program.

INTERNATIONAL EDUCATION

Educational programs for careers in speech-language pathology and audiology are offered in more than 40 countries throughout the world including Canada, Mexico, Argentina, South Africa, Peoples Republic of China, Japan, Australia, Germany, The Netherlands, and Sweden. Educational programs in foreign countries are located in special schools, universities, and hospitals or medical facilities. They are usually 3- or 4-year programs that lead to either a diploma, certificate, registration, or degree. The curricula vary, but generally include coursework in anatomy, physiology, linguistics, language, psychology, and neurology, and considerable clinical practice.

The models of the educational programs vary. For example, in Egypt, a postgraduate program of 12 months in length includes coursework in anatomy, physiology, physical bases of speech and hearing, linguistics, and language development. Two-hundred and fifty hours of clinical practice are necessary for the certificate to be a logopedist or speech-language pathologist. In Germany, 3-year educational programs for logopedists are affiliated with phoniatric departments in university hospitals. In the United Kingdom, there are 3- and 4-year degree courses in universities, polytechnics, and colleges of education. Some courses of study lead to an ordinary degree (also called a pass or unclassified degree) status. An honors degree includes an empirical research project, demands more from the student, and denotes more specialization than an ordinary degree (Stewart, 1991).

Because of Standard I of the standards for the CCC, students who receive their graduate professional education in other countries may not be eligible for the CCC. The ASHA Council on Professional Standards has adopted a program of endorsement of foreign credentials to assist those educated in other countries in obtaining the CCC. In addition ASHA is working with the International Association of Logopedics and Phoniatrics (IALP) to develop commonalities in the education of speech-language pathologists to improve mobility of professionals in the world market. Additional information on education of speech-language pathologists and audiologist in foreign countries can be obtained from the International Association of Logopedics and Phoniatrics (IALP) or the American Speech-Language-Hearing Association. (See Chapter 7 by Wilson for further information on international perspectives.)

CONTINUING EDUCATION

The discipline of communication sciences and disorders is constantly developing new knowledge and new technology. In order for professionals to continue to be competent, it is necessary to obtain current information impacting on practice of the professions. Professionals must make a lifelong commitment to maintain currency in the area of practice. Continuing education is education beyond the minimum required for entry into the professions.

Continuing education may take the form of independent study through directed reading of professional literature, attendance at continuing education activities offered by professional associations, agencies, or institutions, participation in journal or study groups, preparation of coursework, workshops, or visitation to master clinicians, or other experiences that improve the ability to deliver quality service.

The ASHA Code of Ethics, Principle IIC states that "Individuals shall continue their professional development throughout their careers" (ASHA, 1993a). ASHA maintains a program of voluntary participation in a formal continuing education program and awards the Award for Continuing Education (ACE) to persons who complete current requirements for the award. Many states with licensure require evidence of continuing education for renewal of the professional license. Participation in the ACE program provides a mechanism to document continuing education and allows formal recognition for completion of continuing education activities. For information on continuing education contact ASHA's Continuing Education Division.

SUMMARY

Education in communication sciences and disorders is a lifelong process along a continuum of undergraduate, graduate, and continuing education. Undergraduate or pre-professional preparation for careers in speech-language pathology or audiology provides an introduction to the discipline of communication sciences and disorders within the context of a liberal arts education. Graduate education occurs at the master's and doctoral levels. The master's degree level is the minimum level required for entry into professional practice. It emphasizes application of knowledge to the development of research to solve clinical problems. Doctoral education is the highest level of academic achievement. Doctoral study prepares persons for careers in research and scholarship usually related to university teaching or for careers in specialized clinical research and practice. The professional doctorate prepares persons at the highest level for careers in clinical practice.

Educational programs in speech-language pathology are offered throughout the world. There are many different models of international education leading to several different credentials for practice in foreign countries. ASHA is working with the IALP to develop commonalities in educational standards for practice of speech-language pathology and audiology.

DISCUSSION QUESTIONS

1. What are the advantages and disadvantages of enrolling in a preprofessional-only program for the undergraduate degree?

2. Should all graduate programs offer a standardized academic curriculum? Why? Why not?
3. What are the advantages and disadvantages of selecting the thesis option in a master's degree program?
4. What are the advantages and disadvantages of the professional doctorate as a requirement for practice of the professions?
5. Why is continuing education an important component in career development? What continuing education programs are appealing to you and why?

REFERENCES

American Speech-Language-Hearing Association. (1990). *Report of Ad-Hoc Committee in Undergraduate Education.* Rockville, MD: Author.

American Speech-Language-Hearing Association. (1991a). *Guide to graduate education in speech-language pathology and audiology.* Rockville, MD: Author.

American-Speech-Language Hearing Association. (1991b). Report on doctoral education. *Asha, 33*(Suppl. 3), 1–9.

American Speech-Language-Hearing Association. (1993a). Code of ethics. *Asha, 35,* 17–18.

American Speech-Language-Hearing Association. (1993b). Implementation procedures for the standards for the certificates of clinical competence. *Asha, 35,* 76–83.

American Speech-Language-Hearing Association. (1994a). Personal communication from Educational Standards Board.

American Speech-Language-Hearing Association. (1994b). Change in certification standard. *Asha, 36,* 63.

Council of Graduate Schools in the United States. (1969). *The nature and naming of graduate and professional degree programs. The accreditation of graduate and professional degree programs.* Policy statement of the Council of Graduate Schools in the United States. Washington, DC: Author.

Council of Graduate Schools in the United States. (1971). *The doctors degree in professional fields. A statement by the Association of Graduate Schools in the Association of Graduate Schools in the United States.* Washington, DC: Author.

Council of Graduate Schools in the United States. (1977). *The doctor of philosophy degree—A policy statement.* Washington, DC: Author.

Council of Graduate Programs in Communication Sciences and Disorders. (1991). *Report of the Ad-Hoc Committee on Doctoral Education.* Washington, DC: Author.

Creaghead, N., Bernthal, J., & Gilbert, H. (1991). *1990–91 National Survey.* Minneapolis, MN: Council of Graduate Programs in Communication Sciences and Disorders.

Harris, J., Troutt W. E., & Andrews, G. (1980). *The American doctorate in the context of new patterns in higher education.* Washington, DC: Council on Postsecondary Accreditation.

Neidecker, E., & Blosser, J. (1993). *School programs in speech-language: Organization and management.* Englewood Cliffs, NJ: Prentice-Hall.

Stewart, B. (1991). *International directory of education for speech-language pathologists.* Rockville MD: American Speech- Language-Hearing Association.

Terrizzi, A. (1988). Status report on undergraduate education in communication sciences and disorders, *Asha, 30,* 31–33.

RESOURCES

For specific information on undergraduate or preprofessional programs in speech-language pathology contact:

Sandy Salisch, President
National Academy of Pre-Professional
  Programs
Speech Communication Department
Pace University
Pace Plaza
New York, NY 10038
(212) 346-1441

For a listing of all programs in speech-language pathology and audiology accredited by the Educational Standards Board of ASHA see the March issue of *Asha.*

Specific information on the accreditation status of graduate programs is available from the American Speech-Language-Hearing Association Action Line 1 (800) 638-6868.

For information on specific graduate programs consult the

Guide to Graduate Education in Speech-
  Language Pathology and Audiology,
American Speech-Language-Hearing
  Association
10801 Rockville Pike
Rockville, MD 20852

Specific information on financial assistance for graduate study in communication sciences and disorders is available from the Financial Aid Office of your college or university and from the Office of Recruitment and Career Development of ASHA.

Specific information on the scholarships available from the American Speech-Language-Hearing Foundation can be obtained from:

American Speech-Language-Hearing
  Foundation
10801 Rockville Pike
Rockville, MD 20852

For information on federal fellowships and assistantships through personnel preparation grants contact:

U.S. Department of Education
Office of Special Education and
  Rehabilitative Services
Division of Personnel Preparation
Washington, DC 20202

■ CHAPTER 4 ■

Certification and Licensure

■ DOLORES BATTLE, Ph.D. ■

SCOPE OF CHAPTER

The practice of a profession carries with it responsibility. Professional associations and governmental agencies regulate the relationship between the right to practice and professional responsibilities. This chapter provides an overview of the three major types of professional practice regulation: certification, licensure, and registration. It reviews differences between voluntary and mandatory regulation, the primary characteristics of statutes, and standards regulating the practice of speech-language pathology and audiology. Finally, it looks to future trends expected in regulation of the professions of speech-language pathology and audiology.

HISTORY OF REGULATION OF SPEECH-LANGUAGE PATHOLOGISTS AND AUDIOLOGISTS

Although occupational and professional licensing in the United States began in the mid-1850s as a means of protecting the public from untrained physicians (Carthcart & Graff, 1978; Hume, 1985; Shimberg, 1982), regulation of speech-language pathologists did not begin until the 1950s. Persons who provided speech-language services were regulated first through teacher certification under the general category of elementary or special education, rather than speech-language pathology. Through the 1960s, as the federal government became involved in the nation's health and educational systems, most departments of education established certification for persons providing speech-language pathology services in the public schools. In 1969, Florida recognized the need for establishing credentials for the practice of the professions in noneducational settings and established the first state law for the licensing of speech-language pathology and audiology. Between 1969 and 1975, legislation to license speech-language pathologists and audiologists passed in 27 states.

By the end of 1992, 43 states had passed legislation to regulate speech-language pathologists and audiologists (see Table 4–1). Forty states issue a license to practice either speech-language pathology or audiology. Alaska licenses audiologists but not speech-language pathologists. New Hampshire licenses speech-language pathologists but not audiologists. Minnesota

20

regulates speech-language pathologists and audiologists through registration. Seven states do not regulate either speech-language pathologists or audiologists: Arizona, Colorado, Idaho, Michigan, South Dakota, Vermont, and Washington. Washington, DC does not regulate either speech-language pathologists or audiologists.

TABLE 4–1. STATES REGULATING SPEECH-LANGUAGE PATHOLOGISTS AND/OR AUDIOLOGISTS AS OF JANUARY 1994. (ENACTMENT SEQUENCE IN [ ], ENACTMENT DATE FOLLOWS)

Alabama	[27]	12/75	Nebraska	[31]	7/79
Alaska[a]	[37]	5/86	Nevada	[31]	7/79
Arkansas	[20]	2/75	New Jersey	[35]	1/84
California	[6]	12/72	New Hampshire[b]	[43]	5/92
Connecticut	[11]	6/73	New Mexico	[32]	4/81
Delaware	[15]	7/73	New York	[18]	6/74
Florida	[1]	4/69	N Carolina	[26]	3/75
Georgia	[16]	3/74	N Dakota	[22]	3/75
Hawaii	[17]	5/74	Ohio	[25]	6/75
Illinois	[38]	9/88	Oklahoma	[9]	5/73
Indiana	[7]	4/73	Oregon	[13]	7/73
Iowa	[28]	2/76	Pennsylvania	[36]	12/84
Kansas	[41]	5/91	Rhode Island	[10]	5/73
Kentucky	[3]	4/72	S Carolina	[12]	6/73
Louisiana	[5]	7/72	Tennessee	[8]	4/73
Maine	[29]	4/76	Texas	[34]	6/83
Maryland	[4]	5/72	Utah	[21]	3/75
Massachusetts	[33]	1/83	Virginia	[2]	3/72
Minnesota[c]	[40]	2/91	W Virginia	[42]	3/92
Mississippi	[23]	4/75	Wisconsin	[39]	4/90
Missouri	[14]	7/73	Wyoming	[19]	4/90
Montana	[24]	5/75			

Source: Adapted from information provided by American Speech-Language-Hearing Association Governmental Affairs, January 1994; Lynch & Welsh, 1993.

[a] Licenses audiologists; not speech-language pathologists
[b] Licenses speech-language pathologists; not audiologists
[c] Regulates through registration

Note: States that do not regulate speech-language pathologists and/or audiologists; Michigan, Arizona, South Dakota, Colorado, Vermont, Idaho, and Washington, plus the District of Columbia.

WHY REGULATE SPEECH-LANGUAGE PATHOLOGISTS AND AUDIOLOGISTS?

The need to regulate the practice of speech-language pathology and audiology is embodied in the consumer protection movement. The consumer places faith in the knowledge and services of experts. The consumer, however, may not be able to make reasoned judgments about the quality of the service received or the competence of the person providing services. Consumer protection is necessary because young children, individuals with disabilities, and the elderly—the primary consumers of the services of speech-language pathologists and audiologists—are the least able to seek restitution for abuses of professional practices. Regulation serves to protect the consumer from harm caused by improper diagnosis and treatment and helps consumers predict the quality of service (Lynch, 1986).

TYPES OF REGULATION

Professional regulation or credentialing involves the establishment of minimal standards for entry into the general practice of a profession. There are four types of credentials in the professions of speech-language pathology and audiology, each providing different levels of restriction on the ability to practice: licensure, professional certification, teacher certification, and registration.

LICENSURE

Licensing is the process by which a government grants permission to an individual to engage in a given occupation. Permission to practice within a profession is granted on determining that the applicant has attained the minimal degree of competency necessary to ensure that the public health, safety, and welfare will be protected.

Licensure is based on the belief that stringent entry requirements and ongoing scrutiny by government will ensure the protection of the consumer. Such protection is deemed necessary because of the difficulty consumers have in ascertaining the competence of those who purport to be skilled, and because of consumers' inability to recognize when substantial injury has been sustained at the hands of the service provider (Carthcart & Graff, 1978).

Licensure is always a function of a state government. Licensure is established by an act of a state legislature and approval by the governor. Only those who hold the license may practice the profession in the state. Licensure is the most restrictive form of regulation, because its requirements are codified in state law. Professional licensure is characterized by self-regulation managed by members of the profession. By working through a state regulatory agency, the members of the profession establish the requirements for the license and monitor the activities of those who hold the license. This assures that the interests of the public are being served. The ultimate sanctions for violation of the licensure statute are removal of the license and/or payment of fines.

Licensing Laws Versus Rules and Regulations

Although a law contains broad provisions governing the practice of speech-language pathologists and audiologists, more specific rules and regulations are set to implement the law. The law (or statute) can only be changed by a state legislature and approved by the governor. If any part of a licensure law is to be changed, the law must be reintroduced through the legislative process. The entire law is then subject to review. The regulations are changed by the process adopted by a state for altering regulations, such as approval by a board of regents or medical board. Changes in rules or regulations can be made without altering the statute.

Sunset Review

Sunset review is a process in which government agencies are automatically terminated on a specific date unless the legislature reviews their operations and approves their continuation. Although no license in speech-language pathology or audiology has ever been eliminated because of a sunset provision, several have faced reorganization, and one has resulted in an upgrading of the standards.

PROFESSIONAL CERTIFICATION AND TEACHER CERTIFICATION

Certification refers to a credential that recognizes an individual's achievements based on predetermined standards. It is a process by which a governmental or nongovernmental agency grants an individual the authority to use a specific title or to engage in a specific occupation after meeting predetermined qualifications. The governmental or statutory certificate is mandatory for practice of the occupation and often qualifies a professional as a service provider for third-party (insurance) reimbursement. Statutory or governmental certification is usually established and monitored by the government and not by members of the profession.

Teacher Certification

The most common governmental certification is teacher certification, which is granted by the state department of education for identifying persons who have met minimum requirements to provide educational services in the public schools. In some states, such as Massachusetts, there is no teaching certification, because a state license is necessary to practice speech-language pathology in the schools.

Requirements for a teaching certificate vary from state to state. Most states require that the holder have at least a master's degree with educational preparation including a specified amount of professional coursework.

In addition to professional knowledge in speech-language pathology, some states require that applicants have coursework that specifically prepares the applicant for work in the educational setting. Required coursework may include educational pedagogy, school or state history, and/or coursework in human development. In addition, teacher certification may require other specific training. For example, some states require persons holding the teaching certificate to have foreign language training. In New York, applicants for the teaching certificate must have training in drug and alcohol abuse and in recognizing child abuse.

Most states require a school-based practicum or student teaching under the supervision of a person who holds the appropriate teaching certificate. The practicum usually is for a period of at least 8 weeks and must involve experience in assessment and treatment of children with communication disabilities.

Most states require a passing grade on an examination to determine if applicants for the certificate have the necessary knowledge and skills for successful teaching. Many states require the National Teacher Examination Core Battery, which consists of separate tests of communication skill, general knowledge, and professional knowledge. Some states require the National Examination in Speech-Language Pathology. Other states have examinations developed specifically for the purpose.

Many states require applicants to complete a period of supervised work experience before granting the teaching certificate. This may vary from 9 months to 2 years, (as in New York).

In 1986, Public Law 99-457 was passed by the U.S. Congress (U.S. Department of Education, 1986). This law, which amended the Education of the Handicapped Act (PL 94-142), requires that persons who provide services to children receiving special education and related services hold the academic training and degree equivalent to the "highest requirements in the state applicable to a specific profession or discipline." The teaching certificate requirements in most states are equal to those of licensure. Other states are working to upgrade the requirements for certification to be consistent with state licensing laws and, therefore, be in compliance with PL 99-457.

Specific requirements for teaching certification can be obtained from the state commissioner of education or department of education in your particular state. Addresses and state education agency contacts are usually published in the March issue of *Asha*.

Professional Certification

Professional certification is awarded to members of professional associations who meet established requirements or standards established by the association. Such professional certification is a way to build professional identity, improve the quality of service, and to promote ethical behavior by monitoring the professional activity of association members. The ultimate sanction for violation of the voluntary certificate is removal of membership and/or certification.

Professional certification is voluntary. Although professional certification is not legally binding as a qualification for practicing in a particular profession, it may be mandatory for certain members of the association who engage in certain practices. The Certificate of Clinical Competence (CCC) offered by the American Speech-Language- Hearing Association (ASHA), for example, is awarded to its members who engage in clinical practice. It is not mandatory for members of the association who do not engage in clinical practice, nor is it mandatory for persons who are not members of the association. However, the more necessary a nongovernmental credential is perceived to be, the less voluntary holding it becomes. The professional organization may be considered to be engaged in a quasipublic, quasilegal activity which may make it subject to legal regulation under antitrust or other laws (Moll, 1991; Reaves, 1992). To avoid the appearance of violation of antitrust laws, ASHA allows nonmembers to hold the Certificate of Clinical Competence (CCC). Such persons must, however, pay a fee to cover the cost of the certification program as determined by ASHA. Nonmembers who hold the CCC must also abide by the ASHA Code of Ethics.

The practice of voluntary certification is not without its opponents. Some believe that certification programs are inherently misleading because certification represents an implicit claim of quality that cannot be verified. Others believe that it unfairly restricts competition by giving those who hold the certificate a competitive advantage. In June 1990, the U.S. Supreme Court case, *Peel v. Attorney Registration and Disciplinary Commission of Illinois* (Levy & Goldfarb, 1991), addressed voluntary credentialing of professionals for the first time. Based on the First Amendment of the United States Constitution, the case was a challenge to a state restriction on the use of specialty certification by attorneys. The court found that properly structured credentialing programs do provide useful information to the consumers. The decision established the principles that state government agencies cannot forbid professionals from truthfully presenting themselves to the public as certified in a particular specialty or field by responsible certifying associations. States can, however, impose reasonable regulations on specialty certification claims to prevent the public from being confused or misled. The states may also require that associations make public the standards for certification so consumers can evaluate what the certification actually means (Levy & Goldfarb, 1991).

Relationship Between Licensure and Certification

The relationship between licensure and certification can be complementary. A licensing statute may specify a voluntary certificate and certifying body and provide an alternative pathway to obtaining a license. For example, a state licensure statute may state that a person holding the ASHA CCC may be granted a license to practice the profession in that state. The person applying for the license, in the state need only provide evidence of certification to be granted the license.

Requirements for a professional license and a teaching certificate may differ within a state. The provisions of PL 99-457, the Education of Handicapped Children Act Amendments of 1988 require that persons providing educational services to children with disabilities hold the highest qualification for practice of the profession within the state. Most states have altered their certificates governing speech-language pathology to ensure that the requirements for the teaching certificate and the professional license are compatible, or states have required a license for professional practice in educational settings.

REGISTRATION

Registration, the least restrictive form of regulation, permits persons to use certain titles or to engage in certain activities. Individuals may be required to meet minimum practice standards before registering and using the title of a registered practitioner. Nonqualified persons may continue to practice as long as they do not use certain titles or represent themselves to the public as "qualified."

In several states without licensure, such as Arizona, Vermont, Washington, and Idaho, speech-language pathologists and audiologists are required to register. Minnesota has voluntary registration for speech-language pathologists and audiologists.

Many states require registration of hearing instrument dispensers or hearing aid dealers. In some states licensed audiologists must register as hearing aid dealers to dispense hearing aids. Some states register support personnel (e.g., speech assistants).

In some states there is a relationship between registration and licensure. A professional may be issued a license indicating that the minimum qualifications for practice have been met. The license is in effect for life unless it is removed, revoked, or suspended. To practice, individuals must register for the period in which they are to practice the profession. Professionals not engaging in professional practice within the state during a particular period may not be required to register; however, they will continue to be licensed. For example, if persons licensed to practice a profession in a particular state leave the state or will not practice the profession within the state for a period of time, they are not required to register for practice. On their return or when resuming practice in the state, they must reregister to practice the profession legally in the state.

LICENSURE IN SPEECH-LANGUAGE PATHOLOGY AND AUDIOLOGY

COMPONENTS OF LICENSURE LAWS

Although the specific content of licensure laws varies from state to state, each law has certain basic components.

Introduction/Intent of the Legislation

Several licensure laws include a statement that explains the intent of the statute. For example, the Declaration of Policy and Legislative Intent in the Alabama Licensure Law for Speech Pathologists and Audiologists (1975) states:

The practice of speech pathology [sic] and audiology is a privilege which is granted to qualified persons by legislative authority in the interest of public health, safety and welfare, and, in enacting this law, it is the intent of the legislature to require educational training and licensure of any persons who engage in the practice of speech pathology and/or audiology, to encourage better educational training programs, to prohibit the unauthorized and unqualified practice of speech pathology and/or audiology and the unprofessional conduct of persons licensed to practice speech pathology and audiology and to provide enforcement of the chapter and penalties for its violation. To help insure the availability of the highest possible quality speech pathology and/or audiology services to the communicatively handicapped people of the state, it is necessary to provide regularity authority over persons offering speech pathology and audiology services to the public.

Definition: Practice of the Profession

Licensing laws, often referred to as "practice acts," usually establish a "scope of practice" covered by the act. They define what persons

covered by the act are allowed to do in the practice of the profession. For example, the New York State Education Law Article 159 (1974) law licensing speech-language pathologists defines the practice of speech-language pathology as:

The practice of the profession of speech-language pathology shall mean the application of principles, methods, and procedures of measurement, prediction, non-medical diagnosis, testing, counselling, consultation, rehabilitation and instruction related to the development and disorders of speech, voice, and/or language for the purpose of preventing, ameliorating or modifying such conditions in individuals and/or groups of individuals.

The definition of the practice of audiology in the New York State Education Law (1974) is:

the application of principles, methods, and procedures of measurement, testing, evaluation, consultation, counselling, instruction and habilitation or rehabilitation related to hearing, its disorders and related communication impairments for the purpose of non-medical diagnosis, prevention, identification, amelioration or modification of such disorders and conditions in individuals and/or groups of individuals.

Prohibited Acts

Many licensure laws prohibit the use of the professional title by persons not holding the license. This assures that persons who use the title of the profession have met the standards established by the regulatory body. In the Alabama Licensure Law for Speech Pathologists and Audiologists (1975), for example, prohibited acts include "any person who shall use in connection with his name or otherwise assume, use or advertise and title or description tending to convey the impression that he is a speech pathologist or audiologist without being licensed."

In New York State Education Law (1974) anyone not authorized to use a professional title and who uses the professional title shall be guilty of a class A misdemeanor. Anyone who knowingly aids or abets three or more persons not authorized to use a professional title or knowingly employs three or more persons not authorized to use a professional title, or who uses such title in the course of such employment, shall be guilty of a class E felony.

Organization/Structure of the State Board or Committee

Licensure laws usually establish a board of examiners in speech-language pathology and audiology, an audiology and speech-language pathology advisory committee, or a council of advisors in speech-language pathology and audiology. In California, for example, the regulatory functions are conducted by the Speech Pathology and Audiology Examining Committee of the Medical Board of California. A board may be assigned to a department in the state government structure, such as the state's department of health, education, commerce, or consumer affairs.

The state boards or committees are usually made up of members of the profession to be licensed. Thirty-one of the boards for speech-language pathology and audiology have consumer or public members to ensure that the views of consumers are protected and represented in board activity. Twenty-one of the licensure boards have physician members. In Connecticut and Missouri, members of the medical profession serve as members of the speech-language pathology board, with speech-language pathologists and audiologists serving as consultants.

Licensure boards ensure the self-regulatory function of the profession within the state. This may include proposing policy, making final decisions on disciplinary matters, overseeing administrative operations, such as processing applications, recording continuing education credits, handling complaints, and/or providing advice and counsel to the administrative department.

REQUIREMENTS FOR HOLDING THE PROFESSIONAL LICENSE

Licensure defines for the public the minimum qualifications for entry into the practice of the profession (Flower, Ohta, Stephens, Quinn, & Orahood, 1986). The minimum requirements include specification of education, degree, examination, and experience. Twenty-seven states have requirements that are compatible with the ASHA CCC. Several other states differ in either the examination requirement or the minimal passing examination score, the requirements for the clinical fellowship year (CFY), the degree requirement, or the specific coursework or practicum requirements. There is considerable variation from state to state in the areas of reciprocity (recognition of a license issued by another state), interim practice (practice while the license application is in process), and other special provisions.

Education

All state laws regulating speech-language pathologists and audiologists specify the master's degree for receipt of the license. The statute often is stated using general terms with the specific course requirements presented in rules or regulations. For example, in Nebraska Law for the Practice of Audiology and Speech Pathology (1978), the education requirement states, "Every applicant for a license to practice audiology or speech-language pathology shall (1) present proof of a master's degree or its equivalent in audiology or speech-language pathology from an academic program approved by the Board." The specific academic credit is then defined in the Rules and Regulations Governing Audiology and Speech-Language Pathology (1987). Some states, however, specify academic coursework requirements in the statute. For example Alabama licensure law [§34-28A-21], details the specific courses that provide information about and training in the management of speech, hearing, and language disorders and that provide information supplementary to these areas.

Experience

Most states expect applicants for the license to have completed a 9 month, full-time supervised clinical experience, as is required for the ASHA CCC. Some states, however, such as Nevada, North Dakota, and Virginia, have no specific experience requirements.

Examination

All licensure laws require an examination to assess professional knowledge in the area of practice. Licensure laws often do not identify a specific examination in the statute. Rather, the laws require an examination that is "acceptable to the board" or one that "it considers appropriate." All states licensing speech-language pathologists and/or audiologists, however, have adopted the National Examinations in Speech Language Pathology and Audiology as the appropriate examinations.

EXEMPTIONS

Many licensing statutes have provisions that exempt certain persons from holding the license to practice of the professions of speech-language pathology and audiology. Federal employees are exempt from state licensure laws because the federal government has sole jurisdiction over its employees. Further, many states exempt persons certified by the state department of education to provide speech-language pathology and audiology services in the public schools. Although many state licensure laws originally had provisions that gave exemption to persons practicing speech-language pathology in educational settings, the personnel requirements of Public Law 99-457 have led to the elimination of these exemptions in most states. ASHA continues to assist states in eliminating exemption from the professional license for professionals employed in educational settings.

States also exempt for the license in speech-language pathology and audiology other persons who practice professions under other state licensing laws. Most common exemptions include physicians, surgeons, industrial hearing testers, hearing aid dealers, students and trainees, and persons fulfilling postgrad-

uate professional experience requirements. Some states also exempt nurses, teachers of the deaf, and persons with alaryngeal speech who are providing services to other persons with similar disabilities.

CONTINUING EDUCATION AND LICENSURE

The right to continue to practice after initial entry into professional practice is usually regulated by requirement to periodically renew the license. Such renewal may require the licensee to demonstrate continued competence. More than half of the states licensing speech-language pathologists and audiologists require continuing education for license renewal. Continuing education assures that licensees maintain currency and uphold standards of practice acceptable to the profession.

There is considerable variation in the requirements for continuing education across states. For example, Indiana requires 36 clock hours in 2 years, 6 hours of which must be in self-study. Utah requires 30 clock hours all of which must be at the graduate level, related to the area of practice (i.e., speech-language pathology or audiology) and obtained within a 5-year period.

A summary of the characteristics of state licensure laws is available in the March 1993 issue of *Asha* (Lynch & Welsh, 1993). Specific information can be obtained from individual state regulatory agencies. Current addresses and contact persons are listed each year in the March issue of *Asha*.

PROFESSIONAL DISCIPLINE

Licensure laws contain provisions for persons who violate the professional code of conduct. Alleged violation of the statute and/or regulations are reported as complaints of unprofessional conduct. Violations are handled by the board of examiners, the attorney general, or the local district attorney who has jurisdiction where the violation took place. Disciplinary proceedings, procedures, and penalties are defined in rules and regulations. Penalties may include surrender of license, probation and/or fines.

SPECIAL PROVISIONS IN LICENSURE LAWS

Transferability and Reciprocity

A license issued in one state is not directly transferable to allow practice in another state. One must apply for a license to practice in each state before being allowed to practice. Several states have provisions to waive the examination requirement for a license for practice in their state if the person holds either the CCC or a license from a state with equivalent standards. California, New York, Ohio, and Utah do not accept licenses from another state.

Interim Practice or Temporary Licenses

Interim practice provisions allow a person to practice for a period of time before the actual license is issued or while a license is pending. Provision and allowable period for interim practice vary across states. The time period allowed for interim practice varies across states. In several states, a temporary license is issued while the licensure application is being processed. In other states, a temporary license is issued to allow practice if all requirements except passing the required examination have been met. In these cases it is usual for the temporary license to be in effect until the next administration of the required examination.

SUPPORT PERSONNEL LICENSING

Several states have provisions for granting a license or registration to support personnel, speech assistants, or speech aides. Speech assistants or support personnel are persons who provide specified speech-language or audiology support services under the direct supervision of the licensed professional. For example, the Iowa Law Chapter 302 Speech Pathology and Audiology Assistants (1990) defines "speech assistant" as a person who works under the supervision of an Iowa licensed speech pathologist or audiologist, does not meet the requirements to be licensed as a speech pathologist or audiologist, and meets the minimum requirements set forth in these rules.

Qualifications for persons licensed or registered as assistants varies from the requirement of a high school education or equivalency to the holding of an associate's or bachelor's degree with specific content including at least an introductory course in speech-language pathology or audiology.

Support personnel must be supervised by persons who hold the license, according to the statutes. In addition, support personnel's duties and responsibilities are often restricted to those identified in a statute. For example, in California a registered speech aide is a person who assists or facilitates while a "speech pathologist" [sic] is evaluating the speech and/or language of individuals or is treating individuals with a speech and/or language disorder. Similarly, a registered audiology aide assists or facilitates while an audiologist is evaluating the hearing of individuals and/or is treating individuals with hearing disorders.

The duties of the supervisor are usually included in a statute or rules and regulations. In addition there are frequently restrictions on the number of assistants a licensee may utilize at any one time. This restriction ensures proper supervision. In all cases, it is clear that a licensed professional is legally responsible for the actions of support personnel in the performance of assigned duties.

ASHA CERTIFICATION

ASHA first developed standards for its members in 1942. With the growth of the profession in health care and education, the need for more stringent standards emerged. In 1951, two levels of certification were approved: a Basic Certificate awarded to those with bachelor's degrees and 1 year of experience and an Advanced Certificate awarded to those with master's or doctoral degrees in either speech-language pathology or audiology. In 1962, ASHA adopted the master's degree as the minimum requirement for membership. By 1965, certification standards were adopted. These standards required a master's degree in speech-language pathology or audiology or the equivalent, specific course requirements, a full-time paid professional experience called the clinical fellowship year (CFY), and the passing of a national examination in the area of certification. In 1972, the dual certification program was altered to establish a single level of certification—the Certificate of Clinical Competence (CCC). These standards for clinical certification were maintained until 1988, when new standards were adopted effective January 1, 1993. (See Standards for the Certificates of Clinical Competence in Appendix 4A.)

The CCC in speech-language pathology or audiology permits the holder to provide independent clinical services and to supervise the clinical practice of student trainees and clinicians who do not hold certification.

REQUIREMENTS OF THE CERTIFICATES OF CLINICAL COMPETENCE

Applicants for the CCC must meet the five standards adopted by the Council on Professional Standards (See Appendix 4A). Standards are statements of minimum qualification that must be met to be eligible for the certificate. The Clinical Certification Board determines whether applicants have met the standards. Applicants who are denied certification can appeal the decision of the ASHA Clinical Certification Board to the Council on Professional Standards. The decision of the Council on Professional Standards is final.

For further information, see Chapter 5 on standards by Madell in this text. Specific information on obtaining the CCC and the current application forms can be obtained from the American Speech Language Hearing Association, 10801 Rockville Pike, Rockville, MD 20852.

CERTIFICATION OF FOREIGN TRAINED PROFESSIONALS

The standards for the CCC require that after January 1, 1994, graduate professional education and clinical practicum must have been initiated and completed at an institution whose program is accredited by the Educational Standards Board of ASHA. Because ASHA can only accredit educational programs in the United States, persons who receive their professional education in foreign countries are not eligible for the CCC under the 1993 standards.

To allow access to the CCC for persons trained in foreign countries, the Council on Professional Standards has adopted a program to endorse credentials issued by non-US national private credentialing agencies and to allow persons educated outside the United States to submit their credentials for evaluation by the Clinical Certification Board. The details of this program of endorsement are in the process of being developed at the time of this writing.

FUTURE TRENDS IN CERTIFICATION AND LICENSURE

Because speech-language pathology and audiology are evolving professions, the programs regulating the professions can be expected to evolve. In the future, ongoing discussions will ensue regarding specialty certification, mandatory continuing education, and certification of support personnel.

MANDATORY CONTINUING EDUCATION

The right to continue to practice under the CCC requires only that the practitioner pay the required annual certification fee. Although mandatory continuing education has been proposed and is included in the requirements for renewal of the license in more than half of the states, it has not yet been adopted for the CCC. The Award for Continuing Education (ACE) Program continues as a voluntary program of continuing education with ASHA.

SPECIALTY CERTIFICATION

The CCC standards are considered to be minimal standards established for entry into the practice of the professions. Many practitioners develop expertise in a particular area of practice. They believe that it is desirable to hold a specialty certificate that recognizes their area of special expertise beyond the entry level.

Persons who support the idea of specialty certification believe that such a program will increase the competence of persons aspiring to hold the specialty certification, thus increasing the quality of service to the public. Supporters say it will facilitate the ability of the public to choose qualified practitioners and will increase selectivity for referral within the profession.

The opponents of specialty certification believe their scope of practice can be restricted regardless of their holding the CCC. They fear that the public would interpret the qualifications of the person who holds the entry level certificate as less qualified than the person who holds the specialty certificate. Also the view is posited that the public would be confused in attempts to distinguish between a "specialist in voice disorders," for example, versus someone who "specializes in voice disorders." There is some concern that persons who deliver service for which they do not hold specialty certification will be subject to lawsuits for malpractice or other forms of professional discipline. Finally, opponents believe that the higher cost of obtaining the specialty certificate will result in higher costs to the public and possible reduction of payment to persons who do not hold the specialty certificate, especially from third-party payers.

If a program of specialty certification is to be developed, standards will have to be established specifying the educational and practice standards for the specialty certificate. Many related professional organizations or the Special Interest Divisions of ASHA may undertake the granting of specialty certificates to recognize the special interest and expertise of its members.

CERTIFICATION OR REGISTRATION OF SUPPORT PERSONNEL

The use of support personnel has been on the increase throughout the profession. The future may see the development of plans to certify or register support personnel as speech assistants or audiometric technicians. The ASHA Task Force on Support Personnel is studying the many issues surrounding the training, supervision, and use of support personnel. An official ASHA position is expected in the near future.

INTERNATIONAL STANDARDS

At the present time, there is considerable interest in creating mechanisms for persons who are certified in one country to receive reciprocity with other countries having similar requirements for certification. In addition, the International Association for Logopedics and Phoniatrics is in the process of developing standards for international certification. Both activities are necessary because of the increasing mobility of persons throughout the world and the desire to allow access to practice by professionals throughout the international community.

SUMMARY

The practice of speech-language pathology and audiology is regulated by licensure, teacher certification, registration, and professional certification. Regulation is necessary to assure the public that persons providing professional services have the necessary knowledge and skills for practice.

Licensure, teacher certification, and registration are granted by state governments. They are required by law to practice the professions in settings specified in the law. Forty-three states regulate speech-language pathologists and/or audiologists.

Professional certification is awarded by professional associations. It is awarded to members of professional associations according to standards established by the association. The American Speech-Language Hearing Association grants the Certificates of Clinical Competence (CCC) in speech-language pathology and audiology to members and nonmembers who have met established standards.

DISCUSSION QUESTIONS

1. What is the purpose of professional regulation?
2. What harm can be brought about in the practice of speech-language pathology and audiology by persons not properly educated?
3. What are the specific requirements for licensure in speech-language pathology and audiology in your state?
4. How do the requirements for the license in speech-language pathology and audiology in your state differ from the requirements for the Certificates of Clinical Competence?
5. What impact will specialty certification have on the professions of speech-language pathology and audiology?

REFERENCES

Alabama Licensure Law for Speech Pathologists and Audiologists. Acts of 1975, §34-28A-2.

Carthcart, J. A., & Graff, G. (1978). Occupational licensing—factoring it out. *Pacific Law Journal, 9,* 147–163.

Flower, R. M., Ohta, D., Stephens, M., Quinn, P., & Orahood, R. (1986). Perspectives on licensure. *Asha, 28,* 19–23.

Hume, E. (1985). CGS Backgrounder. Council of State Government. Lexington, KY.

Iowa Law of 1990 Speech Pathology and Audiology Assistants §645-302.2(147).

Levy, N. I., & Goldfarb, N. (1991, July). Pinning down certification. *Executive Update*, pp. 22–26.

Lynch, C. (1986). Harm to the public: Is it real? *Asha, 28,* 25–31.

Lynch, C., & Welsh, R. (1993). Characteristics of state licensure laws. *Asha , 35,* 130–139.

Moll, K. (1991, November). *Standards—Who will set them: Basic aspects of professional credentialing.* Paper presented at the annual convention of the American Speech-Language-Hearing Association, Atlanta, GA.

Nebraska Laws Practice of Audiology and Speech Pathology of 1978 §71-1,190; Laws 1985, LB129, §18; Laws 1988, LB 1100, §67.

Nebraska Rules and Regulations Governing Audiology and Speech-Language Pathology. (1987). Nebraska Department of Health/Professional and Occupational Licenses/Regulations. Title 172 Chapter 19 §001.01.

New York State Education Law Article 159 Speech Language Pathologists and Audiologists §8203, 1974, c.1055; §8202 amended L. 1983, c.43.§1.

Reaves, R. (1992, February). *The role of professional organization and licensure boards in standards changes.* Paper presented at the PES Invitational Seminar: Roads to Specialty Certification, Charleston, SC.

Shimberg, P. (1982). *Occupational licensing: A public perspective.* Princeton, NY: Educational Testing Service.

U.S. Department of Education (1986). Public Law 99-457. Education of the Handicapped Act Amendments of 1986, Title I, Handicapped Infants and Toddlers, Washington, D.C., House Congressional Record.

RESOURCES

Information regarding ASHA Certification can be obtained from:

American Speech-Language-Hearing Association
10801 Rockville Pike
Rockville, MD 20852
1 (800) 638-6868 or (301) 897-5700

Information regarding state licensure can be obtained by contacting the state regulatory agency in your state. See the March issue of *Asha* for a current listing.

Information regarding state teacher certification can be obtained by contacting the state education department in your state. See the March issue of *Asha* for a current listing.

APPENDIX 4A: Standards for the Certificates of Clinical Competence[1]

Standard I: Degree

Applicants for either degree must have a master's or doctoral degree.

Standard II: Academic Coursework

Applicants for either certificate must have earned at least 75 semester credit hours that reflect a well-integrated program of study dealing with (a) the biological/physical sciences and mathematics; (b) the behavioral and/or social sciences, including normal aspects of human behavior and communication; and (c) the nature, prevention, evaluation, and treatment of speech, language, hearing and related disorders. The coursework must address issues pertaining to normal and abnormal human development and behavior across the life span and to culturally diverse populations.

Standard II-A: Basic Science Coursework

Applicants for either certificate must earn at least 27 semester credit hours in the basic sciences. At least 6 semester credit hours must be in the biological/physical sciences and mathematics.

Standard II-B: Professional Coursework

Applicants for either certificate must earn at least 36 semester hours in courses that concern the nature, prevention, evaluation, and treatment of speech, language, and hearing disorders. Those 36 semester credit hours must encompass courses in speech, language, and hearing that concern disorders primarily affecting children as well as disorders primarily affecting adults. At least 30 of the 36 semester credit hours must be in courses for which graduate credit was received, and at least 21 of those 30 must be in the professional area for which the certificate is sought.

Standard III: Supervised Clinical Observation and Clinical Practicum

Applicants for either certificate must complete the requisite number of clock hours of supervised clinical observation and supervised clinical practicum that are provided by the educational institution or by one of its cooperating programs.

Standard III-A: Clinical Observation

Applicants for either certificate must complete at least 25 clock hours of supervised observation prior to beginning the initial clinical practicum.

Standard III-B: Clinical Practicum

Applicants for either certificate must complete at least 350 clock hours of supervised clinical practicum that concern the evaluation and treatment of children and adults with disorders of speech, language, and hearing. No more than 25 of the clock hours may be obtained from participation in staffings in which evaluation, treatment, and/or recommentations are discussed or formulated, with or without the client present.

[1]The Standards for the Certificates of Clinical Competence presented here are abstracted from "Implementation Procedures for the Standards for the Certificates of Clinical Competence" published by the Clinical Certification Board of the American Speech-Language-Hearing Association in the March, 1993, issue of *Asha*. Note that these standards were adopted October 23, 1988, effective for applications postmarked on January 1, 1993, and thereafter.

Standard IV: National Examinations in Speech-Language Pathology and Audiology

Applicants must pass the National Examination in the area for which the certificate is sought.

Standard V: The Clinical Fellowship

After completion of academic coursework (Standard II) and clinical practicum (Standard III), the applicant must successfully complete a Clinical Fellowship.

◼ CHAPTER 5 ◼

Professional Standards

◼ JANE R. MADELL, Ph.D. ◼

SCOPE OF CHAPTER

This chapter discusses what professional standards are and why they are needed. Standards programs for the certification of individuals, the accreditation of graduate education programs, and the accreditation of professional service programs will be reviewed. Standards programs developed by the different organizations involved in the certification, licensing, and accreditation of audiology and speech-language pathology are included.

WHAT ARE STANDARDS?

Standards are, primarily, a consumer protection device. They are a way of ensuring the quality, as far as possible, of products and services provided by individuals or organizations. Many governmental, professional, manufacturing, and consumer organizations set standards for what they consider to be the minimally acceptable quality for a product or service. The federal government sets automobile safety and air pollution standards for the production of cars. Under-

writer's Laboratory (UL) sets standards for safety of electrical appliances. State motor vehicle bureaus set performance standards for driving a motor vehicle in their state. Professional organizations, like the American Speech-Language-Hearing Association (ASHA), set standards for provision of services to persons with communication and related disorders and for education of persons providing such services.

WHY ARE STANDARDS NEEDED?

Without standards, consumers are left on their own to determine the quality of services or products they wish to purchase. Most of us are not in a position to determine if a car meets appropriate safety standards, if a school is capable of providing quality education to our child, if a hospital can meet established medical criteria, or if a health care provider is qualified. Although we do not think about it daily, we rely on standards set and evaluated by others when we purchase products and services. As a wise consumer you will inquire if a product or service you are interested in purchasing meets appropriate standards.

If you accept the need for standards to ensure quality you can understand why many professional organizations wish to be involved in the development of standards. Members of a given profession are the best resource for determining what is reasonable in the practice of their profession. In addition, professionals understand that if they do not develop standards, some other governing body will develop standards they will be required to meet. Externally developed standards might be more objective than those developed by a group with a vested interest. An outside group, however, may lack sufficient understanding of all the issues involved to develop standards that at the same time are in the best interest of the consumer and place reasonable requirements on the service or product provider.

In the field of communication disorders there are three types of standards: ① standards for individuals who provide professional services in communication disorders, ② standards for programs providing professional services in communication disorders, and ③ standards for graduate education programs training individuals who will provide services in communication disorders.

THE STANDARDS PROGRAM OF THE AMERICAN SPEECH-LANGUAGE-HEARING ASSOCIATION

ASHA is committed to ensuring that quality speech-language pathology and audiology services are provided to the public. To that end, ASHA has developed an extensive standards program. The program is voluntary. Participation is not a requirement of membership in the organization, and one can participate in the standards program without being a member of ASHA. However, the standards program is so well established that many employers require ASHA certification for employment, and other accrediting bodies look to ASHA standards when reviewing professional services in the area of communicative disorders.

ASHA is a membership organization. Members elect the Executive Board (President and Vice Presidents) for management of the business of the association. Members also elect the Legislative Council that determines the policies of the association. The Legislative Council is made up of members from each state. The number of representatives from a state is determined by the number of ASHA members in the state. The council authorizes the formation of committees and boards and establishes their responsibilities. The executive board appoints committee members. (See Chapter 2 by Williams on professional organizations.)

Standards are developed by the *Council on Professional Standards in Speech-Language Pathology and Audiology*. The council members are appointed by the Executive Board of ASHA but the council itself is autonomous in the development of standards. The *Standards Council of ASHA* develops standards for the certification of individuals, the accreditation of graduate education programs, and the accreditation of professional service delivery programs. It is the policy of the Standards Council to submit any suggested changes in standards to the public for review and comment, but the final decision about setting standards is the sole responsibility of the Standards Council. The council is also responsible for arbitrating appeals of decisions made by the operating boards.

There are three operating boards. The *Clinical Certification Board* (CCB) is responsible for review of applications for individuals seeking certification in audiology and/or speech-language pathology. The *Educational Standards Board* (ESB) is responsible for the accreditation of master's degree programs in speech-language pathology and audiology. The *Professional Services Board* (PSB) is responsible for the accreditation of professional service programs in speech-language pathology and audiology. Implementation of standards is the responsibility of the operating boards. Implementation includes the development of indexes by which standards may be met and the development of policies and procedures for reviewing applications.

STANDARDS FOR INDIVIDUAL PROFESSIONAL SERVICE PROVIDERS

Speech-language pathologists and audiologists are monitored in several ways. ASHA, through the Standards Council, has developed certification standards for individuals who wish to provide services in the area of communication disorders. The standards include minimum academic requirements, clinical practicum requirements, the passing of a national examination, and completing a period of supervised experience. ASHA certification is voluntary. However, many employers will not hire individuals who do not hold ASHA certification, and many insurance companies require ASHA certification for reimbursement.

Individual states have licensing laws for speech-language pathologists and audiologists. In states with licensing laws, the license is the minimum requirement for practice in that state. In some states, licensing laws are identical to current ASHA certification requirements; in others they are not. In some states, certain work settings, such as schools, are exempt from licensure requirements, but individuals who practice in those settings must meet state department of education requirements. Laws vary from state to state and practitioners in each state are required to know and adhere to the laws of that state. (See Chapter 3 by Battle for further information on certification and licensure.)

STANDARDS FOR PROFESSIONAL SERVICE PROGRAMS

There are a number of different standards programs that monitor provision of professional services in communicative disorders.

Professional service programs in communication disorders may be evaluated by the Professional Services Board of ASHA, the Joint Commission on Accreditation of Healthcare Organizations (JCAHO), the Commission on Accreditation of Rehabilitation Facilities (CARF), and State Health and Education Departments, among others.

PROFESSIONAL SERVICES BOARD ACCREDITATION FOR PROFESSIONAL SERVICES IN AUDIOLOGY AND SPEECH-LANGUAGE PATHOLOGY

The Standards Council of ASHA has developed standards for professional service programs in audiology and speech-language pathology. The Professional Services Board (PSB) is the body responsible for implementing these standards. The PSB limits its program review to aspects of the professional program that provide services in communicative disorders. For example, if the communicative disorders program is located in a hospital or school, PSB does not review other departments in the larger institution. It restricts its review to the department of communicative disorders.

Although there are many ways to assess quality, the Standards Council has determined that certain components are essential for quality of service, and the standards reflect those basic components. The standards are used for assessing programs and for guiding program development. They are intended to provide for self-evaluation and future planning and can be used to educate administrators, governing bodies, consumers, the general public, students, and practicing professionals about the essentials required for quality care.

The PSB Standards

The *Professional Services Board Accreditation Manual* (ASHA, 1992) lists eight standards that must be met for a program to receive accreditation. The topics covered by the standards are:

1. Missions, goals, and objectives
2. Nature and quality of services
3. Quality improvement and program evaluation
4. Administration
5. Financial resources and management
6. Human resources
7. Physical facilities and program environment
8. Equipment and materials

Each standard has several subsections that more fully describe the intent of the standard. For example, Standard 1 (ASHA, 1992) has five subsections. The first two are:

1.1 The program has a written mission statement that describes its purpose and scope of practice.

1.2 The mission statement is periodically and systematically reviewed for appropriateness in relation to current needs and modified as may be indicated. (p. B1)

In addition, there are suggestions for implementation (ways in which a program can demonstrate that it meets the standard). The first implementation suggestion for Standard 1 (ASHA, 1992) is:

a. The program has a written mission statement that clearly specifies the purpose of the program and its scope of practice, with evidence that it is reviewed periodically and systematically to reflect client/community needs. (p. B1)

Programs are not restricted to the implementation suggested in the manual. Alternative forms of implementation are acceptable as long as the standards are met. For example, a program that does not have a mission statement may have a description of its goals in a program brochure.

Self Evaluation

The accreditation process begins with a self-evaluation. The program staff reviews the standards and the suggested indicators and attempts to demonstrate how the program meets the standards. Through this process, the program staff should be able to ascertain the likelihood of passing the review. Changes can be made to achieve compliance and proceed with the application process. When program staff believe that they are ready for review, they complete the application and submit it to PSB. The board reviews the application, and if the program appears ready, the board will schedule a site visit. If the program does not appear ready for review, the board may suggest that staff continue the self-evaluation process.

The Site Visit

The site visit is intended to verify the accuracy of the information provided in the application for accreditation. Site visitors are staff members of other PSB-accredited programs who have received training to conduct the visits. They examine the program in detail, meet with staff and administrators, review equipment and client records, speak with consumers and referral sources, and report their observations to the PSB.

Accreditation

The PSB then determines whether the program has demonstrated that it meets the standards. If it does, accreditation is granted for a 5-year period. If it does not, accreditation will be denied. If the program meets most of the standards but needs improvement in some areas, the board has the option to grant accreditation and require improvement in the weak areas within a short period of time. All programs are required to submit annual reports indicating any changes in the program and describing how they have answered any of PSB's concerns. If substantial changes occur in the program during the accreditation period or if PSB's concerns have not been answered, then the program may be required to undergo additional review.

Receipt of accreditation permits programs to advertise that the rigorous standards of their professional accrediting body have been met. This helps assure consumers and referral sources and third-party payers about the quality of the services they are receiving.

COMMISSION ON ACCREDITATION OF REHABILITATION FACILITIES

The Commission on Accreditation of Rehabilitation Facilities (CARF) is a national, private, nonprofit organization founded in 1966. Its mission is to serve as the preeminent standards-setting and accrediting body promoting quality services to people with disabilities. The CARF accreditation manual (Commission on Accreditation of Rehabilitation Facilities, 1993) states that one of its primary purposes is to "develop and maintain current, state-of-the-art standards which can be used by organizations to measure their level of performance, to promote consumer-responsiveness, and to strengthen their programs" (p. vii). The CARF manual describes accreditation as valuable, in that nationally accepted standards promote programs of consistent quality, and that standards and the accreditation process promote an environment that facilitates accountability. The manual states that the commission's activities are directed by persons with disabilities, service providers, third party payers, and national and regional organizations.

Organizations such as ASHA, the American Physical Therapy Association, and United Cerebral Palsy Association who support the goals of accreditation have joined together to become sponsoring members of CARF. The commission's board of trustees is composed of one person appointed by each sponsoring member and an equal number of at-large members appointed by the board based on their areas of expertise. The board is responsible for development and modification of standards and for awarding or withholding accreditation.

CARF accreditation is sought by organizations that offer a variety of services in rehabilitation, including speech-language pathology, physical and occupational therapy, vocational counseling, psychological services, recreation services, and so on. The program reviewers represent different program areas and may not be practitioners in speech-language pathology or audiology.

Each program interested in seeking accreditation must meet certain basic accreditation criteria, which primarily cover ways in which the program is organized. The program must demonstrate that it is accessible to people with disabilities, seeks input from those served, meets all necessary safety requirements, and has a continuous program evaluation system. Section 1 of the standards covers organizational standards and includes the purpose, governance, information management, program evaluation, program and staff development, fiscal management, and physical plant. Section 2 covers program standards and includes specific requirements for different service delivery settings, such as programs for comprehensive inpatient rehabilitation, spinal cord injury, brain injury, chronic pain management, and outpatient medical rehabilitation. Professional services in communicative disorders are not reviewed separately but are included as part of the review of other programs.

Accreditation may be granted for 3 years if the program meets all the accreditation criteria and standards. One-year accreditation is granted to programs that meet most requirements but have some deficiencies the board believes can be corrected within 1 year. If an organization has major deficiencies, accreditation will be denied. Under certain circumstances, the decision about accreditation may be deferred for 6 to 12 months to permit the program to make the necessary improvements.

JOINT COMMISSION ON ACCREDITATION OF HEALTHCARE ORGANIZATIONS

The Joint Commission on Accreditation of Healthcare Organizations (JCAHO) was formed in 1951 as a private, not-for-profit national organization offering voluntary accreditation programs dedicated to improving the quality of health care delivery. Accreditation is provided to acute care hospitals, psychiatric facilities, substance abuse and rehabilitation programs, community mental health centers, organizations providing services for the mentally retarded and other developmentally disabled populations, long-term care facilities, home care, ambulatory health care organizations, and hospice programs. The current standards (Joint Commission on Accreditation of Healthcare Organizations, 1993) contain major revisions and reorganization. Instead of reviewing an organization department by department, the new standards shift the review to the effective performance of important organization-wide functions. It is the belief that this will improve patient outcomes. Each facility is left to determine for itself the most appropriate problem-solving and monitoring processes. The standards are intended to encourage the application of continuous quality improvement across all departments (see Chapter 19 by Frattali on quality improvement). Individual programs are expected to develop indicators of quality improvement and to demonstrate that the program meets the indicators. Programs are also expected to meet the accepted standards for their professional area when such exist. For example, in the area of communication disorders, program staff are expected to meet ASHA certification standards as well as state licensure requirements, to demonstrate compliance with ASHA standards for calibration of equipment, and to demonstrate that the program meets standards of professional practice for the professions of audiology and speech-language pathology. The reviewers for JCAHO are physicians, nurses, and medical administrators. Speech-language pathologists and audiologists are not members of the review team.

STATE REQUIREMENTS

Individual states have program reviews designed to approve provision of services and to allow for reimbursement under state programs. The state health department may perform program reviews for programs wishing to provide services under the state's Medicaid program, program for physically handicapped children, or the division of vocational rehabilitation.

Some states require a state license to operate any type of health care program. The state education department may require program review for programs wishing to provide educational services. Individual state laws will determine what organizations require which reviews.

SUMMARY

Most programs will be reviewed by more than one accrediting body. The communicative disorders program of a hospital may be reviewed by ASHA's PSB, JCAHO (as part of the hospital's accreditation program), CARF (as part of the hospital's inpatient rehabilitation program), and by the state health department. A communicative disorders program in a public school receiving some Medicaid funding may be reviewed by ASHA's PSB, the state education department as part of the general school review process, and the state health department to receive Medicaid funding. A PSB review can be expected to be the most rigorous in the area of speech-language pathology and audiology services because the entire review focuses on those areas and the reviewers are members of the professions. As a result, it can be expected to provide more insight into improving services. On the other hand, a CARF review will focus on team efforts in providing patient care that can have a significant effect on improving patient outcome. All types of accreditation are valuable. Each meets a different need.

ACCREDITATION OF GRADUATE EDUCATION PROGRAMS IN AUDIOLOGY AND SPEECH-LANGUAGE PATHOLOGY

The Standards Council of ASHA has developed standards to evaluate education programs offering master's degrees in speech-language pathology and audiology. In fact, ASHA is the only body that accredits graduate education programs in speech-language pathology and audiology. The ASHA accreditation program is recognized by both the U.S.

Department of Education and by the Council on Postsecondary Accreditation. The Educational Standards Board (ESB) is the operating board responsible for accreditation of master's degree programs. The Standards Council has delineated standards in five areas for accreditation of education programs (ASHA, 1993a). Programs must satisfy all standards as the necessary condition for accreditation. They are:

1. Administration
2. Instructional staff
3. Curriculum
4 Clinical education
5. Program self-analysis

Each standard has several subsections that further describe the standard. For example, the first minimum requirement for Standard 1 is: "1.1. The applicant institution must have regional accreditation" (p. 13). The first minimum requirement under Standard 2 is: "2.1. The instructional staff must be sufficient in number to meet the instructional, clinical, research, and advising responsibilities without carrying a greater load than is traditional for instructional staff in the applicant institution" (p. 9.15).

For a program to be eligible for accreditation it must have been fully functioning for 3 years prior to seeking accreditation and must have graduated a minimum of 6 students. As with PSB accreditation, the initial part of the process is a self-evaluation. The program is expected to complete the self-evaluation, review the standards, and determine for itself if requirements have been met. The program can submit an application to the ESB once the staff believes that the requirements have been met.

The application is reviewed by the ESB to determine if the program is eligible for accreditation and if it appears to be in compliance with the standards. Any concerns of the board are communicated to the program. The program can then decide whether or not to proceed. If the program decides to proceed, a site visit will be scheduled. As with the PSB site visit, the purpose of the visit is to verify compliance with standards as reported in the application. The site visitors will review the physical facilities; meet with the staff to discuss the program; meet with administrators, students, and off-campus supervisors; review students records; and review the materials and records of the clinical program. The site visit team will send its report to ESB, and ESB will determine whether or not to grant accreditation.

If the program is judged to be in compliance, full accreditation will be awarded for a 5-year period. The board may defer accreditation if compliance with standards has not been clearly demonstrated, but the board believes that the program can demonstrate compliance within 6 months. Accreditation will be withheld if the program is seeking initial accreditation, does not meet standards, and the board does not believe that the deficiencies can be corrected within 6 months.

Each program is expected to submit an annual report to the ESB describing any changes that have taken place within the program within the previous year and discussing what it has done to meet the concerns expressed by ESB in previous years. If it is warranted, ESB may change the accreditation status of the program following the annual report.

Until this time, accreditation of graduate education programs providing master's degrees has been voluntary. However, as of 1994, ASHA certification will be granted only to individuals who have graduated from an ESB-accredited program. The Standards Council believes that this will further enhance the quality of the Certificate of Clinical Competence.

FUTURE DIRECTIONS IN PROFESSIONAL STANDARDS

DOCTORAL EDUCATION

Currently, there is no accreditation for doctoral programs in speech-language pathology and audiology. In the past, accreditation of doctoral programs was not considered necessary because almost everyone who entered a doctoral program had already received a master's degree and would be required to meet the standards imposed by ESB. Doctoral programs were considered to be research degrees and did not require the same kinds of practice standards. This is no longer the case. At the 1992 session of the ASHA Legislative Council, the council passed a resolution requiring doctoral education for entry into the practice of audiology by the year 2001. In 1993, the Legislative Council modified its previous resolution requiring a professional doctorate. (See Chapter 28 by Loavenbruck on the professional doctorate in audiology.) Some audiologists may earn master's degrees prior to obtaining a doctorate but many will seek out clinical doctorate programs and will not obtain master's degrees along the way. It can be expected that new standards programs for institutions granting clinical doctorates will be developed in the next few years.

PREFERRED PRACTICE PATTERNS FOR THE PROFESSIONS OF SPEECH-LANGUAGE PATHOLOGY AND AUDIOLOGY

ASHA has developed Preferred Practice Patterns for the Professions of Speech-Language Pathology and Audiology (ASHA, 1993b). They constitute an official policy of ASHA and are intended to provide guidance in the practice of the professions and to enhance the quality of professional services, although they are not official standards. The Preferred Practice Patterns were developed by the Task Force on Clinical Standards and went through extensive peer review. For each professional procedure, the Preferred Practice Pattern specifies which professionals should perform the procedure, the expected outcome, the clinical indications for the procedure, the clinical processes, the setting and equipment required, safety and health precautions, and the required documen-

tation. The practice patterns are expected to apply across all settings in which a given procedure is performed.

At this writing 43 statements have been written covering 35 areas. For example, the area of basic audiologic assessment has two sections: basic audiologic assessment and pediatric audiologic assessment. The area of language assessment has 10 subsections including spoken language assessment, written language assessment, augmentative and alternative communication, and so on. At the end of each section are references to ASHA policy statements, ANSI calibration standards, and so on. Although the preferred practice patterns are not considered standards, they may have the impact of standards over time, as they become the model for professionals to use in providing service.

SPECIALTY CERTIFICATION OR SPECIALTY RECOGNITION

The ASHA Legislative Council has reviewed the concept of specialty certification several times. Up to this time the council has rejected the concept. The current certification has been viewed as the entry to practice into the professions in the same way as a medical license is the entry into the practice of medicine. There has been concern that if specialty certification is developed, referral sources and payment sources might begin to restrict reimbursement to practitioners who held specialty certification. ASHA currently has an Ad Hoc Committee on Specialty Certification that is reevaluating the topic and will make recommendations to the ASHA Legislative Council.

In 1989, the Legislative Council approved the development of Special Interest Divisions. Special Interest Divisions are groups of members who share an interest in an area of practice. There are currently 13 special interest divisions covering such areas as hearing and hearing loss in children, fluency and its disorders, and neurophysiology. Several of these groups have expressed an interest in developing specialty certification and may work toward that end.

SUMMARY

Standards are a vital part of all areas of professional practice and professional education. As consumers and providers, it is our responsibility to participate in standards programs to assure ourselves and the consumers of our services that we are providing them with the highest quality of care. As we seek services for ourselves and as we refer our clients, we should also inquire about adherence to standards. As the scope of practice of the professions change, so do the standards. It is our responsibility as professionals to be certain that we continue to grow with the standards.

DISCUSSION QUESTIONS

1. What are the benefits of certification or accreditation? Why should an individual or an institution seek out accreditation?
2. Should standards be mandatory or serve as a ideal model of service provision?
3. Do standards provide a sufficient basis for an organization to monitor itself?
4. What are the benefits and/or disadvantages for programs or individuals being required to participate in more than one type of standards review?
5. How can a given professional program obtain and maintain sufficient support from a parent institution to meet professional standards?

REFERENCES

American Speech-Language-Hearing Association. (1992). *Professional services board accreditation manual.* Rockville, MD: Author.

American Speech-Language-Hearing Association. (1993a). *Educational standards board accreditation manual.* Rockville, MD: Author.

American Speech-Language-Hearing Association. (1993b). Preferred practice patterns for the professions of speech-language pathology and audiology. *Asha, 35*(Suppl. 11).

Commission on Accreditation of Rehabilitation Facilities. (1993). *Standards manual for organizations serving people with disabilities.* Tucson, AZ: Author.

Joint Commission on Accreditation of Healthcare Organizations. (1993). *Accreditation manual.* Oakbrook Terrace, IL: Author.

RESOURCES

American Speech-Language-Hearing Association
10801 Rockville Pike
Rockville, MD 20852
(301) 897-5700; Actionline 1-800-638-6868

Commission on Accreditation of Rehabilitation Facilities
101 North Wilmot Road, Suite 500
Tucson, AZ 85711
(602) 748-1212

Joint Commission on the Accreditation of Healthcare Organizations
One Renaissance Boulevard
Oakbrook Terrace, IL 60181
(708) 916-5400

■ CHAPTER 6 ■

Ethical Considerations

■ CHARLENA M. SEYMOUR, Ph.D. ■

What do you know about ethics?

I asked myself that question a few years ago when I was first elected to the Executive Board of the American Speech-Language-Hearing Association (ASHA) as a vice president. Because the title of the office that I was to hold was Vice President for Standards and Ethics, the thought of having such a responsibility did make me feel rather insecure. Although I had extensive experience with the standards programs of ASHA, my only experience with ethics was that I was a good person and I presumed, therefore, that I was a good professional, too. Soon the title of the office was changed to Vice President for Quality of Service, but the responsibilities and implications remained the same. I was to represent the conscience of ASHA, Joan of Arc and Don Quixote combined into one lofty anatomy that seemed beyond the reach of my mere mortal qualifications. In my estimation, to take on such a formidable role was not an easy task and my premonitions were proven to be correct. For survival's sake I found it necessary to do some additional research about professional ethics, and my pursuit for knowledge in the area resulted in a continuous desire to know more. Learning about ethics has been one of the most exciting and worthwhile challenges that I have confronted in my career. The information you will be reading is based on my experience monitoring the ASHA Ethical Practice Board and the Council of Professional Ethics, developing instructional classroom materials about ethics with my students, attending numerous presentations about ethics, and reading many articles about ethics. In retrospect, it was a very good choice and I had a very good time.

SCOPE OF CHAPTER

All programs in communication disorders accredited by the Educational Standards Board (ESB) must provide their students with instruction about the Code of Ethics of the American Speech-Language-Hearing Association (ASHA). Ethics education and its application to the professions of audiology and speech-language pathology are the basis for a strong cohesive association and for continuous consumer protection. The scope of practice of the professions is continuously expanding into new arenas. Professionals in the discipline of human communication sciences and disorders are working with new populations, new technologies, and in new settings. All of these circumstances have placed many professionals into situations where decisions about the quality of their service must remain above suspect—otherwise the integrity of their professions would be at stake. Therefore, the primary purpose of this chapter is to provide you with some general information about ethics, the ASHA Code of Ethics, and the importance of the code to each of the professions and to consumers as well. A second purpose of the chapter is to provide some suggestions for infusing the subject of ethics into communication disorders curriculum.

DEFINING ETHICS

When defining *ethics* people often use the words right, good, and moral or associate it with a doctrine like the "golden rule" to explain its meaning . For many of us ethics is simply doing the right thing according to accepted standards of our specific community, culture, or profession. Some people use the words morals and ethics interchangeably although *morals* usually refer to rules that society expects people to obey in all situations and at all times. Both words are associated with the concept of right versus wrong. Ethics is a part of philosophy and uses reason, logic, concepts, and philosophical expla-

nations to analyze its problems and find answers (White, 1988). Actually, ethics can be thought of as a moral philosophy that examines the truths and principles of conduct in a systematic way. Solomon (1984) defined ethics as the part of philosophy that is concerned with living well, being a good person, doing the right thing, and wanting the right things in life. He wrote that "ethics" refers both to a discipline—the study of our values and their justification—and to the subject matter of that discipline—the actual values and rules of conduct by which we live. According to Solomon, the two meanings merge in that we behave and misbehave according to a complex and continually changing set of rules, customs, and expectations; consequently, we are forced to reflect on our conduct and attitudes, to justify, and sometimes to revise them.

Harris (1986, p. 2) provided the following definition of ethics which he took from a dictionary: "ethics: 1. the study of standards of conduct and moral judgment; moral philosophy 2. a treatise on this study; book about morals. 3. the system or code of morals of a particular philosopher, religion, group, profession." If one were to compare the two words, morals and ethics, wrote Harris (1986), morals would imply conformity with the general accepted standards of goodness in conduct or character. In contrast, ethics implies conformity with an elaborated, ideal code of moral principles, sometimes specifically, with the code of a particular profession. The simplest way to explain what ethics does, is to say that it evaluates human actions (White, 1988). These evaluations are usually classified as either positive or negative in nature (e.g., right/wrong, good/bad, just/unjust, fair/unfair, ethical/unethical). White (1988) contrasts the evaluation of human actions from an ethical perspective with those of law, religion, psychiatry, medicine, and business.

Law divides actions into legal and illegal and tells us that if we disobey we'll go to jail, pay a fine, or lose some privilege. Religions advise us what to believe and how to act if we want to please God, achieve eternal happiness, or avoid the fires of Hell. Psychiatry explains the difference between behavior that's normal, neurotic, and psychotic. Medicine gives us a yardstick for deciding how healthy our behavior is—business, how profitable (p. 7).

DEVELOPING AND LEARNING ETHICS

Ethical behavior is learned gradually, beginning in childhood. According to Solomon (1984), we first are taught a system of *do's* and *dont's* such as do talk nice to your teacher and don't break your sister's toys. As we grow older we realize that ethics is not just a varied collection of "do's and dont's" but a system of values and principles that tie together in a reasonable and coherent way to make our society and our lives as "civilized" and as happy as possible. The study of ethics is the final step in this process of education—the understanding of that system as such and the way that all our particular values and principles fit into it (Solomon, 1984, pp. 2–3).

Kohlberg (1969) believed that moral concepts develop naturally in a sequence of six different stages in which the individual applies rules for being fair. The six stages are based on an individual's perception of justice which is the basis for Kohlberg's theory of moral development. He believes that an individual's view of justice helps the person to define human rights and obligations and to solve any moral conflict. The individual's concern for justice is given a different and broader definition at each stage of development. According to Lickona's (1980) review of Kohlberg's work, at Stage 1, the idea of justice is a primitive one: *an eye for an eye and a tooth for a tooth.* At Stage 2, personal viewpoints differ from those of other individuals about issues, and persons are mutually aware of their differences. For justice to prevail it is necessary for individuals to behave reciprocally: *if you help me, then I'll help you; let's make a deal.* At Stage 3, justice means ideal reciprocity by applying the "golden rule" to in-terpersonal relationships and putting yourself in the other person's shoes. During Stage 4 the individual fulfills obligations demanded from a complex society by obeying the law. Doing the right thing is determined not only by one's conscience, but by rules and regulations. *Respect for authority and law* is to be upheld except in extreme cases if rules conflict with other fixed social duties, for example, F.B.I. wiretaps of Martin Luther King, Jr., which supposedly were carried out in the name of national security. Fewer than 20% of adults move beyond this stage. In Stage 5, individuals will act to achieve *the greatest good for the greatest number* in the interest of impartiality. At Stage 6, Kohlberg's highest stage, some individuals, such as philosophers, will articulate *universal ethical principles* underlying the assertion of human rights. This stage is not viewed as a natural psychological stage in moral development, but a proclamation of adherence to higher universal laws of humanity.

FORMAT AND STRUCTURE OF THE ASHA CODE OF ETHICS

A code of ethics is a guideline of principles for professional conduct that is intended to direct the professional in particular situations and roles. Many professions (e.g., law, medicine, engineering, social work, and accounting) also have codes to preserve and safeguard the public's confidence in their services. A code of ethics is used not only by most national professional associations, but also by state and local associations as well. By having a code of ethics, an association protects the consumer from charlatans and incompetent individuals and tells the public that the association's professionals are governed by a set of rules for proper conduct. Schmeiser (1992) stated that, " these codes deliver a clear message that the professions want their members to recognize the ethical dimensions of their work and to adhere to ethical standards in their practice on behalf of the public, clients, and the profession itself" (p. 5).

The ASHA Code of Ethics (*Asha*, 1993b) is a logical starting place to begin discussion about professional ethics. The primary reason for the founding of the American Academy of Speech Correction (later ASHA) in 1925 was to *establish scientific standards and codes of ethics*. There was great concern by the academy members that unscrupulous or fraudulent practitioners would undermine public confidence and destroy the honorable professional reputation of the academy. Therefore, requirements for membership in the academy were based on an individual having an untainted professional reputation and maintaining professional integrity. These specifications were included in the first Constitution of the Academy as the principles of ethics for the selection of new members and for the guidance of present members. It was not until 1952 that the ASHA Code of Ethics was published as an independent document separated from the by-laws of the association. Since the founding of ASHA, the code has gone through only a few substantial revisions, the last major revision producing the current format was published in 1993. However, the code can be amended any time with approval of the Legislative Council of ASHA.

The Code of Ethics retains ASHA's commitment to high personal standards of professionalism. It is introduced with a preamble that explains the intentions of the code and the guiding principles for the formation and structure of the code. The main body of the code has four parts each introduced by a Principles of Ethics (PE) statement and followed by an outline delineating the Rules of Ethics (RE) which apply to the specific preceding principle. The purpose of the Principles of Ethics is to provide an underlying moral basis for professional consideration and frame of reference; with the Rules of Ethics describing minimally acceptable professional conduct and prohibitions related to the preceding principle. Each set of principles has a target audience. Principles of Ethics I and II relate to one's responsibilities to persons served; Principle of Ethics III relates to one's responsibilities to the public; and Principle of Ethics IV relates to one's responsibilities to the professions. All members of ASHA, nonmembers of ASHA who hold certification (CCC in audiology or speech-language pathology), and applicants for membership or certification, as well as clinical fellows, are bound by the code. However, students who are not applicants for membership or certification and who are not clinical fellows are not bound by the ASHA Code of Ethics. A copy of the code can be found at the end of this chapter in Appendix 6A.

The current code contains some stipulations that are different from previously constructed ASHA codes. Probably the most important change is the interpretation of *competence*. This is a key issue discussed in more detail later in this chapter. The code requires that professionals perform within the scope of their *competence* which is based on education, training, and experience (PE II, Rule B). Stromberg (1990) stated that most professionals want to expand their scope of practice. Yet most ethics bodies are obliged to prevent professionals from expanding beyond their actual areas of expertise (p. 26). Professionals have to continually determine the limits of their expertise and to be careful of practicing or assuming responsibility in areas in which they do not possess adequate competence. This means that having ASHA certification is not sufficient to meet the demands of every aspect of the scope of practice of the certification area. *Competence* is a level that exceeds the minimal requirements necessary for certification. ASHA certification means having a credential indicating that the individual has met the minimal entry level requirements to practice as a professional audiologist or speech-language pathologist. These requirements include completing specific coursework and clinical practicum, passing a national examination, and participating in a fellowship plan as specified by ASHA. Other new stipulations of the code are:

Rules of Ethics requiring:

1. Withdrawal from professional practice when either substance abuse or an emo-

tional or mental disability may adversely affect the quality of services rendered, PE I, Rule L

2. Assigning of credit to those who have contributed to a publication, presentation, or product in proportion to their contribution and only with the contributor's consent, PE IV, Rule C

3. Acceptance of the responsibility of the independent status of the professions of speech-language pathology and audiology, PE IV, Rule E

4. Making certain that all equipment used in the provision of services is in proper working order and is properly calibrated, PE II, Rule F

Rules of Ethics prohibiting:

1. Misrepresenting diagnostic information, services rendered, or products dispensed in order to obtain payment or reimbursement, PE III, Rule C

2. Permitting a member of one's professional staff to engage in the provision of services that exceed the staff member's competence considering his or her level of education, training, and experience, PE II, Rule E

3. Misrepresentation of research results, professional services, or products, PE II, Rule D

The ASHA code provides a definition of the term misrepresentation: "any untrue statements or statements that are likely to mislead. Misrepresentation also includes the failure to state any information that is material and that ought, in fairness, to be considered" (*Asha*, 1993b, p. 17).

LICENSURE AND ITS RELATIONSHIP TO ETHICS

Sometimes having a code of ethics is not the only preventive measure for protecting the public from persons who do not have the necessary credentials or experience. Therefore, a regulatory mechanism, such as licensure, is necessary for enforcing the quality of

service provided to consumers. *Licensure* provides the consumer with a legal means by which to remove unqualified and dishonest individuals from practice or press charges against a professional for malpractice. For that reason many states have licensure laws that mandate specific requirements to practice in a professional area. Persons who practice without a license are subject to legal consequences. Many times the requirements for licensure are closely aligned with those established for certification.

All states do not now have licensure laws as a stipulation for practice as an audiologist or speech-language pathologist (see Chapter 4 by Battle on licensure and certification). Both licensure laws and codes of ethics establish and require adherence to a model for professional behavior. Flower (1984) states that consumer protection is the principal goal of both legal and ethical regulation of human service professions. In his chapter, "Legal and Ethical Considerations," he writes that

Legal controls, having the force of law, would seem the more effective [than codes of ethics]. Yet they generally define only the outer limits of acceptable practice. Ethical controls on the other hand, represent efforts towards professional self-regulation. Although carrying less stringent penalties, codes of ethics offer more detailed definitions of acceptable standards of professional practice. (p. 289)

ETHICS EDUCATION AND ENFORCEMENT

ASHA's ethics program for members consists of two synergistic working units: the Council on Professional Ethics (COPE) and the Ethical Practice Board (EPB). COPE and EPB include mostly ASHA members who meet periodically to implement the charges of their specific committees. In 1989, COPE was created to provide ASHA with a mechanism for educating members about ethics. The charge of COPE is to define and propose revisions for the Code of Ethics to the Legislative Council;

to develop educational programs in ethics for distribution to members and certificate holders; and to prepare educational materials for professional educational programs (*Asha*, 1993a, p. 74). With its program of ethics education in place, ASHA intends to make both preprofessionals and professionals more sensitive to the rules for ethical conduct across the scope of the practices.

But, as rules of professional conduct are sometimes violated, it is necessary for ASHA to have a mechanism for investigating these allegations. Providing a peer review of alleged violations is the major responsibility of EPB. The charge of EPB is to formulate and publish procedures that will be used for the processing of alleged violations of the Code of Ethics, including a reasonable opportunity for suspected violators to be heard through counsel of one's own choosing; [determine] sanctions for violations in its discretion including revoking and/or suspending membership and/or certification (*Asha*, 1993a, p. 74).

EPB has the responsibility to interpret, administer, and enforce the Code of Ethics of the association (*Asha*, 1993c, p. 19). To accomplish these functions, EPB has delineated practices and procedures to investigate charges of improper conduct. (The Statement of Practice and Procedures is published annually in the March issue of *Asha* for review by members.) The first step in the process is a review by EPB of the alleged violations. If EPB decides that an investigation is warranted, then EPB notifies the alleged offender in writing about the charges. The alleged offender is called the respondent and has up to 45 days to answer the allegation. As long as the case is pending, the membership and the certification status of the respondent may not change without EPB approval. Furthermore, if the respondent voluntarily resigns membership or surrenders certification, these circumstances do not prevent EPB from continuing to process the case. EPB considers all information obtained during its investigation and the respondent's responses to the charge(s) to make an initial determination. During this step of the process, if EPB finds that there is not sufficient

evidence to continue the proceedings, the investigation is ended. On the other hand , if there is sufficient evidence, EPB determines the nature of the violation, the sanction or penalties for the respondent, and the extent of the disclosure of the final EPB decision to persons other than the respondent. At that point in time, EPB may notify the respondent to stop any practice that violates the code. Failure to comply with the ruling of EPB is considered to be a violation of the code and can result in appropriate sanctions.

The respondent has the right to request a further consideration hearing after EPB has made its initial determination. When the respondent is unsatisfied with the decision of the further consideration hearing about revocation of membership/certification status or disclosure of the violation in *Asha*, the individual can then appeal to the Executive Board of ASHA to overturn the EPB decision. The ruling of the Executive Board about EPB's decision is the final step of the process.

EPB determines the sanctions that it considers to be appropriate for each violation. These sanctions range from a reprimand to the suspension or revocation of ASHA membership and/or certification. All sanctions, except reprimands, are publicly disclosed in *Asha*. Reprimands are disclosed only to the respondent, the respondent's counsel, ASHA's counsel, the complainant(s), designated witnesses, and sometimes other appropriate parties.

KEY PROFESSIONAL ISSUES IN AUDIOLOGY AND SPEECH-LANGUAGE PATHOLOGY

Under some circumstances, there are key professional issues that cannot be easily resolved with the minimal guidelines and instruction provided by the ASHA Code of Ethics. Therefore, to assist readers in the interpretation of some parts of the code, COPE and EPB have developed *Issues in Ethics Statements* (*Asha*, 1992) that expand and clarify aspects of the code. Usually the issues under discussion involve significant predicaments that most professionals face across settings and practice. *Issues in Ethics Statements* are considered educational materials for informing and enlightening professionals about issues that have far-reaching effects and widespread serious implications. Some of the controversial topics discussed in the statements include:

- Appropriate handling of competition and publicity in providing services to clients
- Delivery of services in areas that are common to the scope and practice of both professions
- Supervision of student clinicians by a non-ASHA certificate holder
- Extent and use of power by the clinical fellowship supervisor
- Involvement in clinical practice without any ASHA certification
- Falsification of credentials and use of degrees from unaccredited institutions
- Responsibilities and obligations of researchers to students, colleagues, and subjects
- Referral of clients from the practitioner's primary place of employment to the professional's private practice
- Representation of services for insurance reimbursement and funding

Earlier in the chapter there was a discussion about the interpretation of *competency* as a key issue that was addressed in the present code. The ASHA code stipulates that professionals must not provide services without the proper education, training, and experience in the specific area in which services are being provided. Therefore, if a professional wants to work with persons who stutter, the professional must be prepared for that work by education, training, and experience, not just by the ASHA certification credential. The issue of competence is forcing many professional organizations like ASHA to consider developing programs for specialty recognition. Such a program would allow some professionals to be identified as specialists in a particular practice area according to their education, experience, and training. With a

mechanism in place for specialty recognition, members practicing in an area of specialization without the proper credentials would be in violation of the ASHA code.

A second key ethical issue is acknowledging the professional commitment embodied in the ASHA Code of Ethics to help all who need services regardless of background. The U.S. Bureau of Census predicts that minority populations will become the majority in many U.S. cities by the turn of the century. Birth rates for nonwhite groups consistently are higher than those for whites who will, it is predicted, become the nation's largest minority group by the year 2080. This dramatic shift in demographics has some sobering implications as the United States becomes less European in culture and complexion. Meanwhile, in America today, to be nonwhite too often equates with being part of an underclass that is poorer, less healthy, less educated, and less cared for than the rest of the population. Nevertheless, in an increasingly multicultural society—one with broad social and economic gaps—it is important to ensure accessibility of services to all who need them. Although professional audiologists and speech-language pathologists serve clients regardless of background, there is a tendency, for example, for minority professionals to work with minority clients. Therefore, it is of great concern that the number of minority professionals in ASHA is about 6% of the entire association. This low percentage of available minority professionals is insufficient for the rising number of minority children who will need treatment for communication disorders. Moreover, because most audiologists and speech-language pathologists are not bilingual, many poor children whose first language is not English will be at a great disadvantage for receiving help for communication disorders. (See Chapter 14 by Kayser on multiculturalism and Chapter 12 by Lubinski and Masters on special populations and settings for more discussions of this topic.)

A third key ethical issue for practitioners in all settings is grappling with the pressure dictated by the costs of health care. In many instances, reimbursement policies dictate who receives treatment, how much, how often, and by whom. As costs for health care technology escalate and available resources dwindle, people who need professional services the most—especially children and elderly persons—can least afford to pay for them. At the same time, audiologists and speech-language pathologists have to try to find a balance between professional responsibility, the pressure to meet health care costs, and the need to make a decent salary. In school settings, rising costs and shrinking resources may necessitate a heavy caseload and over-reliance on support personnel. In private practice, hospitals, and clinics, handling high costs and low assets translates into ongoing debates about good business practice, professional accountability, making a livelihood versus personal gain, professional misconduct, and conflict of interest (see Chapter 13 by Kooper on professional liability).

Every day professionals in communication disorders face situations where the rightness or wrongness of an action is not clear. Clarification and resolution about ethical issues may be determined by using the ASHA Code of Ethics and *Issues in Ethics Statements* as resources. If an issue still seems confusing, seek advice from a supervisor, a lawyer, a state licensing board, or the Division of Ethics in the ASHA national office.

INSTRUCTIONAL CLASSROOM MATERIALS FOR TEACHING ETHICS TO STUDENTS

A predicament for educational programs in communication disorders is how to instruct students about ethics. Most educators would agree that it is difficult to teach ethics and that the role of the teacher should be to facilitate discussion about situations that contain opposing viewpoints. Pannbacker, Lass, and Middleton (1993) find that most programs (90.9%) in communication disorders do not offer a course devoted entirely to ethics, although 56.9% of their responding programs believed

that coursework in ethics should be required and 36.8% felt that most programs do not provide sufficient training in ethics. The usual way of providing information to students about ASHA's Code of Ethics has been for the instructor to give each student a copy of the code and ask the student to memorize it. Such a nonmeaningful process results in a lack of appreciation of how critical the study of ethics is to everyday professional practices and the delivery of professional services.

When Ducharme (1992) surveyed a group of students predominantly consisting of communication disorders majors, she found that most students felt that they did not have any exposure to ethics in their curriculum; yet the majority of the students surveyed recognized that they might be confronted with ethical dilemmas sometime in their careers and wanted training in ethical decision making to help them deal with conflicting situations as professionals. In Ducharme's study, 98.2% of the respondents felt it was important to learn about ethics and 76% felt that they would benefit from a course. However, only 40% of Ducharme's respondents said they were aware of the code and most of them knew nothing or very little about information within the code. Ducharme and Seymour (1992) found that students in communication disorders did need more specific exposure to the ASHA Code of Ethics as well as a framework for ethical decision making. Gonzalez (1992) indicated that students preferred the case study approach as the method for teaching ethics and that the student-led case study method would be of greatest assistance in the learning of ethics. Based on these studies, some materials were developed by the author and her students using a student-led case study format with the intent of generating the students' awareness and interest in the ASHA Code of Ethics, stimulating some consciousness-raising about professional ethics, and providing students with suggestions for an ethical decision-making process. The materials include an Ethics Calibration Quick Test, an Ethics Survey, and an Ethics Kit. These materials have been successfully used in an undergraduate communication disorders class to foster classroom discussion and enhance the students' awareness about the ASHA Code of Ethics, professional ethics, and ethical decision making.

Many of the steps in ethical decision making involve knowing one's own mind, making up one's mind, and acting on the decision, even when it may be unpopular or inconvenient. Ethical decision making requires careful deliberation and reasoning to make a choice between opposed values and ideas. It begins with individuals facing a problem, having to make a choice, and not being certain about what to do. Most ethical philosophers hold that ethics is not primarily concerned with getting people to do what they believe to be right, but rather with helping them to decide what is right (Jones, Sontag, Beckner, Morton, & Fogelin, 1977). Trying to decide what to do and what is right often leaves people frustrated, anxious, and/or angry. Mappes and Zembaty (1987) state that the answer to ethical dilemmas involves long rhetorical arguments whose intent is to elicit highly emotional, nonobjective responses.

Ethical decisions should be made within a specific context, which includes changing political, social, and cultural climates. Solomon (1984) posits that:

If we continued to accept whatever values we were taught as children, if there were no disagreements about what is right, the study of ethics might still be desirable but it would not have any decisive impact on our lives. The fact is however, that we live in a society filled with change and disagreements in which each generation is taught to reexamine the values and actions of the [previous] generation. (p. 3)

A *dilemma* is a "situation in which one moral conviction, [value] or right action conflicts with another [conviction/value etc.] and will continue to exist because there is no one, clear-cut right answer [to resolve the situation]" (Hansen, 1990, p. 17). An ethical dilemma represents a situation about confused beliefs, and it is the responsibility of the decision maker(s) to clear up the confusion.

Very often, dilemmas develop because there is a problem about how to resolve legitimate competing claims and not just making a decision between what's right or wrong. Even after a decision is made, there still may be some uncertainty and confusion about whether the choice was proper or wise.

The Ethics Calibration Quick Test (ECQT) is a checklist that contains six suggestions to facilitate classroom deliberation and ethical decision making about dilemmas (see Table 6–1). The suggestions are presented in graduated steps, beginning with the establishment of a dilemma and ending with the resolution of the dilemma. The ECQT has been used to help students resolve preconstructed dilemmas presented to them in a case study format (scenarios) as part of a classroom exercise to study professional ethics. To perform the exercise, the class is divided into small groups of 3 to 4 students. Within each small group, the students designate a *leader* to read the instructions and direct the discussion, and a *recorder* to write down the group's decisions and present them to the class. The instruction to the small group is to read the scenario and resolve the dilemma by progressing through the ECQT. About 15–20 minutes is given for the small group discussion. After each small group has concluded its task, the recorders share the responses with the whole class for intergroup feedback and evaluation.

The ECQT can be used with the *Ethics Kit for Undergraduates* in communication disorders (Jodoin, Konieczny, Martin, & Seymour, 1993). The kit contains 14 scenarios that have ethical dilemmas that would probably be faced by students. Examples of the scenarios can be found in Appendix 6B. The dilemmas involve student/faculty relationships, student/supervisor experiences, student/student situations, and student/client activities. Each dilemma is embedded in a scenario that provides some background information about the issue to be discussed. Following the presentation of the scenario, the students are provided with specific areas of the ASHA Code of Ethics that might apply if a violation occurred, possible solutions for the dilemma(s),

Table 6–1. ETHICS CALIBRATION QUICK TEST (ECQT)

Level	Question
Step 1	What is the problem/conflict/dilemma? Is it a professional violation? Is it a legal violation? Is it a professional and legal violation?
Step 2	What values are in conflict? Under these circumstances, what do I value the most? Will my feelings interfere with my judgment?
Step 3	What evidence is provided by the parties involved? Whose evidence is most convincing? Is there a consistency in the facts? Have I heard all of the facts? What is acceptable practice in this situation? Who is most believable? Have I considered other viewpoints?
Step 4	What courses of action can I take or recommend? Do I need outside consultation? Have I considered the social, cultural, and political impact of the consequences? Have I considered the short term and long term impact of the consequences?
Step 5	In whose best interest is the decision? Will the decision be fair to all parties concerned? If yes, why? If not, why not?
Step 6	How will the decision make me feel about myself today and tomorrow?

and questions for discussion. A set of guiding principles for the development of additional scenarios with related, follow-up activities is also provided in the kit.

Another set of materials, the *Ethics Survey of the University of Massachusetts* (Ducharme, Howard, Santos, & Seymour, 1993) is divided into four main sections. The first section collects demographic data on each student surveyed and information about the student's academic experience with ethics. The second section asks students to answer questions about their own values as they relate to ethics. In this section students have the opportunity to indicate how much they agree/disagree with some statements about ethical principles, such as, women are more ethical than men. In the same section students are questioned about their reactions to

unethical behavior and asked to indicate types of ethical violations that they have observed in classes and in the clinic. The last two sections of the survey ask students to respond to dilemmas encountered by students and those that are encountered by professionals. In the latter situations, students role-play the professional person in the dilemma and then resolve the issue. When using the survey, the instructor asks the students to fill it out, summarize the responses, and share the information as directed by the instructor. Students are then given the opportunity to listen to comments of their peers, react to the comments, and respond appropriately.

Both the survey and kit may be used with graduate students although the materials were developed predominantly on undergraduate student populations. The unique aspect of the survey and kit is that these materials were developed for students mostly by students.

SUMMARY

Ethics is a complex and continually changing area of philosophy. It is used by professional organizations as the basis for developing policy for their members' professional conduct and behavior. One example, the ASHA Code of Ethics, provides principles and rules to help ASHA members deliver services in the best interest of their consumers. When alleged violations of the ASHA code occur, a peer review process determines the settlement of the dispute. Information about ethics and ethical decision making can be provided to students in many different forms (e.g., case study, survey). Learning about ethics and the ASHA Code of Ethics will help professionals to provide a harmonious climate in which to practice.

DISCUSSION QUESTIONS

1. Why is it important for professional organizations to have a code of ethics? Should students in communication disorders be required to follow the ASHA Code of Ethics?
2. How do you learn to be ethical? What factors influenced the development of your ethics philosophy?
3. What are some ethical dilemmas that you have encountered as a student or professional? What steps did you take to handle each situation?
4. Review the ASHA Code of Ethics. What changes would you recommend? Do you think that the procedures for handling alleged violations of the ASHA code are fair?

REFERENCES

American-Speech-Language-Hearing Association. (1992) Issues in ethics. *Asha, 34*(Suppl. 9), 6–21.

American Speech-Language-Hearing Association. (1993a). Boards, committees, and councils. *Asha, 35,* 71–75.

American Speech-Language-Hearing Association. (1993b). Code of ethics. *Asha, 35,* 17–18.

American Speech-Language Hearing Association. (1993c). Statement of practices and procedures. *Asha, 35,* 19–20.

Ducharme, S. (1992). *Ethical trends in communication disorders.* Unpublished manuscript, Honors Track, University of Massachusetts, Amherst.

Ducharme, S., Howard, N., Santos, K., & Seymour, C. M. (1993). The ethics survey of the University of Massachusetts. In *Ethics: Resources for professional preparation and practice* (pp. 3.39–3.46). Rockville, MD: ASHA.

Ducharme, S., & Seymour, C. M. (1992, November). *Ethical trends in communication disorders: A student perspective.* Paper presented at the annual American Speech-Language-Hearing Association Convention, San Antonio, TX.

Flower, R. M. (1984). Legal and ethical considerations. In R. Flower, *Delivery of speech-language pathology and audiology services* (pp. 252–290). Baltimore: Williams & Wilkins.

Gonzalez, L. S. (1992, November). *A survey of student preference of teaching strategies in ethics education.* Paper presented at the annual American Speech-Language-Hearing Association Convention, San Antonio, TX.

Hansen, R. A. (1990). *Lesson 10. Ethical considerations.* AOTA Self Study Series. Rockville, MD: The American Occupational Therapy Association.

Harris, C. E., Jr. (1986). *Applying moral theories.* Belmont, CA: Wadsworth.

Jodoin, J., Konieczny, T., Martin, M., & Seymour, C. M. (1992). *An ethics kit for undergraduates.* Unpublished manuscript, Honors Project, University of Massachusetts, Amherst.

Jones, W. T., Sontag, F., Beckner, M. O., & Fogelin, R. J. (Eds.). (1977). *Approaches to ethics.* (3rd ed.) pp. 6–18. New York: McGraw-Hill.

Kohlberg, L. (1969). Stage and sequence: The cognitive-developmental approach to socialization. In D. Goslin (Ed.), *Handbook of socialization theory and research* (pp. 247–480). Chicago: Rand McNally.

Lickona, T. (1980). What does moral psychology have to say to the teacher of ethics? In D. Callahan & S. Bok (Eds.), *Ethics teaching in higher education* (pp. 103–132). New York and London: Plenum Press.

Mappes, T. A., & Zembaty, J. S. (1987). *Social ethics.* New York: McGraw-Hill.

Pannbacker, M., Lass, N. J., & Middleton, G. F. (1993). Ethics education in speech-language pathology and audiology training programs. *Asha, 35,* 53–55.

Schmeiser, C. B. (1992, Fall). Ethical codes in the professions. *Educational Measurement: Issues and Practice*, pp. 5–11.

Solomon, R. C. (1984). *Ethics: A brief introduction*. New York: McGraw-Hill.

Stromberg, C. D. (1990). *Key legal issues in professional ethics*. In *Reflections on ethics: A compilation of arti-* cles inspired by the May 1990 ASHA ethics colloquium (pp. 15–38). Rockville, MD: ASHA.

White, T. I. (1988). *Right and wrong: A brief guide to understanding ethics*. Engelwood Cliffs: Prentice-Hall.

APPENDIX 6A: Code of Ethics of the American Speech-Language-Hearing Association

Preamble

The preservation of the highest standards of integrity and ethical principles is vital to the responsible discharge of obligations in the professions of speech-language pathology and audiology. This Code of Ethics sets forth the fundamental principles and rules considered essential to this purpose.

Every individual who is (a) a member of the American Speech-Language-Hearing Association, whether certified or not, (b) a nonmember holding the Certificate of Clinical Competence from the Association, (c) an applicant for membership or certification, or (d) a Clinical Fellow seeking to fulfill standards for certification shall abide by this Code of Ethics.

Any action that violates the spirit and purpose of this Code shall be considered unethical. Failure to specify any particular responsibility or practice in this Code of Ethics shall not be construed as denial of the existence of such responsibilities or practices.

The fundamentals of ethical conduct are described by Principles of Ethics and by Rules of Ethics as they relate to responsibility to persons served, to the public, and to the professions of speech-language pathology and audiology.

Principles of Ethics, aspirational and inspirational in nature, form the underlying moral basis for the Code of Ethics. Individuals shall observe these principles as affirmative obligations under all conditions of professional activity.

Rules of Ethics are specific statements of minimally acceptable professional conduct or of prohibitions and are applicable to all individuals.

Principle of Ethics I

Individuals shall honor their responsibility to hold paramount the welfare of persons they serve professionally.

Rules of Ethics

A. Individuals shall provide all services competently.

B. Individuals shall use every resource, including referral when appropriate, to ensure that high-quality service is provided.

C. Individuals shall not discriminate in the delivery of professional services on the basis of race, sex, age, religion, national origin, sexual orientation, or handicapping condition.

D. Individuals shall fully inform the persons they serve of the nature and possible effects of services rendered and products dispensed.

E. Individuals shall evaluate the effectiveness of services rendered and of products dispensed and shall provide services or dispense products only when benefit can reasonably be expected.

F. Individuals shall not guarantee the results of any treatment or procedure, directly or by implication; however, they may make a reasonable statement of prognosis.

G. Individuals shall not evaluate or treat speech, language, or hearing disorders solely by correspondence.

H. Individuals shall maintain adequate records of professional services rendered and products dispensed and shall allow access to these records when appropriately authorized.

I. Individuals shall not reveal, without authorization, any professional or personal information about the person served professionally, unless required by law to do so, or unless doing so is necessary to protect the welfare of the person or of the community.

J. Individuals shall not charge for services not rendered, nor shall they misrepresent,[1] in any fashion, services rendered or products dispensed.

K. Individuals shall use persons in research or as subjects of teaching demonstrations only with their informed consent.

L. Individuals shall withdraw from professional practice when substance abuse or an emotional or mental disability may adversely affect the quality of services they render.

Principles of Ethics II

Individuals shall honor their responsibility to achieve and maintain the highest level of professional competence.

Rules of Ethics

A. Individuals shall engage in the provision of clinical services only when they hold the appropriate Certificate of Clinical Competence or when they are in the certification process and are supervised by an individual who holds the appropriate Certificate of Clinical Competence.

B. Individuals shall engage in only those aspects of the professions that are within the scope of their competence, considering their level of education, training, and experience.

C. Individuals shall continue their professional development throughout their careers.

D. Individuals shall delegate the provision of clinical services only to persons who are certified or to persons in the education or certification process who are appropriately supervised. The provision of support services may be delegated to persons who are neither certified nor in the certification process only when a certificate holder provides appropriate supervision.

E. Individuals shall prohibit any of their professional staff from providing services that exceed the staff member's competence, considering the staff member's level of education, training, and experience.

F. Individuals shall ensure that all equipment used in the provision of services is in proper working order and is properly calibrated.

Principle of Ethics III

Individuals shall honor their responsibility to the public by promoting public

[1]For purposes of this Code of Ethics, misrepresentation includes any untrue statements or statements that are likely to mislead. Misrepresentation also includes the failure to state any information that is material and that ought, in fairness, to be considered.

Source: From American Speech-Language-Hearing Association. (1993). Code of Ethics. *Asha, 35*, 17–18, with permission.

understanding of the professions, by supporting the development of services designed to fulfill the unmet needs of the public, and by providing accurate information in all communications involving any aspect of the professions.

Rules of Ethics

A. Individuals shall not misrepresent their credentials, competence, education, training, or experience.

B. Individuals shall not participate in professional activities that constitute a conflict of interest.

C. Individuals shall not misrepresent diagnostic information, services rendered, or products dispensed or engage in any scheme or artifice to defraud in connection with obtaining payment or reimbursement for such services or products.

D. Individuals' statements to the public shall provide accurate information about the nature and management of communication disorders, about the professions, and about professional services.

E. Individuals' statements to the public— advertising, announcing, and marketing their professional services, reporting research results, and promoting products—shall adhere to prevailing professional standards and shall not contain misrepresentations.

Principle of Ethics IV

Individuals shall honor their responsibilities to the professions and their relationships with colleagues, students, and members of allied professions. Individuals shall uphold the dignity and autonomy of the professions, maintain harmonious interprofessional and intraprofessional relationships, and accept the professions' self-imposed standards.

Rules of Ethics

A.. Individuals shall prohibit anyone under their supervision from engaging in any practice that violates the Code of Ethics.

B. Individuals shall not engage in dishonesty, fraud, deceit, misrepresentation, or any form of conduct that adversely reflects on the professions or on the individual's fitness to serve persons professionally.

C. Individuals shall assign credit only to those who have contributed to a publication, presentation, or product. Credit shall be assigned in proportion to the contribution and only with the contributor's consent.

D. Individuals' statements to colleagues about professional services, research results, and products shall adhere to prevailing professional standards and shall contain no misrepresentations.

E. Individuals shall not provide professional services without exercising independent professional judgment, regardless of referral source or prescription.

F. Individuals who have reason to believe that the Code of Ethics has been violated shall inform the Ethical Practice Board.

G. Individuals shall cooperate fully with the Ethical Practice Board in its investigation and adjudication of matters related to this Code of Ethics.

H. Individuals shall not discriminate in their relationships with colleagues, students, and members of allied professions on the basis of race, sex, age, religion, national origin, sexual orientation, or handicapping condition.

APPENDIX 6B: Examples of Scenarios with Dilemmas

SCENARIO 1

You are a communication disorders major working to complete the required 25 observation hours for ASHA CCC. You have accumulated 20 hours so far and need only 5 more. You are a first semester graduate student, and if you do not meet the deadline for completion in 2 weeks you will not be assigned a client until next semester. During the past five observation sessions, even though you were not supervised according to ASHA's standards, the supervisor signed for those hours. What might you do?

SPECIFIC AREAS OF ASHA'S CODE OF ETHICS WHICH MAY APPLY

Principle of Ethics III Rule A
Principle of Ethics IV Rule A, B, and F

POSSIBLE SOLUTIONS

You could go to the supervisor and express your concerns over the lack of proper supervision in a firm but nonthreatening way.

You could go the supervisor's boss and ask that person to speak to the supervisor.

You could say nothing to anyone and pretend it did not happen.

QUESTIONS FOR DISCUSSION

What if the supervisor continues to behave like this?

What if you say nothing and someone finds out about the lack of proper supervision just as you are completing your final observation hour or just when you begin therapy with your client?

Source: From Jodoin, J., Konieczny, T., Martin, M., & Seymour, C. M. (1992). *An ethics kit for undergraduates.* Unpublished manuscript, Honors Project, University of Massachusetts, Amherst, with permission.

What if you report the supervisor to someone and you have to repeat all of those observation hours that were not properly supervised?

What if you complete your required observation hours and begin your clinical clock hours only to find that you are at a disadvantage because of your lack of supervision during your observation hours?

SCENARIO 2

You are observing your clinical supervisor who is working with a patient and the supervisor tells a joke which you find offensive. The patient laughs at the joke and does not appear to be bothered. Later on you see the patient leave the clinic and the patient tells you that the joke was offensive and that "I will not come back to the clinic until that supervisor is fired." How might you handle the situation?

SPECIFIC AREAS OF ASHA'S CODE OF ETHICS WHICH MAY APPLY

Principle of Ethics IV Rule B
Principle of Ethics IV Rule H

POSSIBLE SOLUTIONS

You could approach the supervisor after work and explain that the joke was person- ally offensive and request that the supervisor refrain from such comments in the future.

You could interrupt the supervisor when the joke was said and explain that the joke was offensive and inappropriate and ask that the supervisor refrain from such comments in the future.

You could approach the supervisor's boss and ask the boss to talk to the supervisor.

You could send the supervisor some materials about defamation of character.

You could ignore the joke and say nothing.

You could seek assistance from an organization in ASHA that represents the defamed group.

QUESTIONS FOR DISCUSSION

What if the this is not the first time that the supervisor has told offensive jokes?

What if you decide to say nothing to the supervisor and the supervisor makes more offensive jokes around other patients?

What if you ask the supervisor to stop using offensive jokes and the supervisor disregards your request.

What if the jokes were sexually offensive? racially offensive? homophobic?

■ CHAPTER 7 ■

International Perspectives

■ MARGO E. WILSON, PH.D. ■

SCOPE OF CHAPTER

The professions of speech-language pathology and audiology have been in existence internationally for more than 65 years. The First International Congress of Logopedics and Phoniatrics was held in 1924 with 65 participants. During the Congress the International Association of Logopedics and Phoniatrics (IALP) was founded. Speech therapy was being provided in 39 schools in Vienna by 1928 (de Monfort, 1990). For more than 30 years, American Speech-Language-Hearing Association (ASHA) members have been publishing reports of research conducted on various aspects of communication disorders in other countries. This research has explored a wide variety of topics, such as treatment of traumatic brain injury in Israel (Katz & Florian, 1991) and in Amerika Samoa (Wallace, 1992), a study of stuttering in the Bantu culture (Aron, 1962), hearing loss in India (Kapur, 1965), hearing screening in the United Kingdom (Davis & Sancho, 1988), and beliefs about communication disorders in an African tribe (Fleming, 1981).

Other reports describe the status of the communication disorders professions in foreign countries. These countries include Belgium, (Hoops, 1972); Brazil, (Navas & Pinho, 1993; Sparks, 1979); India, (Hegarty, 1970; Hegde,1992; O'Neill, Deal, & Kapur, 1972; Stewart, 1970); the Philippines, (Williams, 1971); Singapore, (Ivey & McCafferty, 1975); South Korea (Ries, 1990); Sweden, (Coleman, 1974); and the former USSR (Honeygosky, 1974; Yairi, 1990). ASHA members have also reported on their activities contributing to the development of service programs in such countries as Costa Rica (Norton, 1981), Guam and Micronesia (Stewart & Triolo, 1990), Honduras (Cassie, 1992), Malaysia (ASHA , 1976; Curtis, 1973), Nepal (Werner, 1981), South Korea (Kersting, 1974), South Vietnam (Landis, 1973; Northern, Downs, Hemenway, & Wood, 1972), Ceylon (now Sri Lanka) (Sklar, 1973), Taiwan (Landis, Hwang, & Hsu, 1980), and most recently, Romania (ASHA, 1992). Another group of articles surveys international activities, programs, management strategies, and the training of foreign students. (Curlee, 1974; Li-Rong, 1992; McCavitt, 1971; Pressman & Rudner, 1990).

At the professional association level, ASHA has affiliated with various international groups, most notably the International Association of Logopedists and Phoniatrists. An International Affairs Committee within ASHA was active for many years. After a reorganization within ASHA in 1990, the International Affairs Association (IAA), a related professional organization, replaced the International Affairs Committee. This group is becoming increasingly active in bringing together professionals from a wide variety of countries and in serving as an information source and network for members involved in professional activities internationally.

This chapter focuses on the status of communication disorders internationally, discusses ways of interacting with professional colleagues in other countries, and considers possibilities for increasing the quantity and quality of services for those with communication disorders worldwide. If you are a student, an appreciation of international research and activities will broaden the scope of your professional knowledge. For practicing professionals, this chapter may stimulate your interest in participating in or initiating international professional activities.

STATUS OF COMMUNICATION DISORDERS INTERNATIONALLY

COMMUNICATION DISORDERS: A LOW- (OR NO-) LEVEL PRIORITY INTERNATIONALLY

In 1978, the United Nations, through the World Health Organization (WHO), set the global priority of good health for all by the year 2000, with the emphasis on primary health care activities and early detection. Not until 1985, 7 years after the original proclamation, was hearing loss included in the planning for prevention (Mencher,1988). This occurred only after the Committee for the Worldwide Prevention of Hearing Impair-

ment, formed to coordinate services for hearing disorders worldwide, made a concerted effort. This committee is made up of members of the International Society of Audiology, the International Federation of Oto-Rhino-Laryngological Society (IFOS), the International Federation of the Hard of Hearing, and the World Federation of the Deaf. The most active of these organizations is the IFOS, an internationally based medical group. In 1992 a new, nongovernmental organization (NGO) was formed, called Hearing International. Hearing International is a partnership of the main international nongovernmental organizations working in the area of hearing impairment and deafness. Its mission includes initiating regional and national "ear care" programs. Regional centers for hearing health care have been developed in Bangkok, Thailand, Mexico City, and Bari, Italy. Ear Care Centers are being developed in several countries, including Bangladesh, Indonesia, the Philippines, Kenya, and Egypt. The organization also prepared a resolution for the World Health Organization General Assembly proposing inclusion of prevention and treatment of hearing impairments into existing programs of health and development. Unfortunately, speech and language disorders are not *yet* addressed in the United Nations or WHO programs.

Through the continuing efforts of international professional groups of physicians and audiologists, worldwide activity continues to increase in the area of hearing impairment, with several new organizations being formed. The WHO created a Division for the Prevention of Hearing Impairment (PDH) in 1991, assisting in demographic research, working to raise funds for its work as a nongovernmental agency, and supporting the development of organizations and committees in each country for prevention of hearing impairment and deafness.

TRAINING PROGRAMS WORLDWIDE

The first survey of training programs for speech-language pathology and audiology worldwide was done by Moll (1983), who found 31 countries with some form of professional training. A later survey (Ackerman Stewart, 1990, 1992), found training programs for speech-language pathologists (logopedes) to have increased to 40 countries outside the United States. Most recently, Lesser's (1992) survey identified 42 countries with training programs. The training programs described in these sources range in duration from 2 to 6 years and result in diplomas, degrees, or licenses. Nine of the countries responding offer doctorates in the field.

Among the countries currently offering training programs reported by Lesser and/or Ackerman Stewart are: Argentina, Australia, Austria, Belgium, Brazil, Bulgaria, Canada, China, Colombia, Czechoslovakia (in Bohemia and Slovakia), Denmark, Egypt, Estonia, Finland, France, Germany, Hong Kong, Hungary, India, Indonesia, Iran, Ireland, Israel, Italy, Japan, Jordan, Malta, Mexico, Netherlands, New Zealand, Norway, Peru, Poland, Portugal, Romania, Saudi Arabia, South Africa, Spain, Sweden, Switzerland, Thailand, various parts of the former USSR, countries within the United Kingdom (England, Northern Ireland, Scotland, and Wales), parts of the former Yugoslavia, and Zimbabwe.

Most of these programs are college- or university-based, but others are provided by private physicians or special institutes. Of the 12 countries within the European Community (EC), two (Luxembourg and Greece) currently do not have educational programs. In the other 10 EC countries, 107 programs provide an average annual output of about 1,800 logopedists. (Lesser, 1992).

Audiology training programs are reported in eight countries in addition to the United States: Australia, Canada, Egypt, India, Iran, Japan, South Africa, and Thailand (Ackerman Stewart, 1990). These data are clearly incomplete, because European programs apparently did not respond to this part of the survey. Additionally, in several countries such as India and Brazil, the professions of speech-language pathology and audiology are considered to be one profession and training is given in both areas.

AVAILABILITY OF COMMUNICATION DISORDERS SERVICES INTERNATIONALLY

In the developed nations, communication disorders are recognized, and diagnosis and treatment are available. In some EC countries most children, including those who are hearing impaired, are the responsibility of speech-language pathologists. In other EC countries children who are hearing impaired and other children in special education with speech or language problems are the responsibility of other professions, with speech-language pathologists working primarily in hospitals. In many countries worldwide, physicians are in charge of rehabilitation. The physician is usually a phoniatrist, an otorhinolaryngologist who has taken further training in remediation of voice disorders. The physician prescribes therapy that is provided by trained nonmedical staff. Fully educated and certified speech-language pathologists and audiologists, trained in university systems, are considered subordinate to the physicians.

As Europe moves towards European Community (EC)) objectives, professionals in the various countries are deeply concerned about differences in standards of education and experience (Fawcus, 1993). An EC directive now in effect gives mutual recognition within the EC to any member of the profession whose qualifying "diploma" has been obtained in the EC after at least 3 years of postsecondary study. These professionals are entitled to practice in any EC country. A consortium of EC logopedists has been formed to establish standards of education, training, and practice within the EC. At present there is considerable variability in training and practice among the European countries (Ackerman Stewart, 1992; Lesser, 1992). In most EC countries, it is only work in government-supported services that requires the professional qualification; there are no restrictions on working as a speech-language-pathologist in private practice except in Germany, where 2 years of experience are required. In Denmark the professional qualification is required only for work with adult patients; children are seen by logopedists/special education teachers. The EC Consortium and the Education Committee of the IALP each are considering the development of minimum standards of training to be used within the EC or worldwide. (See Chapter 4 by Battle on licensure and certification.)

The need for communication disorders training or service delivery programs is not officially recognized in many developing nations. Few have requested assistance for services to citizens who are communicatively disordered from the agencies that work with developing nations to provide a variety of health care services (Pleasonton, 1993). A few developing countries are in the initial stages of development of services and may have one or two centers where diagnosis and treatment are available (e.g., Romania and Thailand). These centers are usually focused on the population that is hearing impaired and do not yet include services for speech and language disorders. Others focus only on speech disorders associated with physical causes, such as cleft palate.

EDUCATION, CERTIFICATION, AND LICENSING REQUIREMENTS

As noted in the information about training programs in other countries, there is tremendous diversity in the type and amount of education, clinical practicum, and testing required for recognition as a person who provides speech, language, or hearing services. Even countries that are related by history and language, such as the United States, Canada, Australia, and the United Kingdom, have major differences in their educational programs and certification requirements. Considering how fraught with difficulties the issue of reciprocity between these countries has been, it is not surprising that reciprocity with non-English-speaking countries has seemed unattainable. However, the Clinical

Certification Board of ASHA has developed implementation procedures for review of applications for non-United States national governmental credentialing agencies or from non-United States national private voluntary credentialing agencies to determine whether the agency's credential will be endorsed by ASHA (ASHA, 1993). An applicant holding a foreign credential that has been endorsed by ASHA will not be required to submit documents for individual evaluation, but will be required to complete any requirements that have been stipulated as part of the endorsement. Individuals who successfully complete all requirements will be granted the ASHA Certificate of Clinical Competence (CCC).

ASHA: CAN AND SHOULD WE INCREASE OUR PRESENCE INTERNATIONALLY?

As Mencher (1988) observed when discussing the United Nations initiative for "Health for All by the Year 2000":

If the International Society of Audiology could play so prominent a role where hearing loss and the hearing impaired were concerned, where was (and where is) the International Association of Logopedics and Phoniatrics (IALP), a group representing and speaking for the speech-language impaired at the world level? . . . what role did ASHA play? . . . as a North American audiologist, I am distressed that my profession has contributed so little . . . to this incredibly important world event . . . The Canadian and the American Speech-Language-Hearing Associations had nothing to do with the decision . . . (to eventually include the hearing impaired in the resolution) . . . Let us speak together as people and as professionals. We must shed our provincialism and become national associations with international reputations for leadership, constructive thought, and action. (pp. 8–10)

In the *Asha* issue devoted to the future, the article entitled "We are part of the planet, you know" (Spriestersbach, 1991) notes the increasing world population, the challenge of meeting worldwide health problems, and the need for us, as professionals in communication disorders, to become more aware of other cultures. Additionally, Spriestersbach recommends that professional groups consider how their services will fit into a world for which resources are less plentiful. He suggests that established ways of identifying and serving clients may have to change and that guarding professional turf will be increasingly nonproductive and costly.

Philips (1990) reminds us that, although communication disorders may seem less important than food, housing, and health care, "those who cannot communicate well may have even more difficulty attaining essential food, shelter, clothing, and medical care. Their very survival may be at risk" (p. 51).

What is the status of our professions among the agencies that provide support for health-related services abroad? Pleasonton (1993) conducted a survey of agencies providing health- and education-related services internationally to discover what opportunities were available for overseas work as a communication disorders specialist. Contact with more than 40 agencies produced disheartening results. Most of the organizations were unaware of the professions of speech-language pathology and audiology and of the effect of communication disorders on health, education, and quality of life. When they were aware, they dismissed services as too expensive or unavailable. Pleasonton asks:

What have we done to "sell" the need and value of our services to less affluent countries? . . . Have we forgotton how much we can do . . . to provide diagnosis, training and simple remedies to make life easier for those who suffer (communication) losses? . . . I call on ASHA to take a leadership role in having communication recognized as a basic need; we must sell the world on the value of speech/language/hearing testing and rehabilitation, and on their cost-effectiveness in terms of human quality of life. (pp. 5–6)

It is not an easy task. Even an economically developed country such as ours has only a short history of providing services for disabled individuals. We have no reason to be complacent. Nevertheless, though we are far from having achieved a perfect model of training or service delivery, we are clearly in the forefront and are looked to for help by developing countries of the world. The United States has approximately 5% of the world's population, but around 59% of the world's supply of speech-language pathologists, and 58% of the world's training programs in communication disorders (Lesser, 1992).

We should not be surprised when developing countries are seemingly uninterested in providing speech and hearing services comparable to our standards for their people. Our models and programs are not presently exportable. In fact, given the life and death issues of disease and malnutrition and the basic educational needs that so many countries face, it is surprising that so many developing countries are making a serious effort to begin helping their population with special needs. More than 20% of the affiliates of the International Association of Logopedics and Phoniatrics are countries considered "developing," rather than "developed."

Clearly, we in the United States, where we have the majority of communication disorders professionals and training programs and resources, have not assumed a leadership role at the international level. Despite more than 30 years of individual effort, we have only begun to find ways to foster the development of the professions of speech-language pathology and audiology in developing nations and to enhance the international involvement of ASHA as an association and as individual members.

SOME ACHIEVABLE OBJECTIVES

The ASHA Committee on International Affairs was in existence for approximately 20 years, ending in 1990, as did many ASHA standing committees as a result of committee restructuring. In its last 5 years, the committee greatly broadened its scope and increased its activities. Projects included, but were not limited to: presentations on international topics at the ASHA annual convention; development of the international affairs database, which was accessible on Actionline and provided names of ASHA members who had onsite experience in other countries; preparation of a packet of materials for state associations and others interested in developing a Partnership Program with communication disorders personnel in other countries; and development of a variety of resolutions aimed at increasing ASHA's involvement in international activities.

In 1985, ASHA sponsored a National Colloquium on Underserved Populations. One of the areas of study was "Developing Regions." Many resolutions were approved on international issues and activities (Wilson, 1990). They included proposals for: (a) recruiting students, (b) credentialing standards for students from developing nations, (c) guidelines for conducting basic epidemiologic research, and (d) culture-specific norms. Also proposed was the development of more liaisons with international organizations and a comprehensive database, to include the following kinds of information: (a) funding sources for international professional travel and for foreign student support, (b) training programs developed for foreign students majoring in communication disorders, (c) names of professionals with experience in specific countries, (d) an annotated bibliography, and (e) resource persons in economically developing countries.

IAA members have proposed additional international activities, such as development of a current list of government offices and officials in other countries who oversee programs related to communication disorders, which could be made available to members who are seeking opportunities to consult or teach abroad. Development of more appropriate educational and clinical programs for international students majoring in communication disorders has also been suggested. An ongoing activity that could be expanded is the pairing of professionals from this country with those working in developing countries to share resources, exchange information, and, possibly, visits to one another's work sites.

Working in other cultures and systems of administration is complex and difficult. A set of guidelines for speech-language pathologists and audiologists consulting in developing countries could be developed by a committee of experienced professionals who have learned by trial and error. There is also a need for a document outlining the knowledge and skills needed for effective international consulting. In addition, a list of experienced and culturally sensitive speech-language pathologists and audiologists could be generated and made available to officials from other countries seeking program consultants, just as we now provide a list of bilingual professionals.

A short, interesting brochure could be developed to provide information about communication disorders; how they can be identified, diagnosed, and treated; and about the professions of speech-language pathology and audiology. It should be available in several languages. The brochure could be purchased and distributed by speech-language pathologists and audiologists when they travel to developing countries.

According to the Membership Directory (ASHA, 1992), ASHA has 270 members living and working abroad (not including Canada). In 1986, 760 ASHA members indicated a current involvement in research, teaching, or consultation in 55 different foreign countries. If these professionals worked together, many of these objectives could be met.

In addition to activities seeking to foster the development of the professions of speech-language pathology and audiology worldwide, we need to create opportunities to increase our knowledge of research done in other countries and of the current status of education and clinical service internationally. Almost 20 years ago, Curlee (1974) noted "a special benefit of international involvement (is) the development of an awareness that problems of relevance to speech pathologists {sic} and audiologists exist in similar forms in many places in the world and that advances in scientific knowledge tend to occur in several places at about the same time" (p. 418). Butler (1989), a past-president of ASHA and of the IALP says "International endeavors remain a two-way street, with scientists and professionals in other countries and regions of the world having much to contribute to our knowledge and understanding of the medical, educational, and cultural aspects of human communication and its disorders" (p. 64).

With the exception of a few invited speakers to our national conventions, our professions have not been active in facilitating professional exchanges on an international level through sponsorship of meetings dedicated to exploration of international issues in communication disorders. Canadian associations, however, have sponsored seven meetings. The Seventh International Symposium, held in May, 1987, in Halifax, Nova Scotia, had as its theme: "Human Communication Disorders: A Worldwide Perspective." Participants from Czechoslovakia, Great Britain, Mexico, Malaya, and Thailand, as well as the United States and Canada, reviewed current practices and recent developments in communication disorders. The proceedings of this conference were later published as a book (Gerber & Mencher, 1988).

HOW CAN YOU GET INVOLVED?

What role can you, as an individual, hope to play to further the development of training, research, and service delivery in other countries? Those with experience in the development and accreditation of a university program in communication disorders, with additional experience in working in other cultures and with governmental bureaucracies and with a healthy respect for the competing needs and realities of developing nations, could serve as consultants for universities and colleges wishing to develop training programs. Those with experience in the delivery of clinical services, especially in remote or underserved areas and with adequate understanding of the limitations of a host country can aid in the establishment of services for the communicatively disordered population. Those who are experts in a particular area, and able to adjust their teaching to the cultural values and special needs of other countries, can enhance the knowledge and abilities of existing service providers. Each of you can work as an advocate for increased availability and improved quality of services for individuals with communication disorders worldwide. The following activities provide ways of becoming active and knowledgeable in international affairs and developing contacts that will foster international activities.

The International Affairs Association (IAA), a related professional organization of ASHA, currently has more than 195 members, including members from 27 foreign countries. The association provides an annual directory of members and four newsletters a year. There is an annual meeting during the ASHA Annual Convention. Dues are nominal. To learn more about the organization, read "The International Affairs Association" (Ritter, 1993), or call ASHA's international contact for the name of the current president of the association.

You may also join an international association in your particular area of interest. A partial list of such associations includes the International Society of Audiology, the International Association of Laryngectomees, the International Association of Orofacial Myology, the International Federation of Hard of Hearing People, the International Cleft Palate Association, the International Fluency Association, the International Pragmatics Association, and the International Society of Augmentative and Alternative Communication. Call ASHA for a current contact at these organizations.

The International Association of Logopedics and Phoniatrics (IALP) has a directory of individual members and of Affiliated Societies. Names and addresses of 513 members of the IALP (141 from the United States) are listed. ASHA is one of the 54 Affiliated Societies representing 37 countries listed in this directory.

The IALP has an annual meeting every 3 years. Papers are presented or simultaneously translated into English. Its members are from more than 38 countries, and there are social events at the conference enabling attendees to meet professionals from many other countries.

Communication Therapists International is a group of United Kingdom speech-language pathologists who have worked in developing countries. They have developed an International Register of Therapists, a Resource Pack, and a Reading List. They sponsor Study Days at various locations in the British Isles. Costs for membership and materials are nominal. For information, write Julie Marshall, Centre for Audiology, Education of the Deaf and Speech Pathology, University of Manchester, Oxford Rd., Manchester, M13 9PL, England.

The Overseas Association of Communication Sciences (OSACS) is a professional association with a membership of approximately 100 American ASHA-certified active members, associates, and affiliates. Members are located throughout Europe and work mainly for the United States Department of Defense. In 1989, ASHA voted to recognize OSACS as an official state association, and in 1991, OSACS became a member of the Council of State Association Presidents. OSACS is also recognized as an official Continuing Education sponsor.

One of the purposes of OSACS is to encourage the development of educational opportunities in the overseas area and the interchange of information among European and American speech-language pathologists, audiologists, and other professionals involved in human communication and its disorders. To this end, OSACS holds three conferences annually in Europe. Lecturers are experts in their area of communication sciences and are recruited worldwide. Attendance is open to all professionals and others interested in the field of communication sciences. A current contact for OSACS can be obtained from the ASHA national office to obtain information about upcoming meetings or to locate an ASHA colleague in a foreign country.

A member of the ASHA national office staff has been designated as a contact for information on international affairs. Call the Actionline at 1-800-638-6868 and ask for the "International Desk."

Build a local network of people with international interests by encouraging your state association to form an international committee. A document developed by the Committee on International Affairs (1989), which gives ideas for committee activities such as Partnership Programs, is available from ASHA.

Become a host to an international student at your nearby university. Hosting does not mean the student will live with you; your relationship will be that of friend and advisor. Typical activities might include sightseeing in your area or a holiday dinner at your home. You can gain not only invaluable insights into other cultures, but contacts for future professional visits to other countries.

Travel with a group of communication disorders professionals or other health or education professionals whose tour combines sightseeing with visits to hospitals, schools, or clinics. These are often sponsored by churches, community service clubs, sister city programs, and university departments and provide a completely different experience from the usual tour.

Use every opportunity when you travel to educate health and education professionals and government officials in developing countries about the professions of speech-language pathology and audiology. Such informal education may be reflected in policy enhancement for persons with disabilities and improved services. You can do this by taking along brochures, educational materials, or introductory texts to donate to appropriate educational or governmental contacts.

STRATEGIES FOR FINDING EMPLOYMENT ABROAD

Going to another country for a short time to visit programs, make presentations, or act as a short-term consultant is simply a matter of planning, research, contacts, and finances. Working in another country for an extended period of time is considerably more complicated, requiring not only the basic efforts, but much time and patience in meeting the requirements for a work visa. Most people who have been successful in this endeavor have done so by doing research at home and then communicating with professional contacts in the foreign country. If the possibilities look good, you can travel to the country as a tourist and make the round of employers and governmental offices to facilitate the paperwork required for a work visa.

When you write to agencies asking about professional opportunities, remember to use all of your possible titles, as different agencies use different job titles. Request information for speech therapist, logopedist, speech pathologist, speech-language pathologist, and communication disorders specialist, or audiologist, audiometrician, auditory rehabilitation specialist, and so on. You may also find a niche in special education if you have worked with special populations. You may get a first job as a teacher of English as a Second Language, which will enable you to live abroad while looking for a position in communication disorders.

Whether or not you are presently associated with a university, you can visit its international office. Most are well-supplied with publications and materials that can help you track down job possibilities.

Although few of us are proficient enough in another language to provide direct treatment in that language, there are many ways to share your expertise overseas through teaching, consulting, and research. Speech-language pathologists and audiologists have provided services internationally through the Peace Corps, as Fulbright Scholars, as researchers and lecturers with the World Rehabilitation Fund, as volunteers with Partners of the Americas, World Vision, or the Volunteer Service Organization of the United Kingdom, as employees of the U.S. government working in American schools and hospitals overseas, or in International Schools. Many Americans have established private practices in other countries providing services to English-speaking expatriates. The following resources and strategies are available to help the individual seeking to work in another country.

To begin the process of finding contacts internationally and of learning more about our professions in other countries, you can combine pleasure travel with professional interests and seek out colleagues in countries to be visited. To find out what training programs or clinics exist in other countries or to locate fellow professionals overseas, several resources are available to help you.

PROFESSIONAL PUBLICATIONS

The *ASHA Membership Directory* (ASHA, 1992) has a section that lists ASHA members by geographical area. Included are listings for ASHA members in 56 foreign countries. Their addresses can then be found by consulting the alphabetical listings.

Asha publishes a list of international meetings each month in the "Calendar" section. If there is a conference in a country in which you are especially interested in working, attend the conference and pursue opportunities to meet professionals and learn what job opportunities may exist. *Asha* also publishes a news section called "ASHA Abroad" approximately five times a year. Recent international activities of ASHA members are reported and news of international professional organizations is included.

The May 1990 issue of *Asha* was dedicated to international issues. It contained articles by ASHA members about their work in Korea, Guam and Micronesia, China, the (former) USSR, and two helpful summary articles: "Opportunities for Service in Third World Countries" (Fain, 1990) and the Committee on International Affairs' "Resources." (Committee on International Affairs, 1990).

The new ASHA journals are now including articles with an international emphasis; there is the "World View" section in the *American Journal of Speech-Language Pathology* and the "Perspective" section of the *American Journal of Audiology.*

A joint committee of the IALP and ASHA has compiled an *International Directory of Education for Speech-Language Pathologists (Speech Therapists/Logopedists, Orthophonists) and Audiologists.* (Ackerman Stewart, 1992). This directory, which can be purchased from ASHA, describes the credentialing requirements and professional training for approximately 45 countries and lists a contact person in most countries.

GENERAL PUBLICATIONS

There are a wealth of magazines and books designed for those wishing to work abroad. Although they are not written specifically for communication disorders specialists, they provide valuable information about the general scope of opportunities abroad and resources and strategies for finding employment, as well as reports of living and working conditions in a variety of countries. See the Resources Section of this chapter for addresses.

The International Educator is published four times a year; in July a "Jobs Only" supplement features thousands of vacancies for teachers and administrators in hundreds of the 750 American and international schools located throughout the world.

Transitions Abroad: the Guide to Learning, Living and Working Overseas is published six times a year. Also available, often as a subscription bonus, is a *Guide to Overseas Opportunities*, with names and address of organizations involved in international employment. Each issue of the magazine contains articles about travel, overseas study programs, and overseas employment experiences.

SPECIFIC AGENCIES/PROGRAMS

United States Information Agency

The United States Information Agency (USIA) operates the United States government's programs of educational and cultural exchange, formerly administered by the Department of State. The broad purpose of these programs is to provide citizens of other countries with a better sense of what the United States stands for and why, and to give the American people a more accurate perception of other peoples.

The best known of the exchanges supported by USIA is the Fulbright Scholar Program, or academic exchange program, which operates in 130 countries. Under the Fulbright Scholar Program, approximately 5,000 grants are awarded each year to American students, teachers, and scholars to study, teach, and conduct research abroad and to foreign nationals to engage in similar activities in the United States. There are several types of individual grants under the Fulbright Scholar Program. For example, nearly 1,000 foreign scholars from 125 countries come to the United States every year to lecture and conduct postdoctoral research in fields ranging from biosciences to comparative literature. Some 1,200 American scholars and professionals are sent to 100 nations, generally for 1 academic year, to lecture and conduct research. Approximately 600 American predoctoral graduate students study abroad each year with either full or partial support from the Fulbright program, and more than 3,000 foreign graduate students are supported by Fulbright grants at American universities each year.

In addition, more than 450 elementary and secondary school teachers are exchanged every year, principally between the United States and Western European countries. Although exchanges between speech-language pathologists are rare, they may be created by contacting a colleague in another country directly, with both then applying for exchanges.

The academic exchanges contain many other programs for students, teachers and scholars, including the Hubert H. Humphrey Fellowship Program, under which mid-career professionals from Third World countries receive a year of specially designed graduate-level training at selected U.S. universities, and the Congress Bundestag Exchange Program which provides mutual full scholarships for year-long academic homestay programs between Germany and the United States. These programs are all administrated by the Council for International Exchange of Scholars (CIES).

In response to specific requests from its officers overseas, the USIA sends selected Americans, called "American Participants," abroad for short-term speaking programs. These Americans help inform experts abroad of developments in the United States in economics, foreign policy, political and social processes, the arts and humanities, and science and technology. Some 700 American experts, many of whom take time from their own travel overseas, participate in the program each year.

Peace Corps

A number of ASHA members have served in the Peace Corps over the years. There have been few recent openings specifically for communication disorders specialists, because the host countries have not been requesting them. If you specifically want to be a Peace Corps volunteer, and have a particular country in mind, you may be successful in creating a position for yourself by contacting the in-country director and describing your qualifications and skills and proposing a project.

World Vision International

World Vision International is an organization dedicated to helping people in need throughout the world. Participating in both short- and long-term projects, World Vision International is currently providing child development specialists for the orphanages in Romania, with some ASHA members involved (ASHA, 1992).

International Exchange of Experts and Information in Rehabilitation

The International Exchange of Experts and Information in Rehabilitation (World Rehabilitation Fund) (IEEIR) is funded by the United States Department of Education's National Institute on Disability and Rehabilitation Research. It publishes newsletters and monographs and provides grants for international projects in the area of rehabilitation. Several speech-language pathologists and audiologists have received these grants and authored monographs (Condon, 1990; Katz & Florian, 1991; Peuser, 1984; Sarno & Woods, 1989; Wallace, 1992; Walsh, 1989).

Volunteer Services Overseas

Volunteer Services Overseas is a British organization that places volunteers in 40 countries. They have many requests for speech-language pathologists and audiologists. Their address is 317-325 Putney Bridge Rd., London SW15 2PN, England.

SUMMARY

During the past 30 years we have made a good beginning, usually acting individually, in sharing our expertise and resources overseas. As more countries begin developing education and service programs, opportunities are increasingly available. Advances in technology are making international communication through "information highways" such as E-Mail and Internet fast, easy, and inexpensive wherever there are reliable telephone systems, computers, and modems.

The issues discussed in this chapter require our action to result in specific plans and proposals to facilitate increased, and increasingly effective, international exchanges. We in the economically developed countries have a relative abundance of knowledge and resources; we must discover the best way to share them with countries still in the early stages of health care planning. We must also find ways to avail ourselves of the knowledge and experience of our overseas colleagues.

Using the information and resources in this chapter, we, as individuals, and we, in our professional associations, can have an impact. As Margaret Mead (1992) wrote: "Never doubt that a small group of committed citizens can change the world; indeed, it is the only thing which ever has."

DISCUSSION QUESTIONS

1. Should we, as speech-language pathologists and audiologists and as a professional organization, play a greater role

internationally? What specific actions/projects would you recommend?

2. Should degree programs for international students majoring in communication disorders in the United States be modified for them in any way? Do they need ASHA certification? Should they be required to participate in accent-reduction therapy prior to their clinical practicum?

3. Describe the research you would do before traveling to a foreign country if you were interested in visiting local speech and hearing clinics and educational programs. What sources would you consult?

4. How could you reconcile your concerns about minimum competencies for the practice of speech-language pathology or audiology with a request from a developing country for you to come for 6 months to train paraprofessionals to begin a program of identification and prevention of speech, language and hearing disorders?

REFERENCES

Ackerman Stewart, B. (Ed.). (1990). International directory of education for speech-language pathologists and audiologists (Draft). Rockville, MD: American Speech-Language-Hearing Association.

Ackerman Stewart, B. (Ed.). (1992). International directory of education for speech-language pathologists and audiologists (Revised Draft). Rockville, MD: American Speech-Language-Hearing Association.

American Speech-Language-Hearing Association. (1976). Malaysian speech unit established by ASHA member. Asha, 18, 520.

American Speech-Language-Hearing Association. (1990). International issue. Asha, 32.

American Speech-Language-Hearing Association. (1992). Project ROSES (Romanian Orphans Social Education Services). Asha, 34, 10.

American Speech-Language-Hearing Association. (1992). Membership Directory 1993–94. Rockville, MD: Author.

American Speech-Language-Hearing Association. (1993). New program of endorsement of foreign credentials adopted by Council on Professional Standards. Asha, 35, 128.

Aron, M. L. (1962). The nature and incidence of stuttering among a Bantu group of school-going children. Journal of Speech and Hearing Disorders, 27, 2, 116–128.

Butler, K. (1989). Book review, Asha, 32, 64.

Cassie, D. (1992). A challenge in Honduras. American Journal of Audiology, 1, 9–10.

Coleman, R. O. (1974). Speech science and speech pathology in Sweden. Asha, 16, 310–313.

Committee on International Affairs (1989). Partnership program. Rockville, MD: American Speech-Language-Hearing Association.

Committee on International Affairs (1990). Resources. Asha, 32, 52–53.

Condon, M. (1990). Disability in Kunming, China: An overview of special education and rehabilitation programs. New York: World Rehabilitation Fund; International Exchange of Information in Rehabilitation.

Curlee, R. F. (1974). International involvement of speech pathologists and audiologists. Asha, 16, 416–418.

Curtis, N. W. (1973). Speech and hearing services in Malaysia. Asha, 15, 645–646.

Davis, A., & Sancho, J. (1988). Screening for hearing impairment in children: A review of current practice in the United Kingdom. In S. E. Gerber & G. Mencher (Eds.), International perspectives on communication disorders (pp. 3–10). Washington, DC: Gallaudet University Press.

de Monfort, M. (1990). A brief history of IALP. Asha, 32, 33–35.

Fain, M. R. (1990). Opportunities for service in third world countries. Asha, 32, 45–47.

Fawcus, B. (1993, May). Working within a European context. College of Speech-Language Therapists Bulletin, pp. 11–12.

Fleming, C. A. (1981). Beliefs about speech development in a primitive African tribe. Journal of the National Student Speech-Language Hearing Association, 9, 38–49.

Gerber, S. E., & Mencher, G. (Eds.). (1988). International perspectives on communication disorders. Washington, DC: Gallaudet University Press.

Hegarty, I. E. (1970). A visiting speech pathologist in India. Asha, 12, 18–19.

Hegde, M. N. (1992). A personal journey to a different kind of convention: Speech and hearing in India. American Journal of Speech-Language Pathology, 1, 13–14.

Honeygosky, R. A. (1974). Speech, hearing and language services and professional training in the USSR and Poland. Asha, 16, 142–148.

Hoops, R. A. (1972). A visiting speech pathologist in Belgium. Asha, 14, 445–447.

Ivey, S. M., & McCafferty, M. (1975). The Republic of Singapore's developing speech and hearing program. Asha, 17, 739–741.

Kapur, Y. P. (1965). A study of hearing loss in school children in India. *Journal of Speech and Hearing Disorders, 30,* 225-233.

Katz, S., & Florian, V. (Eds.). (1991). *Returning the individual with traumatic brain injury to the community: An overview of programs and services in Israel.* New York: World Rehabilitation Fund; International Exchange of Information in Rehabilitation.

Kersting, F. (1974). The status of speech pathology and audiology in Korea: A report from the Dong San Medical Center in Taegu, Korea. *Asha, 16,* 423-425.

Landis, P. A. (1973). Training of a paraprofessional in speech pathology: A pilot project in South Vietnam. *Asha, 15,* 342–344.

Landis, P., Hwang, D., & Hsu, S. Y. (1980). Audiology and speech pathology in Taiwan. *Asha, 22,* 21–23.

Lesser, R. (1992). The making of logopedists: An international survey. *Folia Phoniatrica, 44,* 105-125.

Li-Rong, L. C. (1992). Recruitment: Asians and Pacific Islanders. *Asha, 34,* 41–42.

McCavitt, M. E. (1971). International activities of the social and rehabilitation service relating to the field of speech and hearing. *Asha, 13,* 388–390.

Mead, M. (1992). In C. Warner (Ed.), *The last word: A treasury of women's quotes.* Englewood Cliffs, NJ: Prentice-Hall.

Mencher, G. (1988). Speech and hearing disorders: A worldwide problem requiring a worldwide perspective. In S. E. Gerber & G. Mencher, (Eds.), *International perspectives on communication disorders* (pp. 3–10). Washington, DC: Gallaudet University Press.

Moll, K. (1983). Training programs in logopedics. *Folia Phoniatrica, 35,* 198–215.

Navas, D, & Pinho, S. (1993). Speech-language pathology and audiology practice in Brazil. *American Journal of Speech-Language Pathology, 2,* 5.

Northern, J. L., Downs, M. P., Hemenway, W. G., & Wood, R. P. (1972). A project for management of hearing impairment in South Vietnam. *Asha, 14,* 399–401.

Norton, M. (1981). Members aid hearing handicapped in Costa Rica. *Asha, 23,* 615.

O'Neill, J. J., Deal, L. V., & Kapur, Y. P. (1977). Speech pathology and audiology in India: 1975. *Asha, 19,* 420–422.

Peuser, G. (1984). *Language rehabilitation after stroke: A linguistic model.* [Monograph 24], New York: World Rehabilitation Fund; International Exchange of Information in Rehabilitation.

Philips, B. J. (1990). Our international responsibility. *Asha, 32,* 51.

Pleasonton, A. (1993, January). Volunteer opportunities in communication disorders at the international level. *ASHA in the World,* Newsletter of the International Affairs Association.

Pressman, D. E., & Rudner, M. (1990). International service delivery. *Asha, 32,* 48–49.

Ries, J. E. (1990). A view of the profession in South Korea. *Asha, 32,* 35–37.

Ritter, E. G. (1993). The International Affairs Association. *American Journal of Speech-Language Pathology, 2,* 10.

Sarno, M., & Woods, D. E. (Eds.). (1989). *Aphasia rehabilitation in Asia and the Pacific Region: Japan, China, India, Australia, New Zealand.* [Monograph 45], New York: World Rehabilitation Fund; International Exchange of Information in Rehabilitation.

Sklar, M. (1973). Audiology and speech pathology in Ceylon. *Asha, 15,* 421–423.

Sparks, S. N. (1979). Speech pathology and audiology in Brazil, 1978. *Asha, 21,* 280–282.

Spriestersbach, D. C. (1991). We are part of the planet, you know! *Asha, 33,* 34–35.

Stewart, J. L. (1970). Speech pathology in India. *Asha, 12,* 15–17.

Stewart, J. L. & Triolo, D. J. (1990). Development of speech-language-hearing services in Guam and Micronesia. *Asha, 32,* 37–39.

Wallace, G. (1992). *Traumatic brain injury (Ma'i Ulu) in Amerika Samoa: Rehabilitation needs and services.* New York: World Rehabilitation Fund; International Exchange of Information in Rehabilitation.

Walsh, P. (1989). *Recovery from aphasia: Long-term management in New Zealand, Aphasia Rehabilitation in Australia.* New York: World Rehabilitation Fund; International Exchange of Information in Rehabilitation.

Werner, M. S. (1981). Friends of Nepal's hearing handicapped: An outreach by the private sector. *Asha, 23,* 210–215.

Williams, J. D. (1971). Speech and language in the Philippines. *Asha, 13,* 271–274.

Wilson, M. E. (1990). So many worlds. *Asha, 32,* 32–33.

Yairi, E. (1990). Soviet symposium on speech pathology. *Asha, 32,* 43.

RESOURCES

PUBLISHERS

Hearing International: Quarterly newsletter. Dept. of Otolaryngology, Teikyo University School of Medicine, Kaga 2-11-1, Itabashi-ku, Tokyo, 173 Japan.

Intercultural Press, P.O. Box 768, Yarmouth, ME, 04096. Catalog of publications.

International Educator: International Educator's Institute, P.O. Box 103, West Bridgewater, MA 02379. Magazine.

International Exchange of Experts and Information in Rehabilitation (IEEIR): University of New Hampshire, 6 Hood House, Durham, NH 03824. Publishes a newsletter and research reports.

Transitions Abroad: Box 344, Amherst, MA 01004. Magazine.

ORGANIZATIONS

American Speech-Language-Hearing Association (ASHA): 10801 Rockville Pike, Rockville, MD 20852. The Membership Directory has international member and affiliate listings. Call Actionline (800) 638-6868 for current information on international issues.

Council for International Exchange of Scholars (Fulbright Scholar Awards): 3007 Tilden St., N.W., Suite 5M, Box NEWS, Washington, DC 20008-3009. Phone: (202) 686-7877.

International Affairs Committee: No permanent address; consult ASHA for name and address of current President. Publishes quarterly newsletters and Membership Directory.

International Association of Logopedics and Phoniatrics (IALP): No permanent address; consult ASHA for name and address of current President. Publishes *Folia Phoniatrica*, a membership directory, including a directory of affiliated societies, and a newsletter. Conferences held every 3 years: 1995, Cairo, Egypt; 1998, Amsterdam, Holland.

International Exchange of Experts and Information in Rehabilitation (IEEIR): University of New Hampshire, 6 Hood House, Durham, NH 03824. World Rehabilitation Fund Project applications.

International Society of Audiology: The International Society of Audiology meets every 2 years, convening itself as the International Congress of Audi-

ology. No permanant address; consult ASHA for current information.

Overseas Association of Communication Sciences (OSACS): No permanent address; consult ASHA for name and address of current president.

ORGANIZATIONS WHICH MIGHT HAVE A NEED FOR SLPs AND/OR AUDIOLOGISTS:

American Federation of Teachers: 555 New Jersey Ave., NW, Washington, D.C. 20001.

International Foundation for Education and Self-Help: 5040 East Shea Blvd., Suite 260, Phoenix, AZ 85254-4610. Beginning in Fall, 1992, they plan to place 1,000 American educators in African schools, colleges, universities and governmental agencies. Will have openings in the area of health.

International Health Exchange (formerly Bureau for Overseas Medical Services): Africa Centre, 38 King St., London WC2E 8JT, England. Facilitate the provision of health workers to developing countries, through a Register of Health and Management Professionals, and the bimonthly magazine "The Health Exchange." Needs speech therapists {sic} and audiologists.

Project Concern: 3550 Afton Rd., P.O. Box 885323, San Diego, CA 92123. Health care placement service of Project Concern International. Publishes a bimonthly newsletter with openings presently offered by the programs they represent.

Project Hope Health Sciences Education Center: Carter Hall, Millwood, VA 22646. Offers multidisciplinary assistance in health care education at home and abroad. Speech therapy {sic} and audiology are listed.

Asha, May 1990, a list of other service programs, funding sources, exchange programs and educational study-travel programs (Fain, 1990), as well as general resources (Wilson, 1990).

■ CHAPTER 8 ■

Incidence and Prevalence of Communication Disorders

■ CYNTHIA M. SHEWAN, Ph.D. ■

SCOPE OF CHAPTER

To indicate the magnitude of a problem or issue, people often quote statistics. When referring to diseases, disorders, impairments, and so on, these statistics are often referred to as incidence or prevalence statistics. Incidence and prevalence data tell us how many people have a current condition or how many new cases of the condition are expected in a given time period, usually a year.

The first part of this chapter discusses some general issues related to the definition and measurement of incidence and prevalence. Because knowledge of the relevant terminology is crucial to an accurate understanding of incidence and prevalence, the chapter opens with a series of definitions. Data cited from different sources often vary and the reasons for this variability are discussed. The credibility of incidence and prevalence data, also an important issue, is addressed next. The second portion of the chapter addresses the prevalence of hearing, speech, and language impairments, along with data collection issues. Finally, for those of you who wish to explore the area in greater depth, a series of resources for historical and current data are provided.

DEFINITIONS

Incidence rate is the number of new cases of an illness, condition, or disorder that occur in a population in a given period of time, usually 1 year. For example, the incidence rate of stroke in Western countries is estimated at 150/100,000 population/year (McDowell & Caplan, 1985). This means that for 1993, we can expect 384,699 new strokes, based on an estimated U.S. population of 256,466,000 (U.S. Bureau of the Census, 1991).

Prevalence rate is the existing number of cases of an illness, condition, or disorder in a specified time period, often 1 year. For example, the prevalence rate for hearing impairment in 1989 was 83.1/1,000 population (Adams & Benson, 1990).

Prevalence refers to the total number of cases of an illness, condition, or disease present. For example, the total number of individuals with hearing impairment in the United States in 1989 was 20,246,000 (Adams & Benson, 1990).

It is extremely important to distinguish the difference between incidence and prevalence as pointed out by Moscicki (1984). A simple example described by Shewan, Wisniewski, and Hyman (1987) is repeated here to illustrate the point:

Consider, if you will, a country with 5,000 citizens. Within this population two eye colors exist: blue and brown. In 1985 there were 500 people in this country with blue eyes; therefore, the prevalence of blue eyes was 500. The prevalence rate of blue eyes was 10.0% (500/5,000). In 1986, 100 babies were born: 25 with blue eyes and 75 with brown. The **incidence rate** for blue eyes is 25% (25/100). With these additional citizens, the new population of the country is 5,100: 525 blue-eyed and 4,575 brown-eyed. This causes the **prevalence** and **prevalence rate** to increase. The **prevalence** of blue eyes becomes 525, and the **prevalence rate** increases to 10.3% (525/5,100). In this example, reversing the terms **prevalence rate** and **incidence rate** would result in a prevalence rate (25%) more than twice what it should be (10.3%) and an incidence rate (10.3%) less than half of what it should be (25%). (p. 51)

IMPORTANCE OF INCIDENCE AND PREVALENCE STATISTICS

You might wonder why these statistics are important and how they may affect you as a communication disorders professional. Aside from the pain and suffering that people experience as a result of many diseases and disorders, the cost associated with their treatment is tremendous. For disorders that are preventable, adopting health care practices that would prevent these disorders would solve problems of human suffering, loss of life, and cost. Although the United States might be considered to be an industrialized nation with a good standard of health, there are always ways in which the health of Americans could be improved. For example, it was estimated that smoking-related illnesses cost $65 billion annually and that the cost of treating patients with AIDS would be as high as $13 billion by 1992 (*Healthy People 2000*, 1990).

A consortium of almost 300 organizations, state health departments, federal departments and agencies, the National Institute of Medicine in partnership with the U.S. Public Health Service developed a document *Healthy People 2000* (1990) aimed at setting goals to improve the nation's health by promoting health and preventing disease. Achieving these goals will improve the health status of the nation as well as reduce the escalating costs of health care, and focus health care dollars on diseases for which prevention is not yet a possibility, but for which cures or effective treatments can be provided.

The number of people with conditions that require medical services and the nature of those medical services relate, at least to some extent, to the services that are provided. The greater number of people suffering from a condition, the greater the number who will require services and the greater the number of services that are likely to exist. These relationships are not perfect because need for service does not always go hand in hand with the demand or availability of services. This scenario can be applied to the discipline of human communication sciences and disorders. Knowledge of the population of a community and the number of persons likely to sustain a stroke each year and the number of stroke survivors can provide useful information for a hospital looking at establishing an outpatient stroke rehabilitation service. Likewise, a school system can estimate how many speech-language pathologists likely will be needed based on school enrollment and the number of school children who are estimated to have communication disorders.

For those with an entrepreneurial streak, knowledge of prevalence and incidence data will assist in making the decision of whether a community can support a new private practice in communication disorders and also the likely case mix that can be expected, which, in turn, would influence the types of personnel needed to staff the practice.

Grant applications for monies to train qualified personnel to serve individuals with communication disorders and to conduct research in particular disorder areas also require statements to justify granting the money for these projects. Data related to incidence and prevalence can be used to advantage here.

Specifying the prevalence rate or number may sound like a simple task, one of merely counting those with the condition in the case of prevalence number and computing a percentage in the case of prevalence rate. Unfortunately, the matter is not so simple and prevalence data vary widely. Several factors contribute to this variability.

VARIATIONS IN PREVALENCE REPORTING

Different Data Collection Methods

Reported prevalence figures can be influenced by whether the data are gathered from questionnaires or interviews in which persons are asked if they have a certain condition (self-report) or whether persons are actually tested for the condition (test results). Added to this dilemma is that the two methods do not always affect the estimate in the same way. For example, Anderson, Schoenberg, and Haerer (1988) show that the self-report method tended to underestimate the prevalence of Parkinson's disease, but to overestimate the prevalence of stroke when compared with prevalence data obtained from physical examinations.

Different Sampling Populations

The data collected from individuals may differ in the age spans and distributions included in the sample, the socioeconomic strata included, racial/ethnic composition, and if all or only some segments of the population are included. For example, prevalence figures for communi-

cation disorders in the school population will differ from those of the entire population, because prevalence of communication disorders is not constant across lifespans. Another example pertains to stroke. Because hypertension is the most common risk factor for stroke and is more prevalent in the Black population, the prevalence of stroke will differ in White and Black population samples.

Different Definitions of What Is Included in a Disorder Category

People may have different boundaries for what is included in a disorder category. For example, individuals in the communication disorders discipline often refer to the prevalence of communication disorders as 38 million Americans (Adams & Benson, 1992; National Advisory Neurological and Communicative Disorders and Stroke Council, 1989). However, the National Institute on Deafness and Other Communication Disorders (NIDCD) (1992) uses a figure of 44 million. The discrepancy can be explained on the basis that the NIDCD definition includes disorders of taste, touch, and smell, categories that communication disorders professionals exclude from their definition.

Different Criteria for Defining a Disorder or Impairment

Although the use of criteria to define the presence of a disorder is not arbitrary, different criteria or different levels of the same criteria may be used to define the presence of a disorder. Depending on whether the criteria are stringent or lax, the prevalence rate will vary correspondingly. Goldstein (1984) described the variability in the prevalence rate for hearing impairment as a function of the criteria used to define the presence of an impairment (ear, audiometric test stimuli, and test conditions).

Different Test Conditions

Who does the testing and the tests that are used can influence the outcome prevalence data reported. In a survey study, results can vary, based on whether the informant is the person being interviewed or some other party. A self-informant may choose not to reveal the presence of an impairment because of the social stigma in doing so, even if the problem is known to exist. When another party is the informant, how well they know the person may be a factor in whether they accurately report the presence of a condition. Which questions are asked and the format of questions may also influence how people respond to queries. In 1990, the National Health Interview Survey (U.S. Department of Commerce, 1990) changed the questions used to determine presence of hearing impairment. Although one cannot assume cause and effect, the prevalence rate for hearing impairment increased to 9.1% from 8.3% the previous year. When tests are administered, whether the conditions meet "standardized" conditions may influence the results.

FACTORS THAT INFLUENCE DATA RELIABILITY

Several factors that influence the confidence that can be placed in figures quoted are described. Awareness of these issues will help you to make an assessment of the degree to which you can feel comfortable with given data.

Low Prevalence of a Disorder

Because of the low prevalence of certain disorders, the error rate associated with the data can be high and, therefore, reduce reliability.

Timeliness of Data

Because incidence and prevalence data are expensive to collect, the data are often outdated and do not reflect the current population. The most accurate data, as we have seen, come from actual test results or physical examinations. To conduct a widescale investigation sufficient to include a representative sample is a major undertaking, costing millions of dollars. Identifying the presence of a language disorder cannot be done in a minute or two. Therefore, for many communication disorders the identification process is labor-intensive and expensive. For example, the National Health and Nutrition Examination Survey (NHANES) II survey, 1976-1980, collected speech and language sample test data to determine the prevalence rate of speech and language disorders in the child population from ages 4 to 6 years. Due to funding constraints, the data are yet to be analyzed. Even if the data were analyzed tomorrow, the information would be 15 years old and, therefore, suspect as an accurate estimate of the current situation.

Counting Method

When prevalence data are reported for each condition, you can be confident that duplicate counts have not been included. But when the prevalence of an aggregate of disorders is discussed, you must be very careful to avoid duplicate counts. Many conditions co-occur, such as hearing impairment and speech and voice disorders. If you were counting the number of people with a communication disorder, you would not want to count an individual with a hearing impairment with concomitant speech and voice problems three times, once each for hearing, speech, and voice problems. You would want to avoid duplicate counts by counting that individual only once.

The National Health Interview Survey does provide nonduplicated prevalence counts for several categories of multiple impairments, such as hearing and visual impairments only, and visual, hearing, and orthopedic impairments, with or without any other impairment.

Intended Use of Data

Another factor that can influence prevalence data is the purpose for which the data are to be used. For example, different criteria might be used to identify a hearing difficulty, depending on whether the purpose of the test is for screening or for complete diagnosis. Different figures for the prevalence of language impairment would be appropriate to use in determining whether to open an adult rehabilitation center versus determining whether to open a preschool language enrichment program.

FACTORS AFFECTING CHANGING PREVALENCE OF DISORDERS

It is no secret that the U.S. population is aging more rapidly than it is growing. Because aging is associated with an increased prevalence of chronic conditions and because some communication disorders are classified as chronic conditions, we can expect the prevalence of many communication disorders to increase as the aging of the population continues. For example, the prevalence of hearing impairment for those under 18 years is 1.61%; however, this rises to 40.36% for those 75 years and over (Adams & Benson, 1992). Dementias occur primarily in the older segments of the population, with Alzheimer's disease being a well-recognized example. In 1989, of the approximately 3.5 million persons with Alzheimer's disease, some 183,000 were in the 40- to 44-year age range, contrasted with the 2.2 million in the 75 years and over age range (Shewan, 1989). (Dementia is not measured in the population under the age of 40 years.)

The racial and ethnic composition of the U.S. population is also rapidly changing. Populations termed as minorities are growing more rapidly than the White (Caucasian) population. This is of importance in the communication disorders arena, because certain diseases and conditions do not occur with equal frequency in Caucasian and various minority groups. According to the 1991 National Health Interview Survey, the prevalence rate for cerebrovascular disease is higher in the Black population than in the White population across all age groups, with the exception of the group under 45 years (Adams & Benson, 1992). Many differences in prevalence rates among minority groups have been cited related to deafness and hearing loss (*Research and Research Training Needs of Minority Persons and Minority Health Issues,*

1992). Some of these differences, especially the higher prevalence rates, may be related to the poor health status of many minority American groups, which, in turn, may be related to their limited access and/or utilization of health care services. Miyamoto (cited in *Research and Research Training Needs of Minority Persons and Minority Health Issues,* 1992) states that the health status of minority groups, especially African-Americans, is generally poor and that deafness in culturally diverse populations generally mirrors their health status. In addition, many of the risk factors for hearing loss, including congenital infections, low birth weight, and low Apgar scores, are seen more frequently in minority populations in Americas.

Technology in neonatal care has advanced dramatically in the last decade. The introduction of neonatal intensive care units has enabled the survival of many babies who previously would have died. Of course, these infants often have very low birth weights, which puts them at risk for many problems, including communication disorders.

Exposure to toxic substances, substance abuse, and infectious diseases are accounting for increasing numbers of children born at risk for communication disorders. Exposure to toxic substances, such as lead, especially affect the infant and toddler population. Lead exposure is associated with mental retardation and, thereby, with communication disorders. These problems appear to concentrate in the lower socioeconomic strata of the population and arise because of the high lead content of paint and lead solder used in older construction.

Alcohol is the most frequently used and abused substance in American society today (Burke, 1988). In the adult population, alcohol abuse is associated with several disorders, including cerebral dysfunction, which can involve communication disorders. Of great significance is the prevalence of fetal alcohol syndrome (FAS), which is one of the leading known causes of mental retardation in the western world. In addition to mental retardation, FAS is associated with auditory disorders and learning disabilities. Although not all problems are long lasting, the effects of FAS can persist into adulthood. Prevalence rates vary and are especially high in the African-American and American Indian groups (National Institute on Alcohol Abuse and Alcoholism, 1990).

Infectious diseases in the mother may be passed on to the fetus. Although originally thought to be a disease occurring primarily in men, AIDS has become a disease of rising prevalence among women and over 19,000 cases of AIDS in women have been reported to the Centers for Disease Control and Prevention (Report of the National Institutes of Health: *Opportunities for Research on Women's Health*, 1991). In fact, women are the group in which the incidence of AIDS is increasing most rapidly (*Research and Research Training Needs of Women and Women's Health Issues*, 1991). Mothers with HIV infection may infect their children before or during birth. Babies with HIV may show progressive neurologic disease secondary to the infection and therefore may evidence communication problems (American Speech-Language-Hearing Association, 1989).

Maternal cytomegalovirus infection (CMV) is linked with mental retardation and hearing loss. Fully 1% of all babies born in the United States are estimated to have contracted CMV; 10% will probably manifest mental retardation and hearing loss, with another 14% to develop a hearing loss, which may not become evident for many years postnatally (National Institute on Deafness and Other Communication Disorders, 1992).

PREVALENCE OF COMMUNICATION DISORDERS

PREVALENCE OF HEARING IMPAIRMENT

General Statistics

As mentioned earlier in this chapter, prevalence data for communication disorders, including hearing impairment, vary greatly across sources. How this specifically contributes to variability in hearing impairment data is described below.

DIFFERENT DATA COLLECTION METHODS. Some studies have used reports from interviews, such as the National Health Interview Survey (NHIS), with others, such as the National Health and Nutrition Examination Survey (NHANES), basing estimates on actual audiometric test data.

DIFFERENT SAMPLING POPULATIONS. To estimate the true prevalence of hearing impairment, all segments of the population should be included. For various reasons, this has not always been done. Feasibility of such a widescale study is certainly one reason and cost is another. Various studies have included different age ranges, socioeconomic strata, racial/ethnic groups, and population segments. For example, the NHIS includes only the civilian, noninstitutionalized population, although it covers the entire life span. Therefore, these estimates omit those in institutions and the military. The NHANES-II, 1976–80, limited audiometric testing to persons between the ages of 4 to 19 years. Because the prevalence of hearing impairment varies with age, these data cannot be generalized to the entire population.

DIFFERENT DEFINITIONS OF HEARING IMPAIRMENT. Goldstein (1984) described several criteria, discussed below, used to define a hearing impairment. If one or more of these criteria are not consistent across studies, the prevalence figures can vary. Prevalence statistics are directly affected by the criteria and the specific levels of those criteria used in the definition of hearing impairment. "Frequency" refers to the frequencies that are tested when gathering audiometric data for prevalence statistics. Including higher frequencies, such as 8000 Hz, will lead to higher prevalence rates than if the highest frequency tested is 2000 Hz. "Fence" refers to the level in dB above which a significant hearing loss is said to exist. "Ear" refers to whether measurement data from one or both ears are considered in the definition. "Audiometric test stimuli" refers to the type of stimuli used in testing, whether pure tones, speech, and so on. Testing conditions can also affect the data results. Whether a survey informant is providing self-information or about another party may also influence results. For example, a proud 69-year-old grandfather may not report the presence of a hearing loss, although his daughter as informant would report one. When audiometric studies are reviewed, test conditions may not be standard across investigations—another factor that can influence the prevalence data derived.

One of the most frequently cited data sets for the prevalence of hearing impairment comes from the annual National Health Interview Survey (NHIS). Data are self-reports based on a representative sample of approximately 100,000 households in the civilian, noninstitutionalized population in the United States. Although the estimates are probably underestimates because of the omission of the institutionalized population and the potential underreporting, these data are beneficial in their consistency across time and in their comprehensive coverage of the entire age range, geographic distribution, income level, racial composition, and so forth. The most recent NHIS data shown in Table 8–1 (Adams & Benson, 1992) indicate that 22.6 million Americans report a hearing impairment, a prevalence rate of 9.1%. Two important trends to note in hearing impairment prevalence data are the increasing prevalence across the life span and the increasing prevalence across the last two decades. The overall prevalence rate for hearing impairment was 6.9% in 1971 (Gentile, 1975), as contrasted with 9.15% in 1991 and 1992 (Adams & Benson, 1991, 1992).

Another source of data comes from the National Institute on Deafness and Other Communication Disorders (NIDCD) of the National Institutes of Health. At a 1990 NIH Consensus Development Conference on Noise and Hearing Loss, the consensus statement reported that approximately 28 million Americans suffered from some degree of hearing loss (NIH Consensus Development Conference, 1990).

With so many factors influencing prevalence data, it is useful to adopt Goldstein's strategy

TABLE 8–1. PREVALENCE NUMBER AND RATE OF HEARING IMPAIRMENT PER 100 PERSONS IN THE CIVILIAN, NONINSTITUTIONALIZED POPULATION OF THE UNITED STATES.

Age Group (in Years)	Number (in Millions)	Prevalence Rate (in %)
Under 18	1.1	1.6
18–44	5.3	5.0
45–64	6.7	14.1
65–74	4.9	26.6
75 and over	4.8	40.4
All Ages	22.6[1]	9.1

[1]Numbers may not sum due to rounding.

(1984) of providing low, medium, and high estimates. Based on the audiometric data reported by Singer, Tomberlin, Smith, and Schrier in 1982, Goldstein used 7.6% as a low estimate of the prevalence of hearing impairment. Applying this to the 1993 population of the United States (256,466,000), an estimated 19.4 million people are hearing impaired. His middle estimate of 13.5% results in 34.5 million persons with hearing impairment in the United States. The high estimate of 17.4% reveals an estimated prevalence of 44.5 million Americans with hearing impairment.

Prevalence of Hearing Impairment in the Elderly

Of particular importance in the area of hearing impairment is the elderly segment of the population. Hearing impairment is the most prevalent in this group, with estimates of 26.6% in the 65- to 74-year-old age group and 40.4% for those 75 years and over (Adams & Benson, 1992). Also, the elderly group in the population is growing. In 1986, 12.1% of the population was 65 and older, with this percentage predicted to reach almost 22% by 2040. In addition, people are living longer and the "oldest old," those 85 and older, represent the fastest growing segment of the population, both by numbers and percentage. They are predicted to represent 3.7% of the population by 2040 (Brock, Guralnik, & Brody, 1990).

In general, the effects of age on hearing begin to be seen in men in their forties and in women in their fifties. Combining this information, the future holds a larger population who will have hearing impairment and experience its effects for a longer portion of their lives, unless advances are made that will postpone or prevent the onset of hearing loss.

Tinnitus—that is, hearing a ringing, buzzing, or clicking noise in the absence of a stimulus—is a problem also included among chronic health conditions. Tinnitus may occur alone or in conjunction with a hearing impairment. It is reported among 8.2% of those 65 years and older, with the peak prevalence rate (9.5%) in the 65- to 74-year-old age group (Adams & Benson, 1992).

Therefore, in the future, as a practicing audiologist you can expect to see a larger clientele who are elderly and who present with hearing complaints, hearing loss or tinnitus. With the elderly living longer, follow-up with these individuals will also be necessary over a longer period of time. It is crucial that you obtain experience with this population during your graduate academic and clinical training to provide the best quality of service.

Although most individuals 65 years and older live independently in the community, in 1985 approximately 4.6% were living in institutions, primarily nursing homes. This percentage grows with increasing age and grows faster for women than for men. Given the trends described in the above paragraphs, you can expect to find greater numbers of nursing home residents in the future and, according to Diggs (1980), 36% of the residents will have a hearing impairment. Diggs' data may be optimistic. A more recent study screening nursing home admissions revealed the functional hearing status of 22% as definitely hearing impaired and an additional 54% at risk for hearing problems in certain conditions, such as in a noisy background. Sixty percent of the nursing home residents complained of hearing difficulty in daily living situations (Voeks, Gallagher, Langer, & Drinka, 1990).

The clinician of the future needs to be prepared not only to deal with the elderly who present with hearing impairment and/or tinnitus, but also to deal with these individuals in an institutional setting. This will also involve providing appropriate in-service training to staff.

PREVALENCE OF COMMUNICATION DISORDERS

PREVALENCE OF SPEECH AND LANGUAGE IMPAIRMENTS

General Statistics

Similar to the situation for hearing impairment, the data for speech and language impairments are similarly very variable and many of the same factors contribute to this variability.

DIFFERENT DATA COLLECTION METHODS. Data are gathered either by a survey method or from actual testing. Results from these methods can result in different prevalence rates as demonstrated by Anderson, Schoenberg, and Haerer (1988) in their comparison of the prevalence rates of stroke and Parkinson's disease. For Parkinson's disease, self-report resulted in underestimating the prevalence, with the opposite true for stroke. Therefore, methodology is a significant factor to consider when reading the epidemiological literature. For the NHIS survey, the presence of speech and/or language impairments is not pursued if certain other chronic conditions are present. For example, if a stroke is reported, the interviewer proceeds to ask what sequelae followed the stroke, including the presence of speech impairment. However, this does not hold true if Parkinson's disease is the primary condition reported. Therefore, the prevalence number for speech impairment, which is directly influenced by this data collection method, is an underestimate because of omissions such as this.

DIFFERENT SAMPLING POPULATIONS. Studies over the years have covered different populations. Some of this variability occurs naturally because the condition may affect only a certain segment of the population. For example, dementia is not investigated in the population under the age of 40 years because it does not occur in young age groups. Some studies have limited themselves to particular age groups, such as the kindergarten or school populations (Beitchman, Clegg, Nair, & Patel, 1986; Roberts & Baird, 1972).

Because the prevalence of many disorders, for example, stuttering, childhood language disorders, and multiple sclerosis, differs between males and females, it is important to have the data broken out by gender. The NHIS provides aggregate data as well as data by gender, geographic region, racial composition, and socioeconomic strata (income levels). However, it covers only the civilian, noninstitutionalized U.S. population.

For future studies, it is important to gather detailed data for different racial/ethnic groups. With the increasing diversity in the U.S. population, it will be important to know if diseases or conditions are present to greater or lesser degrees in certain racial groups and what the respective distributions are.

DIFFERENT DEFINITIONS OF SPEECH AND/OR LANGUAGE IMPAIRMENT. The criteria used to define the presence of a speech or language disorder differ across studies. One major issue is whether an estimate differentiates speech from language disorders. For example, the NHIS uses the term "speech impairment" to represent a chronic condition that includes both speech and language components. Speech impairment includes various speech disorders, such as articulation problems and stuttering, but excludes the speech problems of cleft palate. It is not known if voice disorders would be included. Some language disorders are subsumed under the speech impairment category, but not all. Excluded are mental retardation, dementia, traumatic brain injury, and so forth. As mentioned previously, the advantages of the NHIS data are consistency across time and comprehensiveness; however, these advantages are counterbalanced by major problems in the scope covered by the term and in the lack of differentiation between speech and language impairments. The most recent data available from NHIS are presented in Table 8–2 (Adams & Benson, 1992).

TABLE 8–2. PREVALENCE NUMBER AND RATE OF SPEECH IMPAIRMENT PER 100 PERSONS IN THE CIVILIAN, NONINSTITUTIONALIZED, POPULATION OF THE UNITED STATES.

Age Group (in Years)	Number (in Millions)	Prevalence Rate (in %)
Under 18	1.1	1.7
18–44	0.9	0.9
45–64	0.5	1.0
65–74	0.1	0.6
75 and over	0.2	1.7
All Ages	2.8	1.1

It is important to note that the overall prevalence of speech impairment is reported as 1.1%, representing 2.8 million Americans. For reasons described above, this number is considered to be an underestimate, which limits the usefulness of the data. However, because of the consistency and comprehensive national coverage, the data can be used to determine trends across time.

A clear differentiation between the separate presence and coexistence of speech and language disorders was made by Beitchman et al. (1986) in their study of the prevalence of speech and language disorders in 5-year-old kindergarten children. The speech/language distinction is important to make, because, as pointed out in this study, speech and language disorders do not always coexist; the conditions can and do occur separately. In the 1991 Annual Report of the National Deafness and Other Communication Disorders Advisory Board (1992), the estimated prevalence of voice, speech, and language impairments was 14 million Americans.

In self-informant studies, informants may employ different internal definitions of what constitutes an impairment. Some people may not consider a lateral lisp as an articulation disorder and therefore would not report it. These different reporting yardsticks will have an effect on the overall data collected.

With multiple factors influencing the statistics, it is useful to develop a strategy of presenting low, medium, and high prevalence estimates. The NHIS data can be used as a low estimate, with a prevalence of 1.1%. If adjusted to include the institutionalized population, this estimate becomes 2.2% (Shewan & Malm, 1990). A middle estimate was derived by Fein (1983) also by adjusting the NHIS data. Fein estimated that the prevalence of speech and language impairments was 3.8 times higher than reported by NHIS. Therefore, his middle estimate prevalence rate was 4.18%, or 10.7 million Americans. Because of the omission of some disorders in the count, Shewan (1988) adjusted the prevalence data reported by the National Advisory Neurological and Communicative Disorders and Stroke Council (1989) to 6.255 to provide a high prevalence estimate.

DIFFERENT TEST CONDITIONS. Whether the prevalence data represent the results of a self-report survey or actual speech-language testing influences the prevalence rate obtained. As seen earlier, people tend to overreport some diseases (stroke) and to underreport others (Parkinson's). This can be the result of lack of knowledge on what constitutes a disorder or intentional bias in reporting or nonreporting. Prevalence figures from actual testing data are available for some speech and language disorders, but no current national data are available for all disorders combined.

Estimating the prevalence of speech and language impairments can be approached in several ways. You can examine the prevalence of different types of disorders, such as articulation disorders, which may cut across several illness, disease, injury, and chronic condition categories. Articulation disorders may be found in patients with HIV and Parkinson's disease and subsequent to traumatic brain injury or stroke, and so forth.

Another approach is to list the prevalence of a disorder for the individual diseases with which it is associated and add the numbers to arrive at an estimate of the total prevalence number. Of course, the challenge is to include all diseases in the count and not to duplicate the counts. Because of the difficulty with and the potential unreliability of this approach, this chapter is limited to presenting broad categories only.

The National Advisory Neurological and Communicative Disorders Stroke Council (NANCDSC) (1989) reported a prevalence number of 8.4 million for speech disorders. Speech disorders in this count would include articulation, fluency, and voice disorders. Hull and Timmons (1971) provided estimates for these subcategories (Table 8–3) in the school-age population 6 to 18 years.

TABLE 8–3. PERCENTAGE PREVALENCE OF SPEECH DISORDERS FROM THE NATIONAL SPEECH AND HEARING SURVEY 1968–1969.

Type of Disorder	Percentage Prevalence
Articulation	1.9
Voice	3.0
Fluency	0.8
Total	5.7

Language disorders have been estimated to be present in 6 to 8 million Americans (National Institute on Deafness and Other Communication Disorders, 1989). Prevalence is higher among preschoolers who are in the process of learning language, drops in the school-age and adult periods, and resumes a higher rate in the elderly population who experience various neurological conditions. Based on a speech and language assessment, language problems were determined to be present in 8.0% of 5-year-old kindergarten children (Beitchman et al., 1986). Aphasia, an impairment or loss of language, caused primarily by stroke, affects an estimated 1 million Americans (Schoenberg, Anderson, &

Haerer, 1986; U.S. Department of Health, Education and Welfare, 1979), primarily those 55 years and above.

SUMMARY

This chapter has discussed many issues surrounding the topic of incidence and prevalence of communication disorders. Although, at first glance, counting persons with communication disorders appears to be an easy task, the material presented demonstrates the difficulties in doing so and the consequences therefrom. Outdated information is a particularly thorny problem, especially in view of changes in the prevalence of disorders.

Discussion of several factors that influence prevalence data provided a background for appreciating the variability among prevalence figures and for the importance of reading prevalence data carefully. Low, medium, and high prevalence estimates were provided for the broad categories of hearing and speech and language impairments. Although some statistics for specific disorders were also provided, the impossibility of providing comprehensive data is managed by including appendixes listing more extensive bibliographic sources. (See Appendix 8A and Appendix 8B.)

DISCUSSION QUESTIONS

1. How would you answer a complaint from a caller who reports having been given erroneous information because of having been given two different figures for the number of hearing impaired persons in the United States?
2. What would you tell nursing home administrators about the numbers of speech, language, and hearing disorders they could expect among their residents?
3. A preschool manager is planning to hire a speech-language pathologist and uses the prevalence rate of 15 to estimate how many children are likely to require speech

and language services. What advice would you give this manager?
4. What implication does the wide variability in incidence/prevalence data have for the delivery of speech, language, and hearing services?
5. What could be the consequences to a research study on the treatment of speech and language disorders of using prevalence data from the early 1980s?

REFERENCES

Adams, P. F., & Benson, V. (1990). *Current estimates from the National Health Interview Survey, 1989.* Vital and Health Statistics, Series 10 (176). National Center for Health Statistics. Public Health Service. Washington, DC: U.S. Government Printing Office.

Adams, P. F., & Benson, V. (1991). *Current estimates from the National Health Interview Survey, 1990.* Vital and Health Statistics, Series 10 (181). National Center for Health Statistics. Public Health Service. Washington, DC: U.S. Government Printing Office.

Adams, P. F., & Benson, V. (1992). *Current estimates from the National Health Interview Survey, 1991.* Vital Health Stat. 10 (184). National Center for Health Statistics. Public Health Service. Washington, DC: U.S. Government Printing Office.

American Speech-Language-Hearing Association. (1989). AIDS/HIV: Implications for speech-language pathologists and audiologists. *Asha, 31,* 33–38.

Anderson, D. W., Schoenberg, B. S., & Haerer, A. F. (1988). Prevalence surveys of neurologic disorders: Methodologic implications of the Copiah County study. *Journal of Clinical Epidemiology, 41,* 339–345.

Beitchman, J. H., Clegg, M., Nair, R., & Patel, P. G. (1986). Prevalence of speech and language disorders in 5-year-old kindergarten children in the Ottawa-Carleton region. *Journal of Speech and Hearing Disorders, 51,* 96–110.

Brock, D. B., Guralnik, J. M., & Brody, J. A. (1990). Demography and epidemiology of aging in the United States. In E. L. Schneider & J. W. Rowe (Eds.). *Handbook of the biology of aging* (3rd ed.). San Diego: Academic Press.

Burke, T. R. (1988). The economic impact of alcohol abuse and alcoholism. *Public Health Reports, 103,* 564–568.

Diggs, C. C. (1980). ASHA recognizes needs of older persons. *Asha, 22,* 401–403.

Fein, D. J. (1983). The prevalence of speech and language impairments. *Asha, 25,* 37.

Gentile, A. (1975). *Persons with impaired hearing, United States, 1971.* Series 10, Number 101, DHEW Publication No. 76-1528. U.S. Department of Health, Education and Welfare.

Goldstein, D. P. (1984). Hearing impairment, hearing aids, and audiology. *Asha, 26,* 25–35.

Healthy People 2000. Conference Edition. (September, 1990). U.S. Department of Health and Human Services. Public Health Service.

Hull, F. M., & Timmons, R. J. (1971). The National Speech and Hearing Survey: Preliminary results. *Asha, 13,* 501–509.

McDowell, F. H., & Capian, L. R. (Eds.). (1985). *Cerebrovascular survey report.* National Institute of Neurological and Communicative Disorders and Stroke, National Institutes of Health, Public Health Service.

Moscicki, E. K. (1984). The prevalence of 'incidence' is too high. *Asha, 26,* 39–40.

National Advisory Neurological and Communicative Disorders and Stroke Council. (1989). *Decade of the brain.* (NIH Publication No. 8802957). U.S. Department of Health and Human Services, Public Health Service, National Institutes of Health.

National Deafness and Other Communication Disorders Advisory Board. (1992). *1991 annual report.* (NIH Publication No. 92-3317). U.S. Department of Health and Human Services, Public Health Service, National Institutes of Health.

National Institute on Alcohol Abuse and Alcoholism (GNAW); Alcohol, Drug Abuse, and Mental Health Administration. (1990, January). *Seventh annual report to the U.S. Congress on alcohol and health.* From the Secretary of Health and Human Services. Public Health Service, U.S. Department of Health and Human Services.

National Institute on Deafness and Other Communication Disorders. (1989, April). *A report of the Task Force on the National Strategic Research Plan.* U.S. Department of Health and Human Services, Public Health Service, National Institutes of Health.

National Institute on Deafness and Other Communication Disorders. (1992). *National strategic research plan for hearing and hearing impairment.* U.S. Department of Health and Human Services, Public Health Service, National Institutes of Health.

National Institutes of Health Consensus Development Conference. (1990, January 22–24). *Noise and Hearing Loss. Consensus Statement.* Volume 8, Number 1.

Report of the National Institutes of Health: *Opportunities for research on women's health.* (1991, September). Office of Research on Women's Health, Office of the Director, National Institutes of Health, Hunt Valley, MD.

Research and research training needs of minority persons and minority health issues. (April 22, 1992). Working group minutes, National Institute on Deafness and Other Communication Disorders.

Research and Research Training Needs of Women and Women's Health Issues (1991, October 3), Report from the Working Group, National Institute on Deafness and Other Communication Disorders.

Roberts, J., & Baird, J. T. (1972). Behavior patterns of children in school: United States. *Vital and Health Statistics.* Series 11, No. 113.

Schoenberg, B. S., Anderson, D., & Haerer, A. F. (1986). Racial differentials in the prevalence of stroke, Copiah County, Mississippi. *Archives of Neurology, 43,* 565–569.

Shewan, C. M. (1988). *ASHA work force study.* Final Report. Rockville, MD: American Speech-Language-Hearing Association.

Shewan, C. M. (1989). Demographic data for cognitive impairments. Unpublished data.

Shewan, C. M., & Malm, K. E. (1990, December). The prevalence of speech and language impairments. *Asha, 32,* 108.

Shewan, C. M., Wisniewski, A. T., & Hyman, C. S. (1987). Disentangling incidence and prevalence. *Asha, 29,* 51.

Singer, J., Tomberlin, T. J., Smith, J. M., & Schrier, A. J. (1982). *Analysis of noise related auditory and associated health problems in U.S. adulthood 1971–75* (Vols. 1 and 2). [Prepared under contract to the Environmental Protection Agency]. Springfield, VA: National Technical Information Service.

U.S. Department of Commerce. (1990). *National health interview survey.* Form HIS-I. Bureau of the Census acting as collecting agent for the U.S. Public Health Service.

U.S. Bureau of the Census. (1991). *Statistical abstract of the United States: 1991* (111th ed.). Washington, DC: Author.

U.S. Department of Health, Education and Welfare. (1979). *Aphasia.* Washington, DC: Author.

Voeks, S. K., Gallagher, C. M., Langer, E. H., & Drinka, P. J. (1990). Hearing loss in the nursing home: An institutional issue. *Journal of the American Geriatrics Society, 38,* 141–145.

APPENDIX 8A: Historical and Current Resources for Incidence and Prevalence Information on Communication Disorders

To provide comprehensive and exhaustive data on the incidence and prevalence of communication disorders by disease, condition, illness, or disorder category is beyond the scope of this chapter. What seems appropriate is to provide a list of resources that can be used to locate the specific material of interest. Again, it is not possible to include every resource that mentions either incidence or prevalence. However, an attempt has been made to include the major resources. Where appropriate, notes have been included to guide the reader about the publication. In addition, the resources have been separated for the areas of speech, language, and hearing. Resources that cut across more than one area are repeated in each appropriate listing.

In 1981, the American Speech-Language-Hearing Association published a review of the literature on incidence and prevalence of communication disorders (Healey, Ackerman, Chappell, Perrin, & Stormer, 1981). This resource (see below) and its bibliography can serve as a foundation and historical view of incidence and prevalence data for communication disorders.

Healey, W. C., Ackerman, B. L., Chappell, C. R., Perrin, K. L., & Stormer, J. (1981). *The prevalence of communicative disorders: A review of the literature.* Rockville, MD: American Speech-Language-Hearing Association.

The following list of resources represents an update from the 1981 ASHA publication. It includes materials that were not included in and materials that have appeared since that publication. The reader should note that some of the resources cited here are also included in the reference section of this chapter. This resource list represents an update of material prepared by the ASHA Research Division in 1988.

HEARING IMPAIRMENT

Brown, S. C., Hotchkiss, D. R., Allen, T. E., Schein, J. D., & Adams, D. L. (1989). *Current and future needs of the hearing impaired elderly population.* GRI Monograph Series B, No. 1. Washington, DC: Gallaudet Research Institute, Gallaudet University.

Fein, D. J. (1983, March). Population data from the U.S. Census Bureau. *Asha, 25,* 47.

Fein, D. J. (1983, November). Projections of speech and hearing impairments to 2050. *Asha, 25,* 31.

Ficke, R. C. (1991). *Digest on persons with disabilities.* Washington, DC: National Institute on Disability and Rehabilitation Research.

Gallaudet Research Institute. (1985, Winter). Today's hearing impaired children and youth: A demographic and academic profile. [Special pull-out section]. *Newsletter.*

Goldstein, D. P. (1984). Hearing impairment, hearing aids and audiology. *Asha, 26,* 24–35.

Healey, W. C., Ackerman, B. L., Chappell, C. R., Perrin, K. L., & Stormer, J. (1981). *The prevalence of communicative disorders: A review of the literature.* Rockville, MD: American Speech-Language-Hearing Association.

Hotchkiss, D. R. (1989). *The hearing impaired population: Estimation, projection, and assessment.* GRI Monograph Series A, No. 1. Washington, DC: Gallaudet Research Institute, Gallaudet University.

Human Services Research Institute. (1985). *Summary of data on handicapped children and youth.* [Prepared under contract to the National Institute of Handicapped Research]. Washington, DC: U.S. Government Printing Office.

Human Services Research Institute. (1986). *Compilation of statistical sources on adult disability.* [Prepared under contract to the National Institute on Disability and Rehabilitation Research, U.S. Department of Education]. Washington, DC: U.S. Government Printing Office.

Hyman, C. S. (1985). PL 94-142 in review. *Asha 27,* 37.

Jensema, C., & Mullins, J. (1974). Onset, cause and additional handicaps in hearing impaired children. *American Annals of the Deaf, 119,* 701–705.

Karr, S., & Punch, J. (1984). PL 94-142 state child counts. *Asha, 26,* 33.

LaPlante, M. P. (1988). *Data on disability from the National Health Interview Survey. 1983–85.* An

InfoUse Report. Washington, DC: U.S. National Institute on Disability and Rehabilitation Research.

Leske, M. C. (1981). Prevalence estimates of communicative disorders in the U.S.: Language, hearing and vestibular disorders. *Asha, 23,* 229–237.

Mathematica Policy Research. (1984). *Digest of data on persons with disabilities.* [Prepared under contract to the Congressional Research Service, Library of Congress]. Washington, DC: U.S. Department of Education, National Institute of Handicapped Research.

Mathematica Policy Research. (1989). *Task 1: Population profile of disability.* (Prepared under contract for the U.S. Department of Health and Human Services, Assistant Secretary for Health and Human Services.). Washington, DC.

National Center for Health Statistics. (1979, July). *The National Nursing Home Survey: 1977 summary for the United States. Vital and Health Statistics.* (Series 13, No. 43. DHEW Publication No. PHS 79-1794). Washington, DC: U.S. Government Printing Office.

National Center for Health Statistics. (1980). *Basic data on hearing levels. 25–74 years. United States. 1971–1975. Vital and Health Statistics.* (Series 11, No. 215. DHEW Publication No. PHS 80-1663). Washington, DC: U.S. Government Printing Office.

National Center for Health Statistics. (1981, February). *Prevalence of selected impairments. United States. 1977. Vital and Health Statistics.* (Series 10, No. 134. DHHS Publication No. PHS 81-1562). Washington, DC: U.S. Government Printing Office.

National Center for Health Statistics. (1986). [Health interview survey data]. Unpublished data, NHIS, 1983–85.

National Center for Health Statistics. (1986, September). *Current estimates from the National Health Interview Survey. United States. 1985. Vital and Health Statistics.* (Series 10, No. 160. DHHS Publication No. PHS 86-1588). Washington, DC: U.S. Government Printing Office.

National Center for Health Statistics. (1986, September 19). *Aging in the eighties: Impaired senses for sound and light in persons age 65 years and over. Preliminary data from the Supplement on Aging to the National Health Interview Survey. United States. January-June 1984.* Advance data from *Vital and Health Statistics.* (No. 125. DHHS Publication No. PHS 8679-1250). Hyattsville, MD: Public Health Service.

Orlans, H. (Ed.). (1985). *Adjustment to adult hearing loss.* San Diego, CA: College-Hill Press.

Punch, J. (1983). The prevalence of hearing impairment. *Asha, 25,* 27.

Punch, J. (1983). Sociodemographic and health characteristics of the hearing impaired population. *Asha 25,* 15.

Schildroth, A. (1986). Hearing-impaired children under age 6: 1977 and 1984. *American Annals of the Deaf, 131,* 85–90.

Singer, J., Tomberlin, T. J., Smith, J. M., & Schrier, A. J. (1982). *Analysis of noise related auditory and associated health problems in U.S. adulthood 1971–75* (Vols. 1 & 2). [Prepared under contract to the Environmental Protection Agency]. Springfield, VA: National Technical Information Service.

SPEECH IMPAIRMENT

Fein, D. J. (1983). The prevalence of speech and language impairments. *Asha, 25,* 37.

Fein, D. J. (1983). Population data from the U.S. Census Bureau. *Asha, 25,* 47.

Fein, D. J. (1983). Projections of speech and hearing impairments to 2050. *Asha, 25,* 31.

Ficke, R. C. (1991). *Digest on persons with disabilities.* Washington, DC: National Institute on Disability and Rehabilitation Research.

Healey, W. C., Ackerman, B. L., Chappell, C. R., Perrin, K. L., & Stormer, J. (1981). *The prevalence of communicative disorders: A review of the literature.* Rockville, MD: American Speech-Language-Hearing Association.

Human Services Research Institute. (1985). *Summary of data on handicapped children and youth.* [Prepared under contract to the National Institute of Handicapped Research]. Washington, DC: U.S. Government Printing Office.

Human Services Research Institute. (1986). *Compilation of statistical sources on adult disability.* [Prepared under contract to the National Institute on Disability and Rehabilitation Research, U.S. Department of Education]. Washington, DC: U.S. Government Printing Office.

Hyman, C. S. (1985). PL 94-142 in review. *Asha, 27,* 37.

Karr, S., & Punch, J. (1984). PL 94-142 state child counts. *Asha, 26,* 33.

LaPlante, M. P. (1988). *Data on disability from the National Health Interview Survey. 1983–85.* An InfoUse Report. Washington, DC: U.S. National Institute on Disability and Rehabilitation Research.

Leske, M. C. (1981). Prevalence estimates of communicative disorders in the U.S.: Speech disorders. *Asha, 23,* 217–225.

Mathematica Policy Research. (1984). *Digest of data on persons with disabilities* [Prepared under contract to the Congressional Research Service, Library of Congress]. Washington, DC: U.S. Department of Education, National Institute of Handicapped Research.

Mathematica Policy Research. (1989). *Task 1: Population profile of disability*. [Prepared under contract for the U.S. Department of Health and Human Services, Assistant Secretary for Health and Human Services]. Washington, DC.

National Center for Health Statistics. (1979, July). *The National Nursing Home Survey: 1977 summary for the United States. Vital and Health Statistics*. (Series 13, No. 43, DHEW Publication No. PHS 79-1794). Washington, DC: U.S. Government Printing Office.

National Center for Health Statistics. (1981, February). *Prevalence of selected impairments. United States. 1977. Vital and Health Statistics*. (Series 10, No. 134. DHHS Publication No. PHS 81-1562). Washington, DC: U.S. Government Printing Office.

National Center for Health Statistics. (1986, September). *Current estimates from the National Health Interview Survey. United States. 1985. Vital and Health Statistics*. (Series 10, No. 160. DHHS Publication No. PHS 86-1588). Washington, DC: U.S. Government Printing Office.

National Center for Health Statistics. (1986). [Health interview survey data]. Unpublished data, NHIS, 1983–85.

LANGUAGE AND LEARNING IMPAIRMENTS

Beitchman, J. H., Nair, R., Clegg, M., & Patel, P. G. (1986). Prevalence of speech and language disorders in 5-year-old kindergarten children in the Ottawa-Carleton region. *Journal of Speech and Hearing Disorders, 51*, 98–110.

Fein, D. J. (1983). The prevalence of speech and language impairments. *Asha, 25*, 37.[1]

Fein, D. J. (1983). Population data from the U.S. Census Bureau. *Asha, 25*, 47.[1]

Fein, D. J. (1983). Projections of speech and hearing impairments to 2050. *Asha, 25*, 31.[1]

Ficke, R. C. (1991). *Digest on persons with disabilities*. Washington, DC: National Institute on Disability and Rehabilitation Research.

Healey, W. C., Ackerman, B. L., Chappell, C. R., Perrin, K. L., & Stormer, J. (1981). *The prevalence of communicative disorders: A review of the Literature*. Rockville, MD: American Speech-Language-Hearing Association.

Human Services Research Institute. (1985). *Summary of data on handicapped children and youth*. [Prepared under contract to the National Institute of Handicapped Research]. Washington, DC: U.S. Government Printing Office.[1]

Human Services Research Institute. (1986). *Compilation of statistical sources on adult disability*. [Prepared under contract to the National Institute on Disability and Rehabilitation Research, U.S. Department of Education]. Washington, DC: U.S. Government Printing Office.

Hyman, C. S. (1985). PL 94-142 in review. *Asha, 27*, 37.[1]

Karr, S., & Punch, J. (1984). PL 94-142 state child counts. *Asha, 26*, 33.

LaPlante, M. P. (1988). *Data on disability from the National Health Interview Survey. 1983–85*. An InfoUse Report. Washington, DC: U.S. National Institute on Disability and Rehabilitation Research.

Leske, M. C. (1981). Prevalence estimates of communicative disorders in the U.S.: Language, hearing and vestibular disorders. *Asha, 23*, 229–237.

Mathematica Policy Research. (1984). *Digest of data on persons with disabilities* [Prepared under contract to the Congressional Research Service, Library of Congress]. Washington, DC: U.S. Department of Education, National Institute of Handicapped Research.

Mathematica Policy Research. (1989). *Task 1: Population profile of disability*. [Prepared under contract for the U.S. Department of Health and Human Services, Assistant Secretary for Health and Human Services]. Washington, DC.

National Center for Health Statistics. (1979, July). *The National Nursing Home Survey: 1977 summary for the United States. Vital and Health Statistics*. (Series 13, No. 43. DHEW Publication No. PHS 79-1794). Washington, D.C.: U.S. Government Printing Office.[1]

National Center for Health Statistics. (1981, February). *Prevalence of selected impairments. United States. 1977. Vital and Health Statistics*. (Series 10, No. 134, DHHS Publication No. PHS 81-1562). Washington, DC: U.S. Government Printing Office.[1]

National Center for Health Statistics. (1986, September). *Current estimates from the National Health Interview Survey. United States. 1985. Vital and Health Statistics*. (Series 10, No. 160, DHHS Publication No. PHS 86-1588). Washington, DC: U.S. Government Printing Office.[1]

National Center for Health Statistics. (1986). [Health interview survey data]. Unpublished data, NHIS, 1983–85.[1]

[1]"Language impairment" is included in the statistics for "speech impairment."

APPENDIX 8B

Some readers may wish to compare the NHIS data across time. For convenience, the NHIS publications containing the speech and hearing impairment data are listed below. The documents are listed in chronological order and cover the data collection years of 1982 through 1991.

National Center for Health Statistics. (1985). *Current estimates from the National Health Interview Survey: United States. 1982. Vital and Health Statistics.* Series 10, No. 150. DHIS Pub. No. (PHS) 85-1578. Public Health Service. Washington, DC: U.S. Government Printing Office.

National Center for Health Statistics. (1986). *Current estimates from the National Health Interview Survey: United States. 1983. Vital and Health Statistics.* Series 10, No. 154. DHHS Pub. No. (PHS) 86-1582. Public Health Service. Washington, DC: U.S. Government Printing Office.

Ries, P. W. (1986). *Current estimates from the National Health Interview Survey: United States. 1984. Vital and Health Statistics.* Series 10, No. 156. DHHS Pub. No. (PHS) 86-1584. National Center for Health Statistics. Public Health Service. Washington, DC: U.S. Government Printing Office.

Moss, A. J., & Parsons, V. L. (1986). *Current estimates from the National Health Interview Survey: United States. 1985. Vital and Health Statistics.* Series 10, No. 160. DHHS Pub. No. (PHS) 86-1588. National Center for Health Statistics. Public Health Service. Washington, DC: U.S. Government Printing Office.

Dawson, D. A., & Adams, P. F. (1987). *Current estimates from the National Health Interview Survey: United States. 1986. Vital and Health Statistics.* Series 10, No. 164. DHHS Pub. No. (PHS) 87-1592. National Center for Health Statistics. Public Health Service. Washington, DC: U.S. Government Printing Office.

Schoenborn, C. A., & Marano, M. (1988). *Current estimates from the National Health Interview Survey: United States. 1987. Vital and Health Statistics.* Series 10, No. 166. DHHS Pub. No. (PHS) 88-1594. National Center for Health Statistics. Public Health Service. Washington, DC: U.S. Government Printing Office.

Adams, P. F., & Hardy, A. M. (1989). *Current estimates from the National Health Interview Survey: United States. 1988. Vital and Health Statistics.* Series 10, No. 173. National Center for Health Statistics. Public Health Service. Washington, DC: U.S. Government Printing Office.

Adams, P. F., & Benson, V. (1990). *Current estimates from the National Health Interview Survey. 1989. Vital and Health Statistics.* Series 10, No. 176. National Center for Health Statistics. Public Health Service. Washington, DC: U.S. Government Printing Office.

Adams, P. F., & Benson, V. (1991). *Current estimates from the National Health Interview Survey. 1990. Vital and Health Statistics.* Series 10, No. 181. National Center for Health Statistics. Public Health Service. Washington, DC: U.S. Government Printing Office.

Adams, P. F., & Benson, V. (1992). *Current estimates from the National Health Interview Survey. 1991. Vital and Health Statistics.* Series 10, No. 184. National Center for Health Statistics. Public Health Service. Washington, DC: U.S. Government Printing Office.

■ CHAPTER 9 ■

Characteristics of ASHA Membership

■ CYNTHIA M. SHEWAN, Ph.D. ■

SCOPE OF CHAPTER

As you embark on your study of the professions of speech-language pathology and audiology, you might wonder who your colleagues will be when you start to work in these professions. This chapter provides you with a sketch of who ASHA members are, what their work characteristics are, and what members might be doing in the next few years.

The first section of the chapter describes the numbers and different types of ASHA affiliates, members and certificate holders. The demographic characteristics, including age, gender, marital status, racial/ethnic background, geographical distribution, and education level of speech-language pathology and audiology professionals follow. Employment and earning characteristics cover the employment status of professionals, as well as who they work for, what their job functions are, and the kinds of facilities in which they work. The earning discussion includes salary data, supplementary income, and fringe benefit considerations.

Predictions about the future size of ASHA affiliates leads into a discussion of ASHA's past growth and how this growth might affect the future. Growth in both speech-language pathology and audiology is described. The chapter closes by considering another approach to forecasting the future—that offered through econometric modeling. Data from such a model are presented.

ASHA AFFILIATES

Before counting ASHA affiliates, it is important to place the ASHA membership in a larger context. One important change in the discipline of human communication sciences and disorders was the separation into the two professions of speech-language pathology and audiology in 1989 (American Speech-Language-Hearing Association, 1993). Another important feature to bear in mind is that ASHA affiliation does not encompass the entire body of persons in the two professions. A comprehensive work force study (Shewan,

1988) indicated that ASHA members represented 51.2% of the current active supply in the work force. Current active supply refers to the number of individuals working as speech-language pathologists and audiologists at a given time. The non-ASHA portion of the professions may seem high; however, it is important to remember that being an ASHA member is not a requirement to practice in the United States. Although all the reasons why an individual might not belong to ASHA are not known, certainly personal choice and ineligibility for membership are among them. ASHA requires a master's degree as one of the eligibility criteria for membership. Consequently, persons with only a bachelor's degree are not eligible for membership.

The term "membership" is one that is used differently by different people. Often it is used in a generic sense to represent people who are associated with ASHA by virtue of membership or certification or both. In a narrower sense, and the one that is precise, membership refers to people who meet the membership criteria and who pay their membership dues. In this chapter ASHA membership is limited to the latter definition, and the term affiliate represents the broader category.

Counts of ASHA affiliates refer to the number of persons affiliated at a given time. Because persons join the association on a continuous basis, the affiliate counts change daily. To provide a stable frame of reference, this chapter uses counts that were made at the end of 1992, otherwise known as 1992 year-end counts.

ASHA MEMBERS

As of December 31, 1992, the membership of ASHA totaled 65,771. This total represents several categories that are defined below and outlined in Table 9–1.

Regular members are individuals who have met the membership/certification eligibility criteria or are in the process of doing so as outlined in the ASHA Bylaws. This category covers the majority of the ASHA membership.

Life members are persons who have applied for life status and have been members of the association for at least 10 consecutive years before reaching the age of 65. **Disability life members** are persons who have applied for disability life status, are totally disabled, and have been ASHA members for at least 5 consecutive years immediately before disability.

Spouse members refer to the so designated member of a wife—husband couple, both of whom belong to ASHA. The other member belongs to another ASHA member category.

Postgraduate student members are members of the association who are students.

Noncertified members are persons who belong to ASHA but who do not hold either of the Certificates of Clinical Competence (CCCs). They are often scientists, researchers, and others who do not engage in clinical practice.

Because membership and certification are important concepts to understand when referring to ASHA affiliates, Figure 9–1 illustrates the relationship between membership and certification. Most ASHA affiliates (92.9%) are both members and certificate holders. A smaller percentage (6.3%) hold a certificate of clinical competence, but are not members. Just less than 1.0% are members who do not hold a certificate of clinical competence.

CERTIFICATE HOLDERS

The other major ASHA affiliate category refers to certificate holders. ASHA awards the Certificate of Clinical Competence (CCC) in speech-language pathology and audiology. Most certificate holders are in the speech-language pathology profession (83.3%), followed by audiology (14.6%), with considerably fewer persons certified in both categories (2.1%) (Figure 9–2). The latter persons are often referred to as dually certified. In addition, at any given time there are many persons who are in the process of obtaining certification. At the end of 1992, that number was 3,401.

NATIONAL STUDENT SPEECH LANGUAGE HEARING ASSOCIATION MEMBERS

Not reflected in these counts are the members of the National Student Speech Language

TABLE 9–1. DEMOGRAPHIC CHARACTERISTICS OF FULL-TIME AND PART-TIME ASHA SPEECH-LANGUAGE PATHOLOGISTS (SLP) AND AUDIOLOGISTS (AUD) (IN PERCENT UNLESS OTHERWISE NOTED).

Demographic Characteristic	Full-time		Part-time		Total	
	SLP	AUD	SLP	AUD	SLP	AUD
Age[a]						
Mean (years)	41	42	40	40	41	40
Median (years)	39	40	39	39	39	39
Gender[a]						
Female	90.9	67.1	98.0	95.6	92.2	67.1
Male	9.1	32.9	2.0	4.4	7.8	32.9
Marital Status[b]						
Single	19.0	24.2	2.2	6.2	16.3	21.6
Married	67.3	65.9	94.2	92.0	71.6	69.7
Separated/divorced/widowed	10.3	6.7	3.6	0.9	9.3	5.8
Other	3.4	3.2	0	0.9	2.8	2.8
Race/Ethnicity[a]						
American Indian/Alaskan Native	0.3	0.2	0.4	0.5	0.3	0.2
Asian/Pacific Islander	1.3	1.8	0.7	1.1	1.2	1.7
Black (Not Hispanic)	2.5	1.2	0.7	1.0	2.1	1.2
Hispanic	1.3	1.1	1.1	1.0	1.3	1.1
White (Not Hispanic)	94.7	95.7	97.2	96.4	95.2	95.8
Census Region Geographic Distribution[a]						
Northeast	24.2	22.6	27.6	28.3	24.8	23.5
Midwest	25.9	26.5	26.5	23.0	26.0	26.0
South	29.6	31.9	25.5	28.2	28.9	31.4
West	20.3	19.0	20.4	20.4	20.3	19.2
Education[b]						
BA/BS	0.4	0.1	1.5	0	0.6	0.1
MA/MS	95.7	87.1	98.5	97.3	96.2	88.6
Doctorate	3.5	12.4	0	2.7	3.0	11.0
Other	0.3	0.3	0	0	0.2	0.3

[a] 1992 ASHA membership year-end counts.
[b] Data from Slater, S. C. (1992b). The 1992 Omnibus Survey: Portrait of the professions. *ASHA, 34*(8), 61–65.

Hearing Association (NSSLHA). NSSLHA is a separate student association that currently has a membership of 12,257. ASHA and NSSLHA enjoy a close and amicable relationship, but because NSSLHA students do not yet meet the eligibility criteria for ASHA membership, they are not included in ASHA counts. However, the majority of NSSLHA members do become ASHA members.

DEMOGRAPHIC CHARACTERISTICS

A description of a population often includes defining characteristics, such as age, education, and so forth. These characteristics, often referred to as demographic characteristics, are outlined for ASHA affiliates in the next section. The data presented stem from two sources, the 1992 ASHA Omnibus Survey and the 1992 ASHA year-end counts. Because characteristics may differ for the two professions and for full- and part-time workers in either profession, both the aggregate and subgroup data are presented.

SPEECH-LANGUAGE PATHOLOGISTS

As seen in Table 9–1, the median age for speech-language pathologists is 39 years. That the mean age is quite similar (41 years) suggests that the age distribution of ASHA's

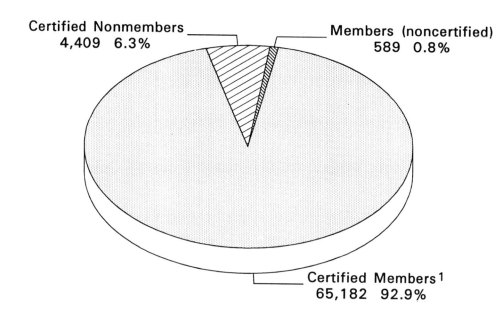

Certified Nonmembers
4,409 6.3%

Members (noncertified)
589 0.8%

Certified Members[1]
65,182 92.9%

[1] Includes members in the process of obtaining certification.

Figure 9–1. ASHA membership and certification.

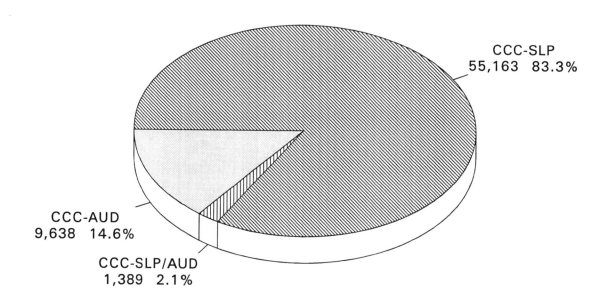

CCC-SLP
55,163 83.3%

CCC-AUD
9,638 14.6%

CCC-SLP/AUD
1,389 2.1%

Figure 9–2. ASHA certification status.

speech-language pathologists is relatively normal. The large majority are married (67.3%) and women (90.9%). Although minority groups are represented in the profession, they compose only a small percentage, approximately 5%. Within the minority groups, Blacks form the largest contingency, representing 2.1% of speech-language pathologists. Hispanics represent 1.3% and Asians and Pacific Islanders represent 1.2%. The smallest minority group is the American Indian and Alaskan Native group, which composes only 0.3% of ASHA affiliates.

The distribution of speech-language pathologists (both members and certificate holders) differs according to geographical area of the country (see Table 9–2). Almost one quarter (24.8%) are located in the Northeast census region, with just over one quarter (26.0%) located in the Midwest. The South census region accounts for the largest percentage of ASHA speech-language pathologists (28.9%). By contrast, the West has only 20.3% of the entire group.

Because the census regions are so large, you might be interested in seeing how the distribution varies more locally, by state, for example. It might also be instructive to see how speech-language pathologists are distributed relative to the resident population in each state, referred to as personnel-to-population ratios. Table 9–2 shows the personnel-to-population ratios for speech-language pathologists by state, census division, and region (Shewan & Slater, 1992). Based on the November 1992 ASHA membership database counts, there were 51,730 certified speech-language pathologists serving the U.S. population, estimated at 254 million (U.S. Bureau of the Census, 1990). These numbers convert to an overall ratio of 20.4 speech-language pathologists per 100,000 resident population. This ratio is not intended to represent any ideal or recommended figure, which would meet the needs of all persons requiring services. It represents only the number available to serve the population. Nor does it take into account that all certified personnel will not choose to pro-

vide clinical services; the figure includes professionals functioning in all roles.

The availability of *certified* speech-language pathologists across the census regions varies considerably, from a high in the Northeast of 24.9 to a low of 17.2 in the South. By state, considerable variability also exists. New Mexico and Wisconsin enjoy the highest ratios, at 34.6 and 32.4, respectively. By contrast, Nevada and Alabama, with ratios of 12.2 and 13.0, respectively, have the fewest speech-language pathologists to serve their populations. The reader is cautioned about viewing a state ratio to be representative of all regions within a state. Remote and rural regions tend to be underserved as compared with metropolitan areas.

Given that the eligibility requirements for ASHA membership include a master's degree, one would expect that a majority of speech-language pathologists have attained this level of education. Fully 96.2% of speech-language pathologists hold a master's degree and 3% hold a doctorate (Table 9–1). Less than 1%, actually 0.6%, have a bachelor's degree only. These are persons who became members of the association before the master's degree became the entry level degree in 1965.

AUDIOLOGISTS

The mean age for audiologists is 40 years, with a corresponding median of 39 years (Table 9–1). The close similarity between the median and the mean suggests that the age distribution of ASHA audiologists approaches a normal distribution. Most audiologists are female, accounting for two thirds (67.1%) of these professionals. A similar percentage are also married (69.7%). The vast majority of audiologists are White (95.8%), with minority groups constituting less than 5% of the professionals. Asians and Pacific Islanders form the largest minority at 1.7%, followed closely by Blacks (1.2%), and Hispanics (1.1%). American Indians and Alaskan Natives form the smallest minority group represented, at 0.2%.

The South and West census regions of the United States contrast in their concentration

TABLE 9–2. CERTIFIED PERSONNEL AND PERSONNEL PER 100,000 POPULATION BY GEOGRAPHIC AREA AND CERTIFICATION STATUS.

Census Division and State	1992 Resident Population[a] (x1,000)	Certified Personnel			Certified Personnel per 100,000 Population		
		CCC-SLP	CCC-AUD	CCC-SLP/A	CCC-SLP	CCC-AUD	Total[b]
UNITED STATES	254,002	51,730	9,052	1,320	20.4	3.6	24.4
NORTHEAST	51,175	12,723	2,034	316	24.9	4.0	29.5
New England	13,309	3,762	576	69	28.3	4.3	33.1
Connecticut	3,302	1,055	120	17	32.0	3.6	36.1
Maine	1,261	234	38	2	18.6	3.0	21.7
Massachusetts	5,963	1,737	308	36	29.1	5.2	34.9
New Hampshire	1,194	284	42	6	23.8	3.5	27.8
Rhode Island	1,007	265	44	5	26.3	4.4	31.2
Vermont	582	187	24	3	32.1	4.1	36.8
Middle Atlantic	37,866	8,961	1,458	247	23.7	3.9	28.2
New Jersey	7,921	1,866	289	40	23.6	3.6	27.7
New York	17,877	4,743	738	114	26.5	4.1	31.3
Pennsylvania	12,068	2,352	431	93	19.5	3.6	23.8
MIDWEST	60,556	13,360	2,374	286	22.1	3.9	26.5
East North Central	42,571	9,046	1,631	187	21.2	3.8	25.5
Illinois	11,731	2,751	464	51	23.5	4.0	27.8
Indiana	5,657	944	212	26	16.7	3.7	20.9
Michigan	9,332	1,746	322	34	18.7	3.6	22.5
Ohio	10,941	2,014	470	51	18.4	4.3	23.2
Wisconsin	4,911	1,591	163	25	32.4	3.3	36.2
West North Central	17,985	4,314	743	99	24.0	4.1	28.7
Iowa	2,777	642	147	19	23.1	5.3	29.1
Kansas	2,538	725	105	18	28.6	4.1	33.4
Minnesota	4,436	1,049	194	18	23.6	4.4	28.4
Missouri	5,269	1,144	174	21	21.7	3.3	25.4
Nebraska	1,599	445	76	11	27.8	4.8	33.3
North Dakota	648	177	28	2	27.3	4.3	31.9
South Dakota	718	132	19	10	18.4	2.6	22.4
SOUTH	88,445	15,218	2,842	453	17.2	3.2	20.9
South Atlantic	45,480	8,287	1,555	251	18.2	3.4	22.2

Delaware	705	144	23	5	20.4	3.3	24.4
Washington DC	596	121	46	11	20.3	7.7	29.9
Florida	13,586	2,280	429	73	16.8	3.2	20.5
Georgia	6,870	1,004	189	15	14.6	2.8	17.6
Maryland	4,934	1,486	287	47	30.1	5.8	36.9
North Carolina	6,892	1,228	192	44	17.8	2.8	21.2
South Carolina	3,648	483	96	11	13.2	2.6	16.2
Virginia	6,443	1,251	219	35	19.4	3.4	23.4
West Virginia	1,806	290	74	10	16.1	4.1	20.7
East South Central	15,755	2,269	494	59	14.4	3.1	17.9
Alabama	4,218	516	115	15	12.2	2.7	15.3
Kentucky	3,750	624	95	15	16.6	2.5	19.6
Mississippi	2,678	373	53	12	13.9	2.0	16.4
Tennessee	5,109	756	231	17	14.8	4.5	19.7
West South Central	27,210	4,662	793	143	17.1	2.9	20.6
Arkansas	2,444	520	66	10	21.3	2.7	24.4
Louisiana	4,334	843	130	38	19.5	3.0	23.3
Oklahoma	3,146	613	92	12	19.5	2.9	22.8
Texas	17,286	2,686	505	83	15.5	2.9	18.9
WEST	53,826	10,429	1,802	265	19.4	3.3	23.2
Mountain	14,028	3,162	601	99	22.5	4.3	27.5
Arizona	3,858	718	147	15	18.6	3.8	22.8
Colorado	3,367	970	210	25	28.8	6.2	35.8
Idaho	1,018	207	26	4	20.3	2.6	23.3
Montana	789	157	25	15	19.9	3.2	25.0
Nevada	1,196	155	25	5	13.0	2.1	15.5
New Mexico	1,579	546	72	13	34.6	4.6	40.0
Utah	1,765	300	76	19	17.0	4.3	22.4
Wyoming	456	109	20	3	23.9	4.4	28.9
Pacific	39,798	7,267	1,201	166	18.3	3.0	21.7
Alaska	537	117	23	6	21.8	4.3	27.2
California	30,304	5,320	796	105	17.6	2.6	20.5
Hawaii	1,182	224	42	6	19.0	3.6	23.0
Oregon	2,857	659	103	23	23.1	3.6	27.5
Washington	4,917	947	237	26	19.3	4.8	24.6

[a]Source: From U.S. Bureau of the Census, Current Population Reports. (Series P-25, No. 1053). *Projections of the Population of States, by Age, Sex, and Race: 1989 to 2010,* U.S. Government Printing Office, Washington, DC, 1990.
[b]In computing the total ratio, the numerator included the dually certified.

of audiologists (members and certificate holders). The South has 31.4% compared with the West, at only 19.2%. Approximately one quarter (26%) of audiologists are located in the Midwest, with the remaining 23.5% in the Northeast. To examine the distribution relative to the population served and for smaller geographical areas, Table 9–2 shows the personnel-to-population ratios for certified audiologists according to census region, division, and also by state. The table shows that there are 9,052 certified audiologists to serve the U.S. population of 254 million, for an overall ratio of 3.6/100,000 persons nationally. As might be expected, this ratio is much smaller than that for speech-language pathologists. This can be explained by the different sizes of caseloads for the two professions. The average monthly caseload size for audiologists is 124, compared with 43 for speech-language pathologists (Slater, 1992b). The New England and Mountain census divisions share the highest ratio at 4.3, with the West South Central region having the lowest ratio at 2.9. The District of Columbia and Colorado have the highest state ratios at 7.7 and 6.2, respectively. Nevada and Mississippi have the lowest ratios at 2.1 and 2.0, respectively. Because the state figures may not be representative of all regions within the state, it is important to use caution when generalizing the data.

Almost 9 in 10 (88.6%) audiologists hold a master's degree, the entry level degree for ASHA members. Another 11% hold a doctorate degree, with very few (0.1%) who have only a bachelor's or some other degree (0.3%).

EMPLOYMENT AND EARNING CHARACTERISTICS

SPEECH-LANGUAGE PATHOLOGISTS

Compared with the nation, the employment status of speech-language pathologists is positive. Only 1.4% are unemployed although seeking employment—that is, job seeking (Table 9–3). Almost three quarters of speech-language pathologists are employed on a full-time basis. Another 16.3% work part-time. A small percentage are on a leave-of-absence from a position, usually for educational or child care reasons, according to the ASHA Work Force Study (Shewan, 1988). An additional 0.2% work on a volunteer basis. Fewer than 1 in 10 speech-language pathologists are not working; 5.6% are unemployed and not looking for a job, with 1.3% retired.

Speech-language pathologists work in a variety of facilities, although the most common facility is a school. More than half (53.7%) of employed speech-language pathologists work in some type of school facility, either a preschool, a special day school, an elementary or secondary school, or in several schools. Just over one third more (34.5%) work in a health care facility. Nonresidential health care facilities include nonhospital rehabilitation agencies; home health agencies, a client's home; private physician's offices; speech-language pathologist's or audiologist's offices; speech and hearing centers or clinics; and other nonresidential facilities. These facilities are the workplaces of 15.2% of ASHA's speech-language pathologists; hospitals follow closely at 14.9%; and 4.4% work in residential health care facilities, including nursing homes. Colleges or universities are the workplace for an additional 6.3% and a small percentage (1.4%) work in various agency, organization, or research facilities. The re-maining 4.1% work in some other kind of facility.

As seen in Table 9–3, the speech-language pathology profession offers its members a variety of roles. This is certainly an advantage of the profession and a feature that no doubt attracts students to select it. Data from ASHA indicate that providing clinical services to clients is the major job function of 75.5% of speech-language pathologists. Less than 10% (8.6%) are involved as educators, either college or university professors or special education teachers. Administrative functions are the primary responsibilities for another 10.5%, who are either administrators of services, programs, or departments, or serve as supervisors. Few speech-language

TABLE 9–3. EMPLOYMENT AND EARNINGS CHARACTERISTICS OF FULL-TIME AND PART-TIME ASHA SPEECH-LANGUAGE PATHOLOGISTS (SLP) AND AUDIOLOGISTS (AUD).

Employment Characteristic	Full-time (in %)		Part-time (in %)		Total (in %)	
	SLP	AUD	SLP	AUD	SLP	AUD
Employment Status[a]						
Employed full-time					73.8	79.5
Employed part-time					16.3	14.2
Unemployed, seeking					1.4	1.5
Unemployed, not seeking					5.6	3.4
Leave of absence					1.6	0.6
Retired					1.3	0.9
Volunteer					0.2	0.0
Type of Employment Facility[a]						
Schools (special, pre-, K-12)	56.4	10.0	41.3	9.4	53.7	9.9
College/university	6.5	9.6	5.6	10.8	6.3	9.8
Hospital facilities	15.0	23.6	14.1	18.2	14.9	22.8
Residential health care facilities	4.3	1.7	5.0	2.0	4.4	1.7
Nonresidential health care facilities	12.7	45.2	25.5	52.6	15.2	46.3
Agencies, organizations, research facilities	1.4	2.8	1.3	1.5	1.4	2.6
All other	3.6	7.1	6.2	5.5	4.1	6.9
Primary Employment Function[a]						
Clinical service provider	74.2	73.7	81.7	80.0	75.5	74.7
Educator	9.4	6.4	4.7	2.8	8.6	5.8
Administrator/chair/ department head/manager	8.4	9.1	1.3	2.8	7.1	8.2
Supervisor	3.6	3.1	2.3	2.9	3.4	3.1
Researcher	0.5	1.7	0.9	1.7	0.5	1.7
Consultant	1.6	2.3	4.4	3.6	2.1	2.5
Other	2.4	3.7	5.1	6.3	2.7	4.1
Employer Category[b]						
Government	58.2	32.2	46.3	19.5	56.3	30.4
Nongovernment	41.8	67.8	53.7	80.5	43.7	69.6
Years of Experience[b]						
Mean (years)	11.2	10.9	10.6	9.4	11.1	10.7
Median (years)	11.0	9.0	10.0	9.0	10.0	9.0
Median Annual Salary[b]	$34,000	$35,782	$20,000	$18,352	$32,500	$34,000
CCC-SLP/A	$44,300		$20,000		$41,000	
Noncertified	$27,000		(N<25)		$26,500	
Salary Period[b]						
9- or 10-month year	48.2	14.6	47.1	16.4	48.0	14.8
11- or 12-month year	51.3	85.1	51.5	81.8	51.4	84.6
Other	0.4	0.3	1.5	1.8	0.6	0.5
Supplemental Annual Income (mean)[b]	$1,915	$3,163	$1,473	$1,509	$1,845	$2,944
CCC-SLP/A	$4,503		$1,610		$4,217	
Noncertified	$1,812		(N<25)		$1,775	

[a] 1992 ASHA membership year-end counts.
[b] Data from Slater, S.C. (1992b). The 1992 Omnibus Survey: Portrait of the professions. *ASHA, 34*(8), 61–65, reprinted with permission.

pathologists report their primary duties as research (0.5%) or consulting (2.1%).

The government, which includes employment in the public schools, employs more than half (56.3%) of ASHA's speech-language pathologists. Nongovernment employment arrangements, which employ the other 43.7%, include those who are self-employed, either running their own practice or independent contractors, and employees of private, for-profit companies, or public or private non-profit organizations.

Speech-language pathology professionals, as a group in the workplace, have considerable experience. The median (50th percentile) number of years of work experience currently is 10.

ASHA collects salary information on an annual basis through its Omnibus Survey. This information is analyzed in depth and published in detail biennially (in even years) in the March reference issue of the *Asha* magazine. Salary data are of great interest to communication sciences and disorders professionals, judging from the number of requests received by ASHA's research division for salary data. The salary data presented here are from the 1992 Omnibus Survey. Although Table 9–3 shows salaries for both full-time and part-time employees, only those for full-time workers are discussed. Here, part-time work can vary from a few hours per week to just under full-time employment, here defined as 30 or more working hours per week. Therefore, one can get a biased view by considering part-time salaries alone or by including them in a total with full-time salaries. For completeness sake, all figures have been calculated in Table 9–3; however, it is the full-time salaries that provide the best representation of the profession. The median annual salary for full-time employed certified speech-language pathologists in 1992 was $34,000. Salaries vary according to many variables such as certification status, length of contract, educational level, years of professional experience, gender, geographical location, work facility, primary job function, and so on. For consideration of this subject in depth, you can refer to the March 1992 *Asha* salary article (Slater, 1992a). Another was published in March of 1994.

Just over half (51.4%) speech-language pathologists' salaries are for an 11- or 12-month period. The large percentage (48.0%) representing a 9- or 10-month period is consistent with the large number of speech-language pathologists working in the schools, where the work year is 9 or 10 months.

Speech-language pathologists have a variety of opportunities to supplement their annual salary. Some have a private practice in addition to a primary job; others provide consulting services; some give lectures and workshops; some write books or produce commercial products; and so forth. Although many speech-language pathologists do not avail themselves of these opportunities, those who do supplement their annual salaries on the average by $1,915. Because the supplemental annual incomes reported here are for 1991, with the basic annual salaries are for 1992, it is not appropriate to add these two numbers. However, presenting both categories provides a more comprehensive picture of the monetary rewards from speech-language pathology as a profession.

Salaries do not tell the whole story of compensation. Also included here is a summary of the types of benefits speech-language pathologists might expect as part of their jobs. The data reported were gathered as part of the 1990 Omnibus Survey (American Speech-Language-Hearing Association, 1990) and because the economic climate may have changed since that time, the reader is advised to view them with caution. Table 9–4 indicates that employers provide a variety of types of leave for employees. Most speech-language pathologists reported receiving sick leave (85.9%) and just over half received either vacation (50.4%) or maternity/paternity leave (51.9%). Insurance coverage spanned life, disability, dental, and health categories. More than half speech-language pathologists indicated that their employers provided health (86.8%), life (65.9%), dental (66.9%), and disability (47.0%) insurance. Much less frequently provided benefits were flextime (14.1%), job sharing (8.5%), and dependent care (2.7%). An additional 7.2% reported receiving some other type of fringe benefit.

TABLE 9–4. FRINGE BENEFITS RECEIVED BY FULL-TIME EMPLOYED SPEECH-LANGUAGE PATHOLOGISTS AND AUDIOLOGISTS.

Fringe Benefits	Speech-Language Pathologists		Audiologists	
Provided by Employer	% cases[a]	% responses[b]	% cases	% responses
Leave				
Vacation	50.4	10.3	78.4	16.3
Sick	85.9	17.6	80.8	16.8
Maternity/Paternity	51.9	10.7	44.6	9.3
Insurance				
Life	65.9	13.5	64.9	13.5
Disability	47.0	9.6	48.7	10.1
Health	86.8	17.8	80.5	16.7
Dental	66.9	13.7	47.2	9.8
Flextime	14.1	2.9	15.0	3.1
Job Sharing	8.5	1.7	5.6	1.2
Dependent care (elder/child)	2.7	0.6	4.3	0.9
Other	7.2	1.5	11.4	2.4

[a]Percent of cases gives results for each response category based on the number of respondents to each question. To obtain results, the number of responses to each response category was divided by the total number of individuals who responded to the question. When respondents indicated more than one response, summation of the percentages was greater than 100%.

[b]Percent of responses is based on total responses to each response category and provides information as to how frequently a response category has been selected relative to other response categories in the same question. To obtain results, the number of responses in each response category was divided by the total number of responses to that question. Summation of the percentages for each response category within a quesiton equals 100%.

Source: American Speech-Language-Hearing Association. (1990). *1990 ASHA Omnibus Survey.* Unpublished data.

AUDIOLOGISTS

Almost 8 of every 10 audiologists works on a full-time basis (Table 9–3). An additional 14.2% are employed part-time and 0.6% are on a leave of absence from a full- or part-time position. Only 3.4% are unemployed and not seeking employment, and an additional 0.9% are retired. Only 1.5% of audiologists are actively in the job market without a current job. Compared with national unemployment rates of over 7.0% in 1992, this rate is low and a good sign of employment opportunities.

Nonresidential health care facilities are reportedly the major employment facility (46.3%) for audiologists. Almost another quarter (22.8%) work in hospitals, which includes general medical, psychiatric, rehabilitation, pediatric, or other types of hospitals. Almost 20% work in educational facilities, either schools (9.9%) or colleges and universities

(9.8%). Few audiologists are employed in agencies, organizations, and research facilities (2.6%) and residential health care facilities (1.7%). The remaining 6.9% of audiologists work in some other type of facility not captured by these categories.

As is the case for speech-language pathologists, almost three quarters (74.7%) of audiologists are employed as clinical service providers (Table 9–3). The next most frequent primary function is administrative, either as a program or department director (8.2%) or as a supervisor (3.1%). Audiologists (5.8%) also serve the role of educator (5.8%), primarily as college or university professors, with fewer as special education teachers. Serving primarily as a consultant is a role assumed by 2.5% of audiologists, and researchers comprise 1.7% of audiologists. The "other" category accounts for the remaining 4.1%.

The primary employers of audiologists are from the private sector (69.6%), with only 30.4% employed by federal, state, or local governments, including the public schools. The median number of years of professional work experience for audiologists is 9, although the mean is 10.7. The difference between these two figures suggests that the distribution is positively skewed by audiologists with a large number of years of experience.

Because salary data are not normally distributed, median salaries are reported here. The median annual salary for full-time certified audiologists was $35,782 in 1992. For the same reasons presented for speech-language pathologists above, part-time and the aggregate of full- and part-time salaries are not discussed, although the reader can readily see the figures in Table 9–3. Most audiologists' salaries are for an 11- or 12-month period (85.1%). This is related in part to the fact that fewer audiologists are employed in school facilities, for which contracts are for a 9- or 10-month annual duration.

Audiologists reported an average supplement of $3,163 to their annual 1991 salaries. Although this figure should not be added to the annual 1992 salary because of the different years represented, the categories together suggest a more optimistic professional income level than from salary alone.

Although salary and income are certainly the major components to a compensation package, consideration of fringe benefits can assume major importance when other factors are equal. The majority of audiologists reported that they received sick (80.8%) and vacation (78.4%) leave in 1990, with a smaller percentage having maternity/paternity leave (44.6%) as a benefit (Table 9–4). More than half received health (80.5%) and life (64.9%) insurance, with disability (48.7%) and dental (47.2%) insurance being less prevalent. Other benefits were enjoyed by small percentages of audiologists: flextime, 15.0%, job sharing 5.6%, dependent care, 4.3%, and other benefits not among the categories listed, 11.4%.

MEMBERSHIP TRENDS

The numbers, types, and characteristics of ASHA affiliates have been described. You have a picture of the present, but what about the future? What can be expected over the next decade? There are several ways of trying to predict the future of ASHA membership. A first method described here is to examine what has transpired in the past and to use these data to estimate subjectively what will be the trend of the future. A second method described to predict future membership is based on economic forces, that is, an econometric model.

By the end of 1992, the ASHA affiliates, including members, certificate holders, and NSSLHA students in the conversion process, had reached 70,180. As Figure 9–3 shows, the ASHA membership has continued to grow over the past several years. The percentage growth rate has varied between 3.8% and 6.8% from 1987 to 1992.

SPEECH-LANGUAGE PATHOLOGY

In absolute terms, the number of certified speech-language pathologists increased by 12,716 from 1987 to 1992 (Table 9–5). This represents growth in both certified members and certified nonmembers (certificate holders only). The rate of growth or percentage change for certified members forms a horseshoe-shaped curve; the largest growth rates occur at each end of the time period (Figure 9–4). The pattern for certified nonmembers is quite different. Although the growth rate was declining from 1987 to 1991, there was still a positive increase in the absolute number of certified nonmembers. However, the precipitous decline in 1992, which might be explained by the new certification requirements, may have motivated applicants to apply for membership concomitant with certification.

Because the largest proportion of affiliates are both members and certified, it is this segment of ASHA affiliates that will, to a large extent, determine what will happen to the numbers in the future. Given the trends for the last several

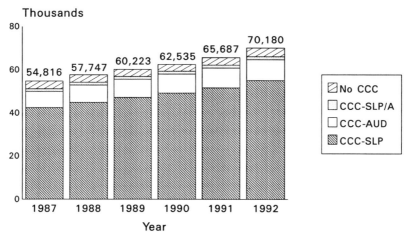

Note: Figures represent ASHA year-end counts.

Figure 9-3. Number of ASHA affiliates by CCC type, 1987-1992.

TABLE 9-5. NUMBER OF SPEECH-LANGUAGE PATHOLOGY CERTIFICATE OF CLINICAL COMPETENCE (CCC) HOLDERS BY MEMBERSHIP STATUS FROM 1987 TO 1992 AND THE PERCENT CHANGE.

Year	Certified Members	Percentage Change	Certified Nonmembers	Percentage Change	Certificate Holders	Percentage Change
1987	38,929		3,518		42,447	
1988	41,281	+6.0%	3,633	+3.3%	44,914	+5.8%
1989	43,541	+5.5%	3,637	+0.1%	47,178	+5.0%
1990	45,542	+4.6%	3,703	+1.8%	49,245	+4.4%
1991	47,975	+5.3%	3,749	+1.2%	51,724	+5.0%
1992	51,600	+7.6%	3,563	-5.0%	55,163	+6.6%

Note: The figures in this table are year-end counts and do *not* include those National Student Speech Language Hearing Association (NSSLHA) members in the process of conversion to ASHA membership. These figures do *not* include individuals holding certification in both audiology and speech-language pathology.

years, it is reasonable to predict that membership will grow at a larger rate in 1993 than previously and then decline to rates in the range of 4.5% to 5.5% annually. Because the number of certified nonmembers is small by comparison, the low positive or negative growth rates will have a small effect on the overall growth of certified speech-language pathologists.

AUDIOLOGY

The number of certified audiologists has increased by 2,141 from 1987 to 1992 (Table 9-6). From a maximum of 7.3% growth rate in 1987-1988, growth rate declined to a low of 3.9% in 1990-1991 and increased to 5.2% in 1991-1992. This pattern mirrors that for certified members as shown in Figure 9-5. Rate of growth for nonmember certificate holders was relatively small until 1989-1990, but increased to 4.7% and 7.3%, respectively, for the 1990-1991 and 1991-1992 periods (Figure 9-5).

If the current trends continue, growth for certified audiologists should continue to be positive for the next few years. A potential negative influence on this growth could be the

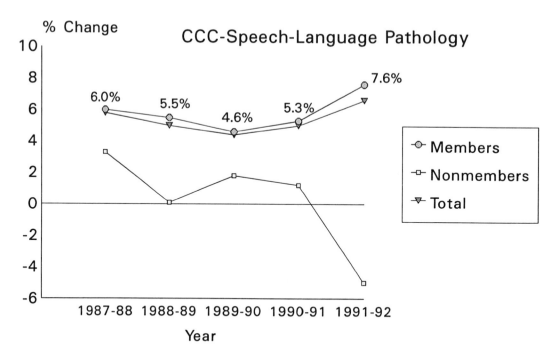

Note: Figures represent ASHA year-end counts.

Figure 9–4. Percentage change from 1987–1988 to 1991–1992 in the number of ASHA certified members, certified non-members, and total certificate holders.

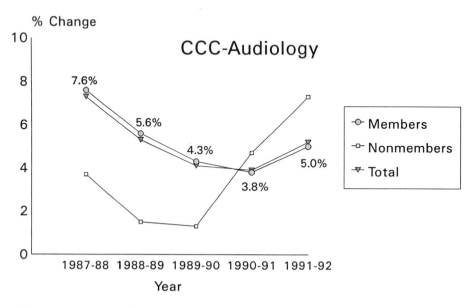

Note: Figures represent ASHA year-end counts.

Figure 9–5. Percentage change from 1987–1988 to 1991–1992 in the number of ASHA certified members, certified non-members, and total certificate holders.

TABLE 9–6. NUMBER OF AUDIOLOGY CERTIFICATE OF CLINICAL COMPETENCE (CCC) HOLDERS BY MEMBERSHIP STATUS FROM 1987 TO 1992 AND THE PERCENT CHANGE.

Year	Certified Members	Percentage Change	Certified Nonmembers	Percentage Change	Certificate Holders	Percentage Change
1987	6,904		593		7,497	
1988	7,432	+7.6%	615	+3.7%	8,047	+7.3%
1989	7,851	+5.6%	624	+1.5%	8,475	+5.3%
1990	8,188	+4.3%	632	+1.3%	8,820	+4.1%
1991	8,500	+3.8%	662	+4.7%	9,162	+3.9%
1992	8,928	+5.0%	710	+7.3%	9,638	+5.2%

Note: The figures in this table are year-end counts and do *not* include those National Student Speech Language Hearing Association (NSSLHA) members in the process of conversion to ASHA membership. These figures do *not* include individuals holding certification in both audiology and speech-language pathology.

introduction of certification by other groups. If this occurs, audiologists would then have the option of being certified by more than one organization. If the economy continues to be weak, audiologists may choose to be certified by only one organization. Choice undoubtedly will be dictated at least partially by the perception of which organization offers the greatest benefits through its certification.

ECONOMETRIC MODEL

The second way to predict ASHA membership described in this chapter is through econometric modeling, that is, by examining the economic marketplace and considering supply and demand. As part of the ASHA Work Force Study (Shewan, 1988), a forecasting model based on economic forces was used to develop long-range estimates of the ASHA membership through the year 2000. This econometric model was based on the principles that supply and demand determine the employment of speech-language-hearing professionals. Because of data requirements, only member data from the 50 states and the District of Columbia were included in the model. Therefore, membership projection numbers will not match the membership data discussed earlier. Although it was desirable to forecast the entire work force of speech-language pathologists and audiologists by

including non-ASHA personnel as well, sufficient data were not available to do so. Restricting the model to the ASHA membership might be a problem if ASHA membership were unrelated to the economic activity in the professions. The model did not omit this link; rather it assumed that the relationship between professional employment and ASHA membership would continue to be what it had been in the recent past.

The model's results projected that in the year 2000 the ASHA membership would be between 80% and 100% larger than in the base year 1985. The 20% variability in the two estimates resulted from the influence of eight states, which were growing either faster or slower than the average. Nevertheless the total sample version was the best forecast to use. Figure 9–6 shows the increases over time, with the total membership predicted to be 83,612 by the year 2000.

SUMMARY

This chapter has presented a portrait of ASHA affiliates, their numbers, their types, their demographic characteristics, their employment characteristics, and their earnings. From the presentation you can deduce that the typical ASHA affiliate is a female member who is a certified speech-language pathologist providing clinical services in a

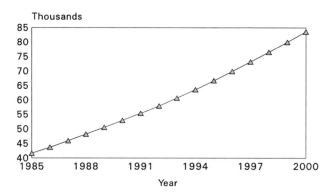

Note: ASHA data includes members and certificate holders for 12/85. The monthly counts have been corrected because dual certificate holders were counted in both speech-language pathology and audiology.

Figure 9–6. Predicted ASHA membership growth (50 states and Washington DC) from 1985 through 2000.

school facility and earning about $34,000 per year. Most of these professionals are married, work full-time, and have an average of 11 years' professional experience.

The membership of ASHA continues to grow annually and various methods can be used to forecast future membership. From a base year of 1985, an econometric model projected that the membership would increase 100% by the year 2000.

DISCUSSION QUESTIONS

1. Explain the reasons why two members calling the American Speech-Language-Hearing Association in the fall of any year might obtain different numbers in response to a question about the membership size of ASHA.
2. Create a demographic profile for a typical ASHA member.
3. Differentiate between the terms ASHA member and ASHA certificate holder.
4. Describe the employment characteristics of ASHA members.
5. Based on the information presented in the chapter, prepare an estimate of the size of ASHA affiliates in 4 years.

REFERENCES

American Speech-Language-Hearing Association. (1990). 1990 Omnibus survey. Unpublished data.

American Speech-Language-Hearing Association. (1993). *Legislative Council resolutions.* Rockville, MD: Author.

Shewan, C. M. (1988). *ASHA Work force study. Final report.* Rockville, MD: American Speech-Language Hearing Association.

Shewan, C. M., & Slater, S. C. (1992). ASHA's speech-language pathologists and audiologists across the United States. *Asha, 34,* 64.

Slater, S. C. (1992a). 1991 salaries on the rise for ASHA members. *Asha, 34,* 13–17.

Slater, S. C. (1992b). The 1992 Omnibus Survey: Portrait of the professions. *Asha, 34,* 61–65.

U.S. Bureau of the Census. (1990). Current population reports. (Series P-25, No. 1053). *Projections of the population of states by age, sex, and race: 1989 to 2010.* Washington, DC: U.S. Government Printing Office.

CHAPTER 10

Work Force Issues in Communication Sciences and Disorders

■ CYNTHIA M. SHEWAN, Ph.D. ■

SCOPE OF CHAPTER

Because members of a profession most often work in that profession, the concepts of membership and work force are related. Therefore, this chapter provides a logical sequel to Chapter 9 by describing the concepts and issues related to the work force in human communication sciences and disorders. Especially important are the concepts of supply, demand, and need. How they are measured is discussed because measurement differences create substantial variability in work force estimates, which, in turn, form the basis of predictions about future job availability in the marketplace.

The chapter continues with a discussion of factors that will affect employment in the professions in the next 10 years. Work force issues, such as predicted occupational growth, demand for services, and shortages are among these factors. Changes in the nature of services needed and, consequently, in the types of services providers needed are also presented.

DEFINITIONS

In a general sense, work force refers to the number of persons employed in a given occupation at a given time. Therefore, the work force in the discipline of human communication sciences and disorders is the number of people employed as speech-language pathologists and audiologists at a given time. As mentioned in Chapter 9, ASHA members represent just over half the entire scope of the professions. Taken together, ASHA and non-ASHA employed personnel constitute the work force. To arrive at a specific number requires counting, which turns out to be an even more complex task than counting the ASHA membership.

Views of the work force have varied. According to the Bureau of Labor Statistics (1974) current supply refers to the number of individuals working or seeking work in an occupation at a given time. Potential supply refers to the numbers of persons "qualified to practice the occupation whether actively practicing or not." (Bureau of Health Planning and Resources Development, 1976, p. 10). Because work force discussions refer to the concepts of supply, demand, and need, these terms are defined below from Shewan (1988).

Supply: The number of individuals working (employed) as speech-language pathologists and audiologists at a given time.

Need: Need refers to the amount of care that experts believe a person should have to remain communicatively effective or to become as communicatively effective as possible, based on current available knowledge.

Demand: Demand refers to the effective request for goods and services in view of their current costs. (pp. 2, 3)

Because these concepts may be unfamiliar, an example will illustrate their meaning. Demand refers to the amount of services people are willing to pay for at a specific price. Although this concept may not appear to be relevant to communication sciences and disorders, some reflection on the matter indicates that it really is. For example, if the economy takes a downturn, a decision may be made to cut certain services in a medical plan. If these cuts include speech-language pathologists' and audiologists' services, to obtain these services people would have to be willing to pay for them out-of-pocket. If the individuals themselves were experiencing economic hard times, they might not be able to afford the services and elect not to obtain them. This would represent a decrease in the demand for speech-language pathology and audiology services. Note that the services are still needed and available, that is, the supply and need are there, but not the demand. If the prices for these services were lowered and people then elected to obtain them, the demand for services would have increased. If service prices are low enough, thereby resulting in low salaries, individuals may not be attracted to the professions of speech-language pathology and audiology, and the supply of personnel would drop. With a drop in supply and a constant need for services maintained, the demand for services rises. As the demand increases, service providers may respond to the market place by raising their prices. If prices go too high, however, we could see a drop in demand. What should be evident is that the relationships among supply, price, and demand are dynamic and that price is the factor that determines the equilibrium between supply and demand.

SUPPLY IN THE WORK FORCE

To estimate the ASHA work force in the United States, you can add the segments of ASHA affiliates who are employed full-time and part-time, who are employed but on a leave of absence, and who work as volunteers. Table 10–1 shows that, using the year-end counts for 1992, this number is 62,905. Remember that this number includes both members and certificate holders. It does not include ASHA affiliates outside the United States, either residing in American territories or in the military abroad, or foreign members. By definition, it excludes those who are not employed and not seeking employment, those who are unemployed and searching for jobs, and those who are retired.

To represent the current active supply of the non-ASHA segment of the work force, the 1988 Work Force Study (Shewan, 1988) estimates were revised. Table 10–1 shows this estimate as 58,391. Adding the ASHA and non-ASHA segments gives a grand total of 121,296 in the current active supply.

This approach used a personnel count to arrive at an estimate of the work force supply. The U.S. Bureau of the Census also uses a personnel count to estimate the work force in communication sciences and disorders. The Bureau of the Census derives its data from the Current Population Survey (CPS), which excludes military personnel, college/university teachers and administrators, and researchers (Table 10–2) (Rones, personal communication 1986).

However, not all groups use personnel counts for their supply estimates. The Bureau of Labor Statistics (BLS) uses a job count to estimate current active supply. BLS counts those in all industries (educational services, hospitals, other health services) and the self-employed. It does not include college/university teachers and administrators. Using the data from the PL 94-142 counts of budgeted positions for speech-language pathologists, teachers of those who are speech impaired, and audiologists, provides another estimate of the work force supply in education. Adjusting this figure for noneducational employment can provide another estimate of supply in the work force. These estimates and the comparative data for 1984 and 1986 are shown in Table 10–2.

TABLE 10–1. CURRENT ACTIVE SUPPLY.

	ASHA[a]		Non-ASHA	
	Percentage	*Number*	*Percentage*	*Number*
Employed full-time	74.8	51,201	75.9	49,518
Employed part-time	15.6	10,678	11.3	7,372
Leave of absence	1.4	958	2.3	1,501
Volunteer	0.1	68	NA[b]	NA
Total	91.9	62,905	89.5	58,391

[a] Excludes foreign affiliates, ASHA affiliates in U.S. territories, and ASHA affiliates in the military abroad.
[b] NA = Not available.

TABLE 10–2. SPEECH-LANGUAGE PATHOLOGY AND AUDIOLOGY ESTIMATES OF CURRENT ACTIVE SUPPLY.

Source	*Characteristics*	*1984*	*January 1986*
ASHA	Personnel count Excludes nonmember and noncertificate holder category MA/MS entry level degree after 1965 (BA/BS group excluded 1965–present) Includes counts in many work settings and activities	40,226	43,455
Bureau of the Census	Personnel count Includes clinical service providers Excludes military and college/university teachers and administrators Large standard error ±8,000	53,472[a]	57,764[a]
Bureau of Labor Statistics	Job count No adjustment for full-time equivalencies (FTE) Includes SLP/A service providers and researchers Excludes college/university teachers and administrators	51,381[a]	55,505
PL 94-142	Budgeted position slots FTEs Includes preschool, elementary and secondary schools only Excludes all other employment settings	62,363[a]	67,369[b]

[a] Figures have been adjusted to represent homogeneous populations.
[b] Figures represent the 1984 estimate brought forward to 1986, using the growth rate (8.02%) of the ASHA current active supply for 1984–1986.

DEMAND

Demand for service may be viewed as the amount of service requested at a given price of service. Demand, then, is affected by several variables, including the incidence and prevalence of communication disorders, cultural (demographic characteristics that affect utilization of services), and economic factors such as income, reimbursement source, and the value of the consumer's time (Shewan, 1988).

Although it is desirable to have a data source that represents demand nationally, no such data source exists for the discipline of human communication sciences and disorders. In the absence of such data, various measures of demand can be applied to those populations for which data are available. Several different approaches to estimating demand are described.

VACANCY RATES

Vacancy rates refer to the number of unfilled, budgeted positions relative to the total num-

ber of positions available. Vacancy rates have been used as an index of the inadequate supply of personnel to provide services. However, you are cautioned about how to interpret vacancy rates and that many questions surround what a vacancy really is. Perhaps the best use of vacancy rates is to track them across time. Their change can signal an alteration in job availability. However, factors such as geography and compensation level, aside from personnel shortages, can influence job availability.

In 1984, the U.S. registered and community hospital vacancy rates for speech-language pathologists and audiologists were 3.6 and 3.5%, respectively, compared with an overall hospital employee vacancy rate of 3.3%. By 1988, the full-time equivalent (FTE) rate for speech-language pathologists was 9%, with 7% being used as the threshold for shortage. This rate represented one of the five hospital personnel categories with the highest FTE vacancy rates (Bloom Kreml, 1989). The vacancy rates varied across the nation: 11

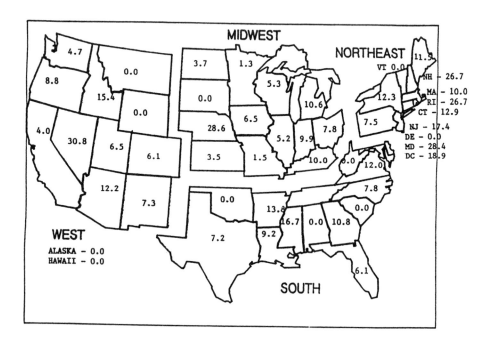

Source: From Survey of Human Resources, American Hospital Association, 1988.

Figure 10–1. Hospital vacancy rates (in percentages) by states and region.

states reported vacancy rates of 0%, with 5 states reporting rates in excess of 25% (Figure 10–1).

Another source of vacancy information comes from the schools. When calculated for the 50 states and the District of Columbia, vacancy rates for personnel to serve persons who are speech or language impaired for the last several years have varied between 7.1 and 8.4%. Vacancy rates for speech-language pathologists were 8% in 1985–1986, 7.1% in 1986–1987, 8.4% in 1987–1988, 7.7% in 1988–1989, and 7.5% in 1989–1990 (U.S. Department of Education, 1988, 1989, 1990, 1991, 1992). Rates for audiologists were generally higher than those for speech-language pathologists: 13% in 1985–1986; 6.4% in 1986–1987; 13% in 1987–1988; 13.3% in 1988–1989; and 12.1% in 1989–1990.

Therefore, available data indicate that vacancies exist in schools and hospitals, which account for approximately 60% of ASHA members' primary employment facilities. Anecdotal reports suggest that vacancies exist in private practice settings and other facilities, although no quantitative data are available to provide an overall picture.

Vacancy rates may also be influenced by geographical factors. Hospital vacancy rates in 1988 were lowest in the North Central region of the West (3.2%) and highest in the New England region (12.9%) (Bloom Kreml, 1989). Therefore, positions may remain unfilled not because of a shortage of personnel but because of a maldistribution of personnel. Generally, positions in rural areas are more difficult to fill than those in larger urban and suburban areas. It is both harder to attract and retain personnel in these areas.

Vacancy rate is one indicator that a shortage of personnel in communication sciences and disorders exists. Another indicator is the increased demand for speech-language pathologists and audiologists in hospital facilities. In 1981, 3,855 full-time equivalent speech-language pathologists and audiologists were employed in U.S. registered hospitals. By 1988, this number was 5,937, representing a 54% increase. An even greater increase of 76.5% was seen in community hospitals (Bloom Kreml, 1989).

Another factor that may contribute to a reduced supply of professionals in communication sciences and disorders is the increased job opportunities in other professions for women, starting in the 1980s. During this period, salaries in other professions were higher than those in speech-language pathology and audiology, and this salary differential may have attracted potential speech-language pathology and audiology personnel.

PERSONNEL-TO-POPULATION RATIOS

Another approach to estimating demand is to use a ratio approach. In Chapter 9, Table 9–2 shows the personnel-to-population ratios by state, census division, and region for certified speech-language pathologists and audiologists. These ratios can be compared with a standard, a ratio representing an ideal balance between the personnel to provide services and the population to be served. In this method, available supply of personnel is assumed to be in equilibrium with demand and the ratio serves as a proxy for demand. There is no standard available; however, if the overall national ratio were adopted as a standard, then 20 states would undershoot this ratio and be deemed to have shortages.

Several problems surround using this method to estimate demand. Non-ASHA personnel are not included and their inclusion might alter ratios differentially across states. The national average may not represent an adequate or ideal standard. A state ratio may not accurately represent all regions of the state. The ratios do not take into account any changes in the productivity of personnel, which influences demand.

UTILIZATION OF SERVICES

Although several measures of utilization are possible, this chapter limits itself to a single method. How much service is utilized can be viewed as the realized or, effective, demand. 1992 year-end counts of ASHA affiliates indicated that 75.5% of full-time and part-time speech-language pathologists reported their primary employment function as providing clinical services. With a mean yearly caseload of 120 and 37,525 clinical service providers, the estimated total number clients served by speech-language pathologists is 4.5 million. Using the same approach for audiologists, 93.7% of whom work part-time or full-time, 74.7% of whom report their primary professional function as clinical service providers and who have a mean yearly caseload of 1,242, the number of clients served is estimated to be 8.4 million. Combined, almost 13 million persons annually utilize clinical services provided by speech-language pathologists and audiologists.

DECREASED SUPPLY

A decreased supply of personnel reduces the services available and creates a demand for the remaining services. Therefore, declining stu-dent enrollments in the communication sciences and disorders discipline could create a greater demand. Education and other "helping" professions experienced a decrease in the number of students enrolling in personnel preparation programs in the 1980s. Clearly, this was the case for communication sciences and disorders for the years between 1982–1983 to 1988–1989 when undergraduate and master's degree enrollments declined (Figure 10–2). However, the trend reversed in the 1990–1991 year, which reported increased student enroll-ments (Creaghead, Bernthal, & Gilbert, 1991). From the few years' data available, it would appear that enrollments wax and wane, some-times reducing supply and, in the face of increased demand, creating shortages. Other times, when demand is constant or declining, the reduced supply does not have the ultimate effect of creating a shortage. What is important to recognize is that supply and demand are related and how they vary from low to high describes various market place results. Figure

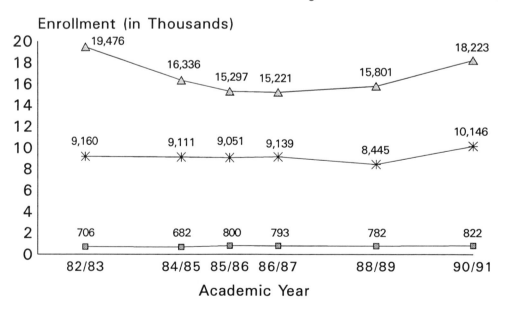

Source: From Creaghead, Bernthal, and Gilbert (1992).

Figure 10–2. Undergraduate, master's, and doctoral student enrollments for academic years 1982–1983 to 1990–1991.

10–3 shows that a shortage is created when supply is low and demand is high. Relative equilibrium is reached between supply and demand when both are low or both are high. A glut (oversupply) on the market is created when supply is high and demand is low.

NEED

Need for speech-language pathologists and audiologists is probably the concept most familiar to you. You hear about persons who need certain services and are not receiving them. Most frequently heard about these days are the needs of the uninsured or under-insured. They either do not have health insurance or have insufficient coverage. To examine the need for speech-language pathologists and audiologists, you can develop estimates by examining the prevalence and incidence of communication disorders, how much service a single speech-language pathologist or audiologist can provide, and determining how

many speech-language pathologists and audiologists are required to supply these services. In fact, this was what was done for the ASHA Work Force Study (Shewan, 1988). The figures have been updated to reflect 1992 population data and current speech-language pathology and audiology caseloads, respectively. Low, medium, and high estimates are provided to incorporate the wide variability in incidence and prevalence statistics reported in the literature. In addition, both average total yearly caseload sizes and reported productivity level methods have been used to estimate the number of full-time equivalent personnel required to serve the population with communication impairments.

Table 10–3 provides the need estimates for speech-language pathologists. As you see, the estimates vary greatly from a low of 24,977 to a high of 356,902. The medium estimate series, based on caseload size (88,900) and productivity levels (239,838), would appear to provide a reasonable estimate of current clinical service needs.

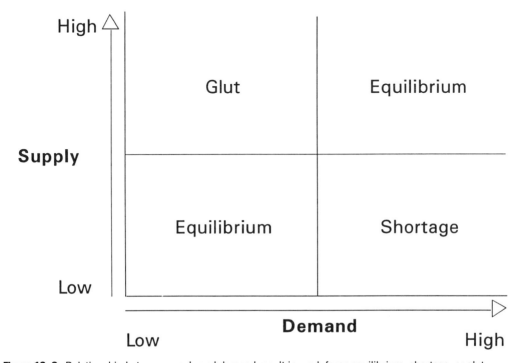

Figure 10–3. Relationship between supply and demand result in work force equilibrium, shortage, or glut.

TABLE 10–3. ESTIMATES OF THE NUMBER OF FULL-TIME SPEECH-LANGUAGE PATHOLOGISTS REQUIRED TO SERVE THE POPULATION WITH SPEECH-LANGUAGE IMPAIRMENTS.

Prevalence	Rate[a]	U.S. Population[b] (in millions)	Number of Speech-Language Impaired	Service Provision by One Speech-Language Pathologist[c]	Number of Full-time Equivalent Personnel Required
			Low Estimate Series		
Low	1.18%	254.0	2,997,200	120.00 cases/yr.	24,977
				44.48 clients/yr.	67,383
			Medium Estimate Series		
Medium	4.20%	254.0	10,668,000	120.00 cases/yr.	88,900
				44.48 clients/yr.	239,838
			High Estimate Series		
High	6.25%	254.0	15,875,000	120.00 cases/yr.	132,292
				44.48 clients/yr.	356,902

[a]The low prevalence rate is from Dawson & Adams (1987). The medium prevalence rate is from Fein (1983), and the high estimate is the rate reported by the National Advisory Neurological and Communicative Disorders and Stroke Council (1988), adjusted to include disorders that were omitted from their count.
[b]U.S. population figure is taken from U.S. Bureau of the Census, *Statistical Abstract of the United States: 1992* (112th ed.), Washington, DC, 1992.
[c]The cases per year data represented the average total yearly caseload size reported by speech-language pathology clinical service providers on the 1986–1987 Omnibus Survey. The numbers of clients per year was calculated by using a yearly productivity level of 0.50 [(37.5 hours per week × 0.50 direct clinical contact hours) × 52 weeks per year] and dividing by the number of service hours estimated for speech-language clients (21.92 or 43.83 one-half hour sessions). Refer to the Ohio Department of Mental Health Transmittal No. Sub. 3, January, 1983 for the productivity levels and to the Ohio PRSO Plan for Hearing and Speech Services Manual (1977) for the average number of visits for clients who are speech-language impaired.

Table 10–4 provides comparable need estimates for audiologists. As was the case for speech-language pathologists, the medium estimate series provides a reasonable estimate of the current clinical need for audiologists. Based on caseload size, the requirement is 27,609 audiologists versus 35,460 using a productivity level approach.

It is important to recognize that these figures represent the need for clinical service providers only and do not include the need for faculty in academic programs or researchers to increase the knowledge base on which the professions are based. For the interested reader, approaches to these estimates are found in the ASHA Work Force Study (Shewan, 1988).

FACTORS AFFECTING EMPLOYMENT PROSPECTS IN THE NEXT 10 YEARS

Those of you who are students and will enter the work force within the next few years are concerned about the prospects of employment. This section describes the predicted occupational growth, the demand for services, the nature of the services needed, and the suppliers of these services.

PREDICTED OCCUPATIONAL GROWTH

Although not listed among the 30 occupations with the fastest projected growth rates,

TABLE 10–4. ESTIMATES OF THE NUMBER OF FULL-TIME AUDIOLOGISTS REQUIRED TO SERVE THE POPULATION WITH HEARING IMPAIRMENTS.

Prevalence	Rate[a]	U.S. Population[b] (in millions)	Number of Hearing Impaired	Service Provision by One Audiologist[c]	Number of Full-time Equivalent Personnel Required
			Low Estimate Series		
Low	7.6%	254.0	19,304,000	1,242 cases/yr.	15,543
				967 clients/yr.	19,963
			Medium Estimate Series		
Medium	13.5%	254.0	34,290,000	1,242 cases/yr.	27,609
				967 clients/yr.	35,460
			High Estimate Series		
High	17.4%	254.0	44,196,000	1,242 cases/yr.	35,585
				967 clients/yr.	45,704

[a] The prevalence rates for hearing impairment were taken from Goldstein (1984) and are based on Singer, Tomberlin, Smith, & Schrier (1982) data using audiometric testing.
[b] U.S. population figure is taken from U.S. Bureau of the Census, *Statistical Abstract of the United States: 1992* (112th ed.), Washington, DC, 1992 .
[c] The cases per year data represented the average total yearly caseload size reported by audiology clinical service providers on the 1986–1987 Omnibus Survey. The numbers of clients per year was calculated by using a yearly productivity level of 0.50 [(37.5 hours per week × 0.50 direct clinical contact hours) × 52 weeks per year] and dividing by the number of service hours estimated for hearing impaired clients (975 or 975 one hours visits). 1986–1987 Omnibus data revealed that 74% of audiologists' time was spent in evaluation sessions on the whole averaging approximately 47 minutes. Based on the assumption of one evaluation per client per year, 962 clients would be seen in one year. The remaining 26% of audiologists' time was devoted to treatment, with a visit averaging 40 minutes in length. Based on an average of 74 visits per year for aural rehabilitation, reported in the Ohio PRSO Plan for Hearing and Speech Services Manual (1977), 5.11 clients could be accommodated. This would bring the total to 967.11 clients per year for each audiologist.

speech-language pathology and audiology are expected to grow more rapidly (medium estimate of 34%) than the average for professional specialty occupations (32%) between 1990 and 2005. Two factors related to this predicted growth are the greater demand predicted for workers with higher levels of education and the generally high growth predicted for the health services professions (Silvestri & Lukasiewicz, 1992).

DEMAND FOR SERVICES

Several factors will impinge on the professions of speech-language pathology and audiology to affect the demand for services. The aging of the population and its increased longevity will increase the need for services.

You will recall that the prevalence of communication disorders is greater in the older segments of the population. This especially affects the audiology profession because the prevalence of hearing loss among the elderly is high. For speech-language pathologists, the increases from aging stem primarily from neurogenic communication disorders, especially stroke and dementia. (See Chapter 12 by Lubinski and Masters on special populations.)

Substance abuse in America also creates a greater demand for speech-language pathology and audiology services. In the younger population, fetal alcohol syndrome is one of the leading causes of mental retardation and is associated with auditory disorders and learning disabilities. Infections, such as human immunodeficiency virus (HIV), the virus that causes Acquired Immune Deficiency

Syndrome (AIDS) and cytomegalovirus, are linked with communication disorders. To the extent that these diseases increase, there will be an associated increase in the need for speech-language pathology and audiology services. (See Chapter 21 by Lubinski on infection prevention.)

From 1985 to 1990, the number and rate of births increased in the United States. Concomitantly, the number and rate of infant deaths decreased, as did the total death rate. These statistics combine to produce a large population, which, based on constant incidence figures for communication disorders, predicts greater numbers at risk for communication disorders and greater numbers requiring services (U.S. Bureau of the Census, 1992).

At the time of this writing, health care reform proposals were being debated at state and national levels. If speech-language pathology and audiology services are included in state or national plans, to the extent that people are not receiving services currently, the demand will increase. If services are not included or are included in a limited way, the demand for services may decrease because the public will be unwilling or unable to pay for these services out-of-pocket.

SHORTAGES

Taking an economic approach to the work force, it is apparent the work force is a dynamic entity. Therefore, you cannot expect it to remain the same from year to year or that a situation of 5 years ago will apply today. The situation described in the ASHA Work Force Study (Shewan, 1988) has changed. Shortages are now described that were not present then. Although no national data representing all work facilities exist and no one indicator definitely indicates a shortage, several sources of data discussed earlier suggest this is the case. Over the past few years, vacancy rates in hospitals have risen dramatically and the number of speech-language pathology and audiology professionals employed in rehabilitation facilities has grown. The marketplace will need to be carefully monitored to deter-

mine the length and regularity in supply cycles. Perhaps, then, some prediction for the situation 10 years hence will be possible.

NATURE OF SERVICES NEEDED

With the advent of PL 99-457, provision of special services in the schools expanded to include infants and toddlers (0 to 2 years) and preschoolers (3 to 5 years). Although the effect is not dramatic, this law resulted in a shift from service delivery by hospitals and private practices to the schools.

Immigration trends are also having a dramatic impact on the schools. With increased immigration, the school system is faced with educating increasing numbers of students with limited proficiency in English and with communication disorders in their native language, which is not English. This situation has created a great demand for professionals who can provide services in languages other than English. These service providers also need to be sensitive to the cultural differences in these populations as well as the language differences. The situation was recently summarized by Shewan and Blake (1992):

If the past 5 years are compared, the rate at which minorities have been entering the professions of audiology and speech-language pathology has not equalled the growth rate of the nation's minority population (2.9%). The difference in these rates creates a larger gap between the professional population available to deliver services and the population in need of these services than is present for the nonminority population. This gap is likely to increase further for Asian and Hispanic minority groups because most of their growth is not as a result of increased birthrate but primarily attributable to immigration (Vobejda, 1991). (p. 76)

Serving the older population will require the services of speech-language pathologists and audiologists with expertise in treating the geriatric population. Service delivery will occur in a variety of settings. If the trend to community-based care continues, provision of home health services will grow. The increase in the population 85 years and older will necessitate increased services in nursing homes because this population segment is most likely to be ill and unable to live independently. The trend of discharging patients earlier will shift care from hospitals to a variety of other institutions, such as skilled nursing facilities, hospices, intermediate care facilities, and so forth.

SERVICE PROVIDERS

Employment prospects will be affected by the numbers of persons qualified to provide services in communication disorders as well as the number of jobs available for these persons. For ASHA, qualified providers refer to certified speech-language pathologists and audiologists. As you have seen, the number of these professionals has been increasing over the past few years. Whether there is an adequate number of these professionals is a complex question addressed earlier in this chapter.

The types of providers in greatest demand by employers will be persons who have the competencies necessary to provide services to the elderly, the birth to 5-year population, and multilingual/multicultural populations. This does not mean that other providers will not be required, for they most certainly will. What it does mean is that providers with these qualifications will be especially in demand and may have the ability to be selective in their employment choices.

SUMMARY

Because most professionals in speech-language pathology and audiology work within the professions, the concepts of membership and work force are related. The chapter described supply in the professions as well as demand for services and the role that price of services plays in balancing supply and demand. When the need for professionals to serve persons with communication disorders was estimated, even the lowest estimates exceeded the available supply. However, it is idealistic to think that these needs will ever be totally met, given the economic climate and the attempts to contain health care costs.

Although speech-language pathology and audiology are not among the fastest growing occupations, they are predicted to grow more rapidly than the average for professional specialty occupations for at least the next decade. Demand for services is likely to increase because of both a growing and aging population, increased substance abuse, and a rise in maternal infectious diseases.

Service provision will change due to the disproportionate growth in minority populations from both increased birth rates and immigration, especially for the Asian and Hispanic minority groups. Professionals who are competent to provide services to the very young, the geriatric, and multilingual/multicultural populations will be the best positioned to compete in the marketplace.

DISCUSSION QUESTIONS

1. Explain the differences between the terms *need* and *demand* as they relate to the ASHA work force and give an example to illustrate.
2. What are some indexes of a personnel shortage and how might a shortage affect the work force?
3. Describe three factors that will affect the future employment of speech-language pathologists and audiologists.
4. Explain why estimates of supply differ depending on the source used for the estimate.
5. How might using a state vacancy rate for speech-language pathologists in hospitals be misleading to a local community health official?

REFERENCES

Bloom Kreml, B. (1989). *Survey of human resources—1988: A report.* Chicago, IL: American Hospital Association.

Bureau of Health Planning and Resources Development, U.S. Department of Health, Education, and Welfare. (1976). *Methodological approaches for determining health manpower supply and requirements: Volume I. Analytical perspective* (DHEW Publication No. HRA 76-14511). Washington, DC: U.S. Government Printing Office.

Bureau of Labor Statistics, U.S. Department of Labor. (1974). *Occupational supply: Concepts and sources of data for manpower analysis* (Bulletin No. 1816). Washington, DC: U.S. Government Printing Office.

Creaghead, N. A., Bernthal, J. E., & Gilbert, H. (1992). *1990–91 national survey of undergraduate and graduate programs*. Minneapolis, MN: Council of Graduate Programs in Communication Sciences and Disorders.

Dawson, D. A., & Adams, P. F. (1987). *Current estimates from the National Health Interview Survey: United States, 1986* (Vital and Health Statistics, Series 10, No. 164, DHHS Pub. No. [PHS] 87-1592. National Center for Health Statistics. Public Health Service). Washington, DC: U.S. Government Printing Office.

Fein, D. J. (1983). The prevalence of speech and language impairments. *Asha, 25*, 37.

Goldstein, D. P. (1984). Hearing impairment, hearing aids and audiology. *Asha, 26*, 24–35.

National Advisory Neurological and Communicative Disorders and Stroke Council. (1988). *Decade of the brain*. Report submitted to Congress.

Ohio Council of Speech and Hearing Executives PSRO Task Force. (1977). *Ohio PSRO plan for and speech services manual.*

Ohio Department of Mental Health Transmittal No. Sub. 3. (1983).

Shewan, C. M. (1988). *ASHA Work Force Study. Final report.* Rockville, MD: American Speech-Language Hearing Association.

Shewan, C. M., & Blake, A. (1992). Demographic characteristics of minority, nonminority ASHA affiliates. *Asha, 34*, 76.

Shewan, C. M., & Slater, S. C. (1992). ASHA's speech-language pathologists and audiologists across the United States. *Asha, 34*, 64.

Silvestri, G., & Lukasiewicz, J. (1992, May). Outlook: 1990–2005. Occupational employment projections.

Monthly Labor Review. Washington, DC: U.S. Government Printing Office.

Singer, J., Tomberlin, T. J., Smith, J. M., & Schrier, A. J. (1982). *Analysis of noise related auditory and associated health problems in U.S. adulthood 1971–75* (Vols. 1 and 2) [Prepared under contract to the Environmental Protection Agency]. Springfield, VA: National Technical Information Service.

U.S. Bureau of the Census. (1992). *Statistical abstract of the United States: 1992* (112th ed.). Washington, DC: U.S. Government Printing Office.

U.S. Department of Education. (1988). *Tenth annual report to Congress on the implementation of the Education of the Handicapped Act.* Washington, DC: U.S. Government Printing Office.

U.S. Department of Education. (1989). *Eleventh annual report to Congress on the implementation of the Education of the Handicapped Act.* Washington, DC: U.S. Government Printing Office.

U.S. Department of Education. (1990). *Twelfth annual report to Congress on the implementation of the Education of the Handicapped Act.* Washington, DC: U.S. Government Printing Office.

U.S. Department of Education. (1991). *Thirteenth annual report to Congress on the implementation of The Individuals with Disabilities Education Act.* Washington, DC: U.S. Government Printing Office.

U.S. Department of Education. (1992). *Fourteenth annual report to Congress on the implementation of The Individuals with Disabilities Education Act.* Washington, DC: U.S. Government Printing Office.

U.S. Department of Health and Human Services. (1986). *Trends in hospital personnel, 1982–1984* (ODAM/report No. 9-86). Washington, DC: Bureau of Health Professions.

Vobejda, B. (1991, June 12). Asians, Hispanics giving nation more diversity. *The Washington Post*, p. 3.

■ CHAPTER 11 ■

Preparing for Employment

■ ROSEMARY LUBINSKI, Ed.D. ■

SCOPE OF CHAPTER

Professional employment is the natural culmination of several years of academic coursework and clinical practicum in your area of specialty. This chapter discusses how to undertake the important process of obtaining employment in a productive manner. The chapter begins with a discussion of the paths a career in speech-language pathology or audiology may take. The body of the chapter focuses on how you can research potential work settings, prepare a resume and cover letter, interview effectively, and accept a final offer. The chapter concludes with a discussion of how to approach a change in employment settings.

CAREER DEVELOPMENT

The search for professional employment as an audiologist or speech-language pathologist is actually the beginning of a career development ladder. An exciting and challenging aspect of becoming a communication disorders professional is that there are many settings in which to work, a variety of types of clients across the age span, and numerous opportunities for branching upward and outward within the professions. Although many of you will remain in your first professional position, it is likely that for a variety of reasons you will move vertically within your profession into supervisory positions, change jobs within your field to a different setting or client population, become self-employed, or continue your education and move into academia, research, or management. A small percentage of you will switch to a related field such as education or medical administration or take time off for family care. In a study of career development characteristics within our professions, Shewan (1987) found that only 5% of professionals took extended leaves of absence after entering and working in the field for a time. Shewan also reported that a vast majority of individuals (94.5%) were employed in their chosen field, and more than 80% worked full time.

This high rate of employment likely reflects the number of positions available throughout the United States. According to the Research Division of the American Speech-Language and Hearing Association (ASHA) (1992), there is about a 9% vacancy rate for hospital positions and as much as a 25% vacancy rate in school settings in some states. In a workforce study done by ASHA (Shewan, 1989), it was predicted that the need for speech-language pathologists and audiologists will "continue to grow and to outstrip supply in the near future, at least to the year 2000" (p. 63). Professionals in communication disorders tend to remain in their positions and change jobs on an average of every 5 years. Shewan (1987) states that, "employment stability provides for continuity in the workplace, an environment conducive to continuous development, and a committed work force" (p. 29).

JOB SEARCH

SELF-ASSESSMENT AND JOB ANALYSIS

Finding and securing the best job involves a series of steps. The first phase begins with a self-assessment of skills, motivations, and constraints. This is followed by an analysis of potential employment settings. Job candidates who know themselves and their target agency are better able to market themselves to a potential employer.

Self-analysis

The search for employment is affected by personal, economic, and job availability factors. Some of you are restricted geographically in the job search because of family reasons, personal preference to remain in a particular area, or limited finances to support a relocation. Others may live in areas that have few available work settings, lack opportunities to complete a Clinical FellowshipYear (CFY), or have no appropriate positions available when you are ready to be employed. Such factors may necessitate a move. Some new graduates

may have a commitment to a sponsor of personal graduate education to work in a particular setting or area.

The search for first employment begins with answering several critical questions:

1. What is my career goal at this time? What do I see myself doing in the field of audiology or speech-language pathology in 3, 5, and 10 years?
2. What type of setting(s) and clientele attracts me at this time?
3. How does my immediate career goal affect my long-range career aspirations?
4. What special experiences and skills do I have that will make me attractive to employers of desired settings?
5. What special skills and experiences would I like to acquire?
6. What geographic areas are attractive to me as sites of employment?
7. What employment settings in those areas match my career goals?
8. What personal, economic, and job availability factors limit my search for employment either in my home area or in a relocation area?
9. What personal, economic, and job availability factors enhance my opportunities to seek employment away from my home area?

During serious consideration of these questions and others that arise during this prejob analysis stage, some geographic areas and settings will naturally be eliminated. For example, one person may feel that options to relocate are limited until a fiancé completes law school. Another person may feel the need to work in an area geographically close to a frail and elderly mother. Some of you may have few personal restrictions regarding relocation, but lack the finances needed to support a move to another area, to meet the costs of housing in that particular area, or simultaneously to repay outstanding loans while incurring the costs of relocation. Some of you may be willing to incur financial debt to pursue an especially challenging and professionally fulfilling position in a desired setting, with a special population, and in a geographically ideal area. Yet others of you may literally be in the "right place at the right time."

Targeting a Position

As this prejob, self-analysis reveals your employment options, certain settings and geographical areas will emerge as best suited for you at this point in your career. The next step is to learn more about the reality of meeting individual personal employment goals in those settings and areas. This can be done in several ways. A first and basic resource in the early preemployment search is to discuss career goals and personal assets and limitations with graduate faculty. Both academic and clinical faculty are likely to be aware of the scope of positions that match a job seeker's goals. In addition, through their participation in local, state and national organizations and committees, they may know of positions available beyond the immediate area of the college or university setting. A similar discussion with off-campus graduate practicum supervisors may reveal present or potential employment opportunities. Although many times these individuals will not know of specific positions available in other areas, they may know of professionals in those areas who could be of assistance. This is called "networking" and is an invaluable means of entry into the professional world. Such discussions with faculty and supervisors will also be helpful to these individuals in writing recommendations.

A second source of employment opportunities includes the employment listings in journals, bulletins, and newspapers, such as *Asha*, the monthly journal of the American Speech-Language-Hearing Association; *Advance*, a biweekly publication for speech-language pathologists and audiologists in health care settings; listings offered by local and state professional organizations; special employment bulletins posted in an academic department; national newspapers such as the *New York Times* (Sunday edition); and community newspapers. Each year at the annual convention of the American Speech-Language-Hearing Association there are special oppor-

tunities to peruse employment listings, list one's name under "Employment Wanted," and meet with potential employers on-site. Similar employment opportunities occur at conventions of state speech-language-hearing associations and meetings of other professional organizations, such as the American Academy of Audiology. Be sure to review the employment section of professional journals in related areas such as education, physical therapy, occupational therapy, and hospital administration. Job seekers interested and prepared for a position in academia might review possible listings in the *Chronical of Higher Education*. Finally, listings of governmental job positions are available through individual state departments of labor and the U.S. Civil Service Commission. See the Resource Section at the end of this chapter for more sources of employment.

A third option for identifying employment in a target geographic area is to do some preemployment research on settings that match your goals and skills. For example, if you are interested in working in an acute care hospital in Chicago, check that area in a listing of settings accredited by the Professional Services Board of ASHA; obtain a list of hospitals accredited by the Joint Commission on Accreditation of Healthcare Organizations; the directory of hospitals published by the American Hospital Association or your state health department; contact the local professional organization for a listing of hospitals; obtain lists of hospitals from the local Chamber of Commerce; check the Sunday edition of major metropolitan newspapers for position announcements; and finally inspect the listings of hospitals in the telephone book. An excellent resource is the *Guide to Professional Services in Speech-Language Pathology and Audiology* published by ASHA (no date).

Yet a final option for seeking potential employers is to join with a search firm. Not common in the field of communication disorders, particularly at the entry level, this is a more likely avenue for professionals seeking high-level clinical administration positions and those willing to change geographic areas. Two types of search firms are available: those that work specifically for you and those that are retained by client hospitals or agencies to fill specific vacancies. Should you choose to work with a search firm, it is prudent to have all details regarding expectations and results in writing prior to any payment for this service. It is also wise to consult with an attorney or the Better Business Bureau before signing a contract with a search firm.

Preemployment Research

Doing some preemployment research on potential employers will be invaluable in clarifying career goals, preparing a resume, and asking for references to tailor recommendations to a potential employment setting. The primary goal of this research is to optimize a match of a job seeker's skills, experiences, and career objectives with the particular institutional and departmental objectives, programs, and needs. This research begins by making a list of standard questions to be answered about each setting so that a careful analysis of options can be made. Some areas to include on an analysis sheet are:

1. Name of setting
2. Address
3. Telephone number of setting, personnel department, and communication disorders department
4. Specific name of person(s) heading the communication disorders department
5. Number of positions currently filled in the communication disorders department and number of openings
6. Description of the communication disorders program—such as pediatric head trauma, adult neurogenic disorders, central auditory processing disorders, and so on.
7. Gaps in the program that you could fill— such as assessment of patients with dementia, dysphagia assessment and treatment, instrumental procedures to assess respiratory and laryngeal functioning, hearing aid assessments, balance system assess-

ment, augmentative communication system selection and training, and so on.
8. Availability of a CFY position with the necessary supervision to meet ASHA certification or state licensure requirements

Although it will not be possible to visit all potential employers for a preapplication visit, inspection of the analysis sheet should reveal several settings that match your goals, skills, and experiences and that potentially have available positions. You may be able to arrange an "informal" site visit of these settings, thus giving more opportunities to know how to tailor an eventual cover letter and resume to that particular institution (Baker, 1989). The site visit may also help eliminate the setting as a potential place of employment.

These site visits have a dual objective: you discover more about the program and the program representative begins to know more about you as a potential job candidate. Even in times of economic constraints on communication disorders programs, there may be potential employment opportunities. It is essential to call ahead and make an appointment with the director/co-director of the communication disorders program, the director of rehabilitation, or the director of the specific division in which the communication disorders program is located. In educational settings the director of speech-language pathology or the director of pupil personnel services is the likely professional to interview. In some very large settings communication disorders may be located in more than one branch of the setting, for example, in some hospitals speech-language pathology may be located in outpatient rehabilitation, neurology, and/or ENT; in educational settings, communication disorders may be a separate program or subsumed under special education, special services, or some other department. Audiology may be associated with speech-language pathology, ENT, or rehabilitation. You should never arrive unexpectedly and after the visit you should send a typed thank-you letter to the host.

Continued Self-analysis

After selecting a list of potential employers, you need to continue your preemployment self-analysis. This will involve objective, critical consideration of assets and deficits versus the skills needed to work successfully in the target setting(s). For example, should visitation to a large metropolitan hospital reveal that 50% of the current case load is dysphagia and you have no academic or clinical experience in that area, this setting should be eliminated as a potential place of employment or continuing education and further experience in that area should be sought. Although potential employers generally realize that few applicants, particularly those entering their Clinical Fellowship Year, can be prepared in all areas, they will want to hire someone who can best fulfill the job requirements with minimal immediate on-the-job training.

At this point, you have identified through advertisements, networking, or site visits a number of agencies that are potential employment settings. This is the time to prepare a cover letter and resume.

COVER LETTER

Your cover letter is equally important as the resume in marketing yourself to a potential employer. This is the *first* impression an employer has of you as a job applicant and is a powerful tool in sparking interest in the resume. A well-prepared cover letter and resume are instrumental in obtaining an interview—the situation in which you actually "sell" yourself. Beatty (1989) maintains that the cover letter reflects an applicant's motivation, organization, and knowledge about the agency. Employers may use the cover letter as a critical screening device even before reviewing a resume. Considerable time should be spent in the preparation of each individual letter. Beatty (1989) in *The Perfect Cover Letter* says that you will have between 20 and 40 seconds to attract the employer's attention and stimulate interest in the resume.

Detailed suggestions for preparing the cover letter can be found in numerous publications, in a library or book store, and also in materials found in a college or university's career planning and placement office. These suggestions can be divided into those focusing on style and content. Because this business letter is highly critical in projecting you as a potential employment candidate, spend **extra** time in ensuring that it is "**letter perfect**." See Appendix 11A for a sample letter.

STYLE SUGGESTIONS

1. Confine the letter to 1 page.
2. Professionally type the letter or work with a word processor to guarantee that the layout and design are stylistically appropriate for a business letter.
3. Use good quality 8.5 × 11-inch, neutral-color bond paper and matching envelopes.
4. All letters should be original—never duplicated—copies.
5. Use appropriate business letter style, for example, full block style: return address, date, agency address, salutation, body of letter, closing, signature, and typed name.
6. Each letter should be personalized to the specific person who is responsible for making hiring decisions in your target department. Be sure to have the correct full name, spelling, title, and address.
7. Address the person by the appropriate title, such as Dr., Mr., Mrs., Ms.
8. Check, then check again, for typographical, grammatical, and spelling errors.
9. A copy of all letters should be kept and filed appropriately.

CONTENT SUGGESTIONS

Generally, the letter contains 3 or 4 paragraphs:

Paragraph 1 introduces the applicant, states the target position, how the applicant learned of the position, and excites the reader about this potential employee.

Paragraph 2 focuses on the applicant's experiences and assets and how these might meet the needs of the target department. This is the applicant's opportunity to highlight how he or she can enhance the organization.

Paragraph 3 is the "action" section in which the applicant requests an interview, tells the employer to expect a call to arrange an appointment for an interview at a convenient time, and states a willingness to provide additional information. Applicants should mention when they are available for an interview and how they can be reached.

The final paragraph offers appreciation for considering the letter and resume.

RESUME

The resume or curriculum vitae is the second important tool for marketing you to a potential employer. For job seekers entering first professional employment, this document will be an initial presentation of their academic and clinical background. Experienced professionals will need to review and update their resumes regularly to ensure that career developments such as additional clinical or administrative responsibilities, teaching, and supervision are captured. Eubanks (1991) states that a resume should be readable, truthful, and polished. Focus is on both functional and chronological information. Again, as in the cover letter, the suggestions for preparing a resume can be divided into style and content suggestions. Many bibliographic resources are available for more in-depth suggestions, and some are presented at the end of this chapter. Finally, the resume should reflect you as an individual and not be a sterile, dull document. Several drafts may be necessary until one clearly, concisely, and creatively reflects you, the job seeker.

STYLE SUGGESTIONS

1. Some job applicants may want to work with a commercial resume preparation expert to enhance resume style. Job applicants should research and clarify the scope of services provided and all expenses. The work done by someone else reflects only on the job applicant, not the preparer.

2. The resume should be limited to one or two pages, particularly for individuals entering the field. Persons with extensive experience **may** require more space.

3. Preparation of an outline helps to organize the major information to be presented. The major words of the outline become the bold headings of the resume. These headings easily alert the reader to important information.

4. A consistent chronological format should be used to present the history of education and employment. The advantage of listing the most recent data first is that the reader knows immediately where the applicant is and present qualifications.

5. A resume must be "readable" (Eubanks, 1991). This means that type is of appropriate size, there are 1-inch margins on all sides, headings are in bold or all-capital type to focus the reader, and indentations are used to separate information.

6. Prudent use of varying typefaces is crucial. Headings should stand out, but not distract the reader.

7. A resume that is dense with information prevents the reader from quickly scanning the document and finding information.

8. The resume must be checked several times on separate days for typographical, grammatical, spelling, or content errors.

9. Someone else should proofread the resume for both style and content. Good people to do this include faculty and supervisory staff, a college or university's career planning and placement office, previous employers, and colleagues. Check a grammar book or dictionary for additional help.

10. High quality, neutral, 8.5 × 11-inch-paper, as in your cover letter, should be used. Unusual colors should be avoided as a means of attracting attention.

11. All copies prepared by commercial duplicating should be checked carefully. Ink

smudges and torn or missing pages reflect negatively on the job applicant.

CONTENT SUGGESTIONS

Identification Section: The first section of the resume should include identifying information including name; current and permanent address; telephone number for the applicant to be reached during business hours of job search time; and business address and telephone number if appropriate to be contacted at that setting.

Job/Career Objective: Resources differ as to whether a career objective should be included in the resume or the cover letter. Many potential employers feel this is very important. If this is included it should briefly but generically and comprehensively describe the type of position desired. It should be no longer than two sentences.

Education: List in chronological or reverse order earned degrees, full name of college or university where obtained, city and state, and dates.

Experience or Work History: This section lists relevant paid professional positions or, in the case of new entrants to the workforce, practicum positions. The purpose of this section is to describe the quantitative and qualitative results of each accomplishment. For example, employers are interested in programs developed, revenues generated, and individuals served. Information can be presented in chronological or reverse order: dates of employment/participation, setting name and address, and job title. The candidate should list job duties, highlighting special components of the program; for example, development of a kindergarten language screening program in an inner city public school, implementation of an in-service program on hearing problems of elderly residents for nursing staff, and so on.

Publications: Any published books, monographs, chapters, or articles should be included here with full bibliographic referencing as seen in professional journals or what is commonly

referred to as American Psychological Association (APA) format. This is the place to include the title of dissertations or theses.

Honors: Included here are professional or academic awards or scholarships/traineeships.

Presentations: This section focuses on presentations to professional associations, including title, name of conference, date, location, and whether invited or competitive.

Professional Affiliations: This segment of the resume lists the name(s) of any professional local, state, national, or international associations to which the applicant belongs. Included also are special roles in such organizations, including committee chairing, conference organizer, and so on.

References: The job applicant must decide ahead of time if references will be provided on request from individuals or included in a "College Credential File." Only the name of persons who have given explicit approval can be listed on the resume. Recommendations for obtaining references will be discussed later in this chapter.

Personal Data (OPTIONAL): Resources differ on whether to include personal information such as age, ethnic background, marital status, number of children, and so on. On the positive side, this information reflects the job applicant more personally and often is the "ice breaker" during an eventual interview for the employer. Conversely, such information may be used to discriminate in subtle ways. This is a good topic to discuss with a faculty advisor or supervisor prior to preparing the final version of the resume.

LETTERS OF RECOMMENDATION

Students and even professionals may be unsure of who serves as a good reference for employment and how to go about securing that recommendation. Good written or oral recommendations are essential in separating one from many other applicants with similar or even superior backgrounds. In choosing references, you should consider what the employer wants to know. Although employers are interested in academic achievements, they are more interested in clinical and personal characteristics. Through these letters the employer should see a well-rounded, multidimensional person. Employers want to know the following types of information:

1. Do you have the professional skills to carry out the target job? What professional or student experiences do you have that will support these statements?
2. What particular professional skills do you have? How have they been exhibited? How have these skills enhanced your present employment/practicum?
3. What will you be like as a professional? Employers want to know about your ability to communicate orally and in writing, your reliability and punctuality in completing tasks, your ability to initiate without direction, your creativity, and your commitment to your position.
4. What is your self-initiative growth potential? Do you demonstrate a sense of independent career development, such as attendance at workshops, creative problem solving, participating in journal groups, and so on.
5. How flexible are you? Are you eager to grow professionally and learn new skills? How have you demonstrated these characteristics?
6. What are your communication skills like with families, for example, parents, spouses, or children of patients?
7. What will you be like as a colleague? Are you appropriately assertive? Do you know how to work on a team? How well do you take direction and criticism?
8. What are you like as a person? Some reference to family or personal background helps the potential employer know you better.

Thus, applicants need to carefully consider both the number and types of individuals who can serve as personal references. Students entering the employment field for the

first time generally rely on academic and clinical faculty as well as outside placement supervisors. It is advantageous to have a balance of academic faculty and clinical supervisors who can reflect on both professional and personal skills. Generally, most applicants have between three and five references. "Family or friend" type references who attest to your positive qualities, but who have no credibility as a professional reference, should never be submitted.

Be prepared when approaching someone to be a reference. This involves calling ahead and, if necessary, making an appointment to discuss reference needs. You should provide the individual with a copy of (a) your cover letter, (b) your resume, (c) name of target agency(s) and intended individual(s) to whom the reference should be sent, and (d) a brief description of the target position(s). This information helps to individualize the reference letter for a particular agency. Students should generally include a listing of courses taken with a professor, grades earned in those courses, and overall grade point average. Clinical supervisors might like to see copies of semester clinical evaluations. This is the time to accentuate clinical and academic accomplishments.

If you are using a college or university's career placement reference forms, these should be given to your reference person. These forms usually have a place for the applicant to waive the right to seeing the reference. If you are asking for letters to individual employers, provide typed names, full addresses, and stamped envelopes. Applicants must discuss forthrightly if the reference person is prepared to offer a positive recommendation. A note of appreciation should be sent to those offering a letter of recommendation.

Job applicants, who are not currently in a college setting but who wish to ask an academic or clinical faculty member for a recommendation, may need to "refresh" the individual's memory. This can be done by describing courses taken or clients seen with the faculty member and any special experiences with that individual. Potential employers are most interested in information relevant to the target position.

Similarly, professionals seeking new employment may find it difficult to obtain references for several reasons. First, the applicant may not want supervisors or colleagues to know about potential change of jobs. Second, colleagues may not be in a position to comment on all of your skills. Other sources of recommendations include former employers and other supervisory staff with the proviso that the current job search be kept confidential. If at all possible, references should be sought from your current supervisor, or you should be prepared to discuss in an interview why this information is not available.

INTERVIEW

PREINTERVIEW

Preparation for the interview is critical. This is when you really have the opportunity to sell yourself to a potential employer. Review of the preapplication analysis is essential along with information gathered from professors, supervisors, colleagues, or friends. Such an information base provides you with confidence to make knowledgeable and constructive comments about the program.

You should critically review your clinical assets and deficits with a mind to the target position, leading to a clear concept of what you can or cannot do. Be prepared to answer questions about these areas in a pressure situation. Edis (1989b) states that overestimation of abilities is likely to encumber, although "openness about your faults may also suggest that you are a self-aware and honest person" (p. 55). You must be prepared to articulate how your skills and experiences can match or enhance the target position and setting. Although you do not want to present yourself as a false master of all skills, this is not the time to assume that the employer knows your special skills and assets.

Role-playing with a fellow student or colleague is an excellent preparation and desensi-

tizing strategy (Davis, 1989). Role-playing gives you an opportunity to "think on your feet" and answer questions that might never be considered otherwise. It also gives you an opportunity to prepare questions for the employer during the interview. Your questions reveal a great deal about your preparation, interest in the position, and insight into the programs of the agency.

Video- or audiotaping the simulated interview provides opportunities to review and refine problem areas. On the other hand, you do not want to be so "programmed" for the interview that you appear robot-like and cannot easily adjust to unexpected questions. The interviewer is trying to get a sense of how you think, problem solve, and relate to people. Below is a list of potential questions for role-playing. This list is not exhaustive, but the very act of role-playing both the employer and interviewee is likely to generate more questions.

POSSIBLE QUESTIONS FROM EMPLOYER

1. What are your primary professional interests? What clinical populations are you interested in? How did you develop these interests?
2. What are your long-term career goals? Where do you see yourself in 5 years? 10 years?
3. Why are you interested in the position of _____?
4. What types of clinical skills do you have that will fulfill this position?
5. How would you plan an assessment for _____?
6. What intervention methods do you find appropriate for a _____ case?
7. Tell me about your writing skills.
8. What would you do if . . .? Have you ever . . .?
9. In what ways might you make a contribution to our agency?
10. Tell me about your most recent job? Why are you leaving it?
11. What is your salary requirement?
12. What questions do you have for me?

POSSIBLE QUESTIONS TO EMPLOYER:

1. What are the responsibilities of this position?
2. How does this position fit into the overall goals of the agency?
3. Is the position permanent? What happens at the end of the CFY?
4. How is the agency or department funded? How stable is this funding?
5. What type of team programs are included in the agency or department?
6. How is patient scheduling handled?
7. To whom would I report?
8. What problems might I encounter with this position?
9. Does the agency have a continuing education program? Is there an education budget for each person?
10. What opportunities are there for advancement within this department?
11. Can you tell me about benefits? (This includes vacation, sick time, pension plans, health care benefits, child care options, and flexible time.)

You should be prepared to discuss salary expectations. For new and even experienced professionals this may be an uncomfortable area. Other professionals in the target geographical area may provide data on beginning or range of salaries. New employees are not likely to get salaries above the average for that position and geographical area. Individuals with more professional experience need to factor in their experience and expectations. Be sure to impress the employer of your value and worth before you enter into salary negotiations.

Finally, consider how you will successfully present yourself during the interview. It is critical to project an image of professionalism and competence. This involves tasteful classic clothing, shoes, and accessories and immaculate personal grooming. It is best to dress conservatively in a suit (skirted for women) and to avoid conspicuous colors, patterns or fragrances.

Before the interview you should check the location of the agency, parking availability or needed travel and time arrangements. A 10-to 15-minutes early arrival gives you time to refresh, introduce yourself to the receptionist, review materials about the agency, or complete further application forms provided at that time. All of these preparations for the interview will give you a sense of confidence to participate in the interview in a meaningful and positive manner.

INTERVIEW

The interview should be perceived as a conversation, dialogue, or information exchange between you and the employer. Consideration has already been given to the cover letter, resume, and letters of reference; so this is your opportunity to convince the employer that you are the best person for the job and will "fit in" to the culture of the program. Krannich and Krannich (1990) state that impressions made of the applicant during first 5 minutes of the interview are *critical* in obtaining the position.

The interview will progress through stages. The first part of the interview usually consists of a few preliminary remarks or "chit-chat" comments focusing on the weather, travel to the interview, common personal interests, and so on. This leads to the opening questions from the interviewer that may focus on: "Why are you interested in this position?" Another direction an interview may take is to encourage you to talk about why you are interested in speech-langauge pathology or audiology and your relevant experiences. Some interviews may begin with the most open of comments "Tell me about yourself." The underlying agenda of the questions focuses on answering the questions: What kind of person are you and what kind of employee will you be? Edis (1989a) states that interviewees should be aware of the style of questions being presented and the focus of the interview. Do the questions tend to be open and allow you a great deal of freedom to answer? Are the questions closed, requiring yes or no responses with little room for elaboration or explanation? There may be some "leading questions" that suggest the expected response such as "how would you deal with a confrontational mother during an interview?"

Applicants should be aware that employers are not allowed by federal law to ask personal questions such as age, health, marital status, children, child care needs, and religion. "To be legally acceptable a question has to be related to the job and asked of all candidates, irrespective of sex" (Edis, 1989a, p. 47). You should be prepared to deal with such questions, however, because they may occur in both direct and indirect ways. For example, during the preliminary informal remarks, questions about personal life may appear in innocuous ways. Applicants should tailor their answer to their own advantage by discussing the job-related quality the interviewer is seeking. Unfortunately, not answering such a question may be subtly held against an applicant.

During the interview you should be sensitive to your own and the interviewer's nonverbal behavior. Interviewers will be aware of eye contact, body posture, gestures, tone of voice, and rate of speech. Firmly shaking the interviewer's hand on entrance along with clear articulation of the person's name, tends to make a positive first impression. Active listening skills during the interview are also essential. You need to pay attention to both the overt question and what may be the underlying message. The interviewer expects appropriate feedback through nods and smiles and relevant responses and questions. This is not the time to let one's mind wander away from the topic or situation.

WHAT IS THE INTERVIEWER EVALUATING?

According to ASHA's (no date) manual *How to Achieve Success in Your Job Interview*, the interviewer is assessing an applicant's (1) mental effectiveness, (2) motivational characteristics, (3) personality strengths and limitations, and (4) knowledge and experience. In addition to being professionally competent and a critical problem solver, the *ideal employee* is honest, responsible, stable, confident, enthusiastic, accepts direction but relies on self-evaluation, friendly, and expresses ideas clearly, precisely, and sensitively. You are being evaluated as much on personal skills as on professional knowledge base and experience. Employers are likely to have numerous equally qualified applicants for a position, and thus, in addition to strong clinical skills, the interviewer will be searching for the best fit: an employee who will blend with existing staff and capably implement the agency's goals. The employer wants to hire an individual who will enhance the organization and will search for the individual who comes as close to the ideal as possible. The employer is seeking to determine not only professional interests and skills, but also longevity as an employee and desire for promotions. Having significant career aspirations, increases an applicant's value as an employee. Thus, your goal is to project these qualities.

END OF INTERVIEW

The closing of the interview gives you an opportunity to express appreciation for the interview and briefly summarize your strengths as they relate to the target position. This is when you tell the interviewer where and when you can be reached for further discussion about the position. For example, a student's permanent address may be more useful than a college address. Currently employed applicants must tell the employer the best methods for correspondence. For example, this applicant may want to give a home phone number, for a message to be left on a telephone message machine. This method allows the applicant to return the phone call from a convenient location and time.

POSTINTERVIEW FOLLOW-UP

Within a week after the interview you should send a typed thank-you letter to your interviewer. Again, appropriate business letter style should be used on 8.5 × 11-inch good quality bond. This letter gives the applicant a chance to express appreciation for the interview, to renew interest in the position, to briefly restate major qualifications, and to explain any unresolved issues raised during the interview. Allen (1992) suggests that if an applicant has not heard from the employer within 1 week of sending a follow-up letter, a telephone call to the interviewer is appropriate. You should prepare for this telephone call as carefully as you did for the interview through practice, role playing, and analysis of tape recordings. This call shows that you are sincerely interested in the position and willing to go a step further to obtain the job. Monday is not a good time to make such a call as it tends to be the busiest day of the week. Should the interviewer state that the position has been given to someone else, express appreciation for the interview and solicit future consideration.

SECOND INTERVIEW

In some agencies a second (or third) interview will be offered to those candidates who appear most qualified for the position (sometimes called the "short list"). It is likely that the applicant will be called to schedule this appointment. This interview may be with the program director or another individual in an administrative capacity in the organization. For example, when applying to an educational setting, the applicant now may be interviewed by the director of pupil personnel services or director of special education; in a hospital , the meeting may be with the director of rehabilitation or the head of Otolaryngology. In some cases, the second interview will also include an opportunity to meet either formally or informally with a select group of current employees.

FINAL OFFER

Once the decision to hire an applicant has been made, a formal offer will be made. Although many offers will be made by telephone, a written offer is essential. Tammelleo (1989) states, "To avoid misconceptions, disappointments or possibly even a lawsuit, get the job offer in writing " (p. 74). The written offer should explicitly state the title of the

position, the period of employment, the duties expected, the salary, steps for salary increments, the beginning date of employment, the benefits package, and any other conditions of employment. Such conditions include supervision of the Clinical Fellowship Year, necessary certifications or licensure, preemployment physical, employee evaluation procedures, continuing education opportunities, and expectations. Some of this information will be presented in an employee manual or handbook. Details presented in this document serve as an agreement between the newly hired individual and the agency (Allen, 1992). The more you know about conditions of employment, the easier it will be to make an informed decision regarding acceptance or rejection of that position.

Consider the offer for a few days (not too long) before accepting. An offer should be accepted with a sense of confidence that this is the best position and that all aspects of the position are clear. You might discuss the position and offer with respected colleagues or individuals who wrote your letters of recommendation. Issues to consider at this time include quality of life in the environment in which you will live and work, challenges inherent in the position, and opportunities for advancement and continuing education. These factors become even more important when an applicant receives more than one offer.

After you have accepted an offer, a thank-you letter should be sent to those individuals who wrote letters of recommendation. Krannich and Krannich (1990) also suggest that applicants periodically keep in contact with these individuals, because they may be helpful in a future career move.

ADVANCEMENT

Once employed, you may find that opportunities for advancement are possible within the current program, within the larger organization, or even within other settings. Individuals become aware of available positions through professional publications, networking, or direct solicitation to apply for a position. Advancement can take the form of moving upward to positions of more direct program responsibility such as supervisory roles, or it can be laterally in which the individual remains in a similar position but has new responsibilities. For example, in some programs, individuals may become team leaders or have special duties such as coordinator of student practica. Advancement both vertically and laterally can be challenging and contribute to a more fulfilling career.

Before advancement, some basic questions arise. What duties does the new position entail? What are prerequisite technical and personal skills and credentials for fulfilling the position? Will the new responsibilities be positively challenging or constitute a professional or personal burden? Will the prestige or financial reward be adequate to compensate for increased or new responsibilities? For example, if you might be promoted to a position that requires considerable travel, would this be possible in your current lifestyle? What personal accommodations would need to be made to fulfill this position successfully?

Should an advanced position be attractive, the application process will be similar to that already described in this chapter: preapplication analysis, preinterview preparation, interview(s), and final offer. A major difference in seeking an advanced position within a present organization is that the interview will be with familiar individuals. Careful preparation is no less important for the long-time employee of the organization. In some cases, a current employee may be competing with individuals from outside the organization whose credentials and experiences are equal to or superior to your own.

CHANGING EMPLOYMENT

An employee may decide to change employment settings for any number of reasons. These include job loss, relocation, unreasonable demands in current position, lack of opportunities for professional growth, infrequent raises, boredom or burnout, lack of employer appreciation, or readiness to assume new or increased responsibilities associated with a different position (Raudsepp, 1990). Regardless of the circumstances, the suggestions for securing employment remain the same. There are, however, some special questions you will need to consider.

The new job search may begin while you are employed at an agency, or the process may begin after resignation from a position. Securing a new position while currently employed presents some challenges. If you are presently employed, you may not want your employer to know that a job search has begun. Should the job search become public, how will this knowledge affect your current position? How available can you be for interviews? Should you feel that you do not want your current employer to know about a potential move, options for references will change. You also must be prepared to take time off from work to attend an interview. In the case of a relocation or a mutually agreeable job change, your current employer will be the best possible reference in securing new employment.

In the situation in which a position has ended before beginning a job search, you again have to evaluate the helpfulness of a former employer. Target agencies will want to know the circumstances of why you left the last position and generally will want some reference from that employer. It is very important to consider that a current employer is the most important reference for the future, and, therefore, conditions under which the applicant leaves should be positive—"a graceful exit "(Kroner, 1989). A present employer must receive sufficient notice of termination, usually 4 weeks, all work should be summarized for a successor, and client reports must be completed. Some applicants offer to help train a replacement. How a departure is handled can positively or negatively affect the tone of future references from the employer.

For applicants who have been unemployed for an extended time, the prospective employer will want to know why and how you have kept your clinical skills up to date. Applicants need to provide clear, concise, and honest answers to these questions. All attempts should be made to redirect the interviewer to the applicant's interest in and qualifications for the present position.

SUMMARY

The focus of this chapter has been on how to secure employment. Key concepts in the chapter include "know thyself," "research," "networking," "preparation," "practice," "style," and "follow-up." Securing fulfilling employment is a deliberate process that begins with self-evaluation and employment setting research. These analyses allow a job applicant to tailor and prepare the cover letter and resume-marketing tools that hopefully will solicit an interview. Careful preparation for the interview gives confidence and helps to project a winning image. Contacts made during interviews can serve as networks for future career moves. Securing employment can be considered a challenging experience that results in a fulfilling contribution to our profession and society.

DISCUSSION QUESTIONS

1. What are the steps involved in securing a meaningful job?
2. What are the hallmarks of a good cover letter and resume?
3. What are the key ingredients in a successful interview?
4. How should you follow up after an interview with an employer?
5. What are the differences in the job search process for someone seeking first employment versus an experienced professional?

RESOURCES FOR SECURING EMPLOYMENT

Check your local library or bookstore for the section on Employment or Business. There are dozens of texts on topics such as interviewing, resume preparation, follow-up methods, and so on.

Most college or university departments receive notices of job vacancies. These may be posted or available in a department administrator's office. Check your local communication disorders department for such information.

The monthly publication *Asha* has a section on employment opportunities.

For Your Life After Graduate School is published by ASHA and describes the job market in communication disorders, resources, and resume and interview preparation. ASHA also publishes a manual entitled *How to Achieve Success in Your Job Interview*. Contact ASHA, 10807 Rockville Pike, Rockville, MD 20852.

ASHA Employment Referral Service. Contact the Membership and Career Development Division at ASHA or call ACTIONLINE 800-638-6868 for information about assistance available for seeking employment.

The *Guide to Professional Services in Speech-Language Pathology and Audiology* (American Speech-Language Hearing Association, no date) lists the names, addresses, and telephone numbers of most nationwide facilities, with the exception of public schools, and the names and addresses of key state education and health agency persons.

Federal Government Uniformed Services Positions. For information about employment through the U.S. Public Health Service, contact the U.S. Public Health Service Recruitment, Suite 600, 8201 Greensboro Drive, McLean, VA 22102. 800-221-9393.

REFERENCES

Allen, J. (1992). *The perfect follow-up method to get the job*. New York: John Wiley.

American Speech-Language-Hearing Association. (no date). *How to achieve success in your job interview*. Rockville, MD: Author.

American Speech-Language-Hearing Association. (no date). *Guide to professional services in speech-language pathology and audiology*. Rockville, MD: Author.

American Speech-Language-Hearing Association. (1992). *1992 Update on personnel shortages* (prepared by Research Division). Rockville, MD: Author.

Baker, J. (1989). Preparing a curriculum vitae. *Nursing Times, 85*, 56–58.

Beatty, R. (1989). *The perfect cover letter*. New York: John Wiley.

Davis, W. (1989). Simulated job interviews as learning devices. *Academic Medicine, 64*, 438–439.

Edis, M. (1989a). The interview: 2. Games people play. *Nursing Times, 85*, 45–47.

Edis, M. (1989b). The interview: 1. Rules of the game. *Nursing Times, 85*, 54–55.

Eubanks, P. (1991). Experts: Making your resume an asset. *Hospitals, 65*, 74.

Krannich, C., & Krannich, R. (1990). *Interview for success*. Woodbridge, VA: Impact Publications.

Kroner, K. (1989). Take the gamble out of changing jobs. *Nursing, 20*, 111–118.

Raudsepp, E. (1990). Knowing when to look for a new job. *Nursing, 20*, 136–140.

Shewan, C. (1987). Some characteristics of career development in the speech-language-hearing profession. *Asha, 29*, 27–29.

Shewan, C. (1989). ASHA work force study. *Asha, 31*, 63–67.

Tammelleo, A. D. (1989). Ways to pin down an employer's promise. *Registered Nurse, 52*, 74–78.

APPENDIX 11A: Sample Cover Letter

1134 Prescott Avenue
Amherst, NY 14260
November 15, 1993

John Adams, Ph.D.
Director, Audiology Services
Buffalo Rehabilitation Center
436 Main Street
Buffalo, NY 14226

Dear Dr. Adams:

I am writing to apply for the position of audiologist that was listed in the November 1993, issue of the *Asha* journal. I am very much interested in this position and would appreciate your consideration as a candidate. I have recently completed my Clinical Fellowship Year at the Veterans Administration Medical Center in Batavia, New York, and have met all requirements for both ASHA Certification and New York State licensure.

During my master's degree program at the University at Buffalo, I had clinical experiences with a wide variety of adult and pediatric clinical cases, including basic tests, central auditory processing, hearing aid assessment and fitting, and interoperative monitoring. I also had the opportunity to develop a hearing screening program for a local senior citizens' facility.

While at the Veterans Administration Medical Center, I was responsible for hearing evaluations and hearing aid assessments and fittings on all inpatients and residents of the long-term care facility associated with the medical center. I presented the results of my nursing home hearing screening program to the regional association of audiologists and at the annual convention of the American Speech-Language-Hearing Association in 1992.

I believe that I am well-qualified for the position of audiologist in your agency and would appreciate an opportunity to meet with you during a personal interview. I can be reached at 716-699-5555 during the day or at 716-384-5555 during evening hours.

Thank you for your consideration. I hope to be hearing from you in the near future.

Sincerely,

John Adams, M.S.

APPENDIX 11B: Sample Resume

RESUME

JENNIFER PATTERSON

23 Fairview Drive
Buffalo, NY 14226
(716) 666-5555

EDUCATION:	State University of New York at Buffalo, Buffalo, NY; M.A. in Speech-Language Pathology, 1993.
	Cornell University, Ithaca, NY; B.A. in Spanish and Linguistics, 1990.
PROFESSIONAL EXPERIENCES:	**Speech-Language Pathologist** at Greenville Elementary School Buffalo, NY; March–June 1993.
	Conducted communication assessment and remediation services for preschool and early elementary children with severe language and speech disorders. Developed an in-service program for classroom teachers on how to use facilitated communication with children who have autism.
	Speech-Language Pathologist at Language Center, Niagara Falls, NY; September–December 1992.
	Provided assistive communication assessments for children aged 2–10 with severe neurological impairments. Responsible for parent program entitled "Using Communication Technology at Home."
	Speech-Language Pathologist at University at Buffalo Speech-Language and Hearing Clinic; September, 1991–August, 1992.
	Provided comprehensive diagnostic assessments and therapy for adults with aphasia, motor speech disorders, voice disorders, and stuttering. Assisted with intensive 6-week school-age language/learning disabilities summer program. Participated in hearing screening program at Amherst Senior Facility.
	Communication Assistant at Summer Fluency Program for Adults at University at Buffalo Speech-Language and Hearing Clinic; June–August, 1991.
	Assisted certified speech-language pathologists with social programs associated with summer fluency program. Transcribed and analyzed videotaped conversations of fluency clients using the SALT program.
PROFESSIONAL MEMBERSHIPS:	National Student Speech-Language and Hearing Association; Speech-Language and Hearing Association of Western New York
PRESENTATIONS:	Patterson, J., & Murphy, G. (1993, April). *Using communication technology at home: A program for parents.* Paper presented at the annual convention of New York State Speech-Language and Hearing Association, Rochester.
SPECIAL TALENTS:	Fluent in Spanish, French, and German
REFERENCES:	Will be sent on request.

CHAPTER 12

Special Populations, Special Settings: New and Expanding Frontiers

■ ROSEMARY LUBINSKI, Ed.D. ■
■ M. GAY MASTERS, Ph.D. ■

SCOPE OF CHAPTER

Many of you were attracted initially to the profession of speech-language pathology or audiology by an interesting, gratifying, or perplexing experience with an individual who had some type of communication problem such as stuttering, aphasia, or hearing loss. One of the truly remarkable features of your professional work is the broad scope of individuals and communication problems encountered as well as the settings in which you exercise your professional and personal skills. Today, not only do speech-language pathologists and audiologists work with traditional clients in educational and hospital settings, but also with clients who have an extended range of communication difficulties in a wide spectrum of agencies and programs. Audiologists and speech-language pathologists have carved out new and challenging

roles with clients from infancy to old age. In addition, rapid technological advances related to communication disorders and current and proposed changes in health care funding further affect how you serve your clients. Therefore, this chapter will introduce you to *some* of the client populations served and special settings in which speech-language pathologists and audiologists provide these services. This introduction should expand your professional horizons to possibilities beyond the more traditional ones. For example, although not covered in this chapter, other special populations that receive innovative communication services include those with multiple sensory impairments, the severely communicatively impaired, recipients of cochlear implants, and users of assistive communication devices. The chapter begins with a discussion of several special populations you may serve as an audiologist or speech-language pathologist. It then turns to a description of three special settings: nursing homes, home health care, and private practice. It is important to remember that, although these populations are discussed as separate entities, in reality there are numerous special subgroups created when the groups overlap, such as the person who is elderly and of a linguistic minority with trauma or dysphagia and the child who is learning disabled from a rural/remote area.

SPECIAL POPULATIONS

THE ELDERLY

Perhaps the fastest growing group of potential clients whom audiologists and speech-language pathologists will serve in the next 20 years are those above 65 years of age. In 1991 there were almost 32 million individuals 65 years of age and older in the United States, constituting 12.5% of the population (*Statistical Abstracts of the United States*, 1992). By 2040 there will be more than 69 million elderly persons representing close to one quarter of the population (Brock, Guralnick, & Brody, 1990). Elderly individuals 85 years and older are among the fastest growing age group and are evidence of the greatest number of physical, sensory, psychological, and emotional changes affecting on communication. The increases in the older population are "unprecedented" in United States history and should continue until at least the middle of the next century (Brock, Guralnick, & Brody, 1990).

Ninety-five percent of the elderly reside in the community (*Statistical Abstracts of the United States*, 1992). "Few statistics are available regarding the incidence or prevalence of speech disorders among the elderly in the community. Fein (1983) estimated that there would be about 1 million older individuals in 1990 with a speech problem, most likely related to stroke, progressive neurological disorders, and laryngectomy. The prevalence of communication problems among older individuals living in the community with dementia is undocumented.

Statistics compiled through the National Health Interview Survey for 1989 reveal that hearing impairments rank number three behind arthritis and hypertension as a chronic condition among the elderly individuals residing in the community (*Statistical Abstracts of the United States*, 1992). The prevalence rate of hearing impairments was 23% for those 65–74 years of age, 33% for those older than 75 years, and 48% for those older than 85 years. The prevalence of hearing loss was consistently higher for males as compared with females (Brock, Guralnick, & Brody, 1990). Epidemiological studies conducted by Gallaudet University predict that by the year 2015, there will be 13 million elders with a hearing impairment (Bebout, 1989). According to National Institute on Aging estimates (1987) at least 11,800 audiologists will be needed in 2015 to serve the hearing needs of the elderly.

The remaining 5% of the elderly reside in long-term care facilities. In 1985 this percentage translated to about 2 million individuals in about 25,000 nursing homes and related care facilities (National Center for Health Statistics, 1989). Residents of such facilities tend to be very old, with an average age of 82 years. Women, usually widows, outnumber men 2 to 1. Most residents are white, reside in the nursing home for at least 1 year, and will die there. A majority have four or more chronic disabilities, are mentally impaired, and are nonambulatory.

Again, current and reliable statistics regarding the number of nursing facility residents with communication problems are scarce. Mueller and Peters (1981), in a study of the prevalence of communication problems in Wisconsin nursing homes, found that approximately 60% of the population had a communication problem. In a retrospective study of the types of communication problems referred to the speech-language pathology department in a nursing home, O'Connell and O'Connell (1978) found that the most frequent problems included aphasia, dysarthria, oral and verbal apraxia, laryngeal pathology, confusion, and impaired memory. More current studies would likely indicate that dysphagia (swallowing disorders) constitutes a high proportion of the case-load in many nursing facilities. Schow and Nerbonne (1980) found that 70 to 90% of nursing facility residents had some degree of hearing impairment. A discussion of the communication services offered in this setting is given later in the chapter.

In 1988 the American Speech-Language-Hearing Association (ASHA) published a position paper regarding the roles of the speech-language pathologist and audiologist in working with older persons. These roles include those related to provision of speech-language pathology services, professional roles associated with working with older clients, and adaptations needed in assessment and treatment to meet the needs of the elderly. Delivery of services may go beyond traditional approaches and focus on assessing the physical and psychosocial environment (Lubinski, 1981,1991; Lubinski, Morrison, & Rigrodsky, 1981), providing in-services to family members and facility staff (Koury & Lubinski, 1991), counseling elders and their families, utilizing new individual and environmental communication technology, and increasing involvement with other clients such as those with dementia.

HIGH-RISK INFANTS AND TODDLERS

About 2% of the more than 3.7 million children born in the United States each year have disabling conditions (*Statistical Abstracts of the United States*, 1992). Public Law (PL) 99-457, passed in 1986, formalized a previously recognized need to provide services for the very young, those from birth through 2 years. It also mandated services under PL 94-142 for 3- to 5-year old children. PL 99-457 mandates that, beginning in 1993, states must provide services for children who have a recognized developmental delay in one of five developmental areas or who have a diagnosis typically associated with a developmental delay. States have the option of providing services for children who are at-risk for a developmental delay.

Children may demonstrate or be at-risk for demonstrating a developmental disorder in one of the following areas: cognitive development, physical development (including vision and hearing), communication development, social/emotional development, and adaptive development. According to the Language Subcommittee on Speech-Language Pathology Service Delivery with Infants and Toddlers (ASHA, 1989), communication disorders include delays in speech production and perception and receptive and expressive language, as well as oral-motor disabilities such as feeding. Numerous factors may contribute to a young child being considered at high risk for communication disorders, including medical conditions such as Down syndrome, biological factors such as low birth weight, respiratory distress syndrome, severe asphyxia, fetal alchohol syndrome, severe brain hemorrhage, and environmental factors such as teenage mothers and parents who are substance abusers or have emotional or mental disturbances.

PL 99-457 contains key provisions in the traditional areas of assessment, intervention, and consultation that challenge all health care-based and school-based professionals (Houle & Hamilton, 1991). All early intervention services must be comprehensive, multidisciplinary, culturally unbiased, community based, and family directed. These services are coordinated by state identified agencies that ensure all provisions are met. At least two disciplines pertinent to the child's known or suspected developmental delay must be involved in the assessment of the child, development of an Individualized Family Service Plan (IFSP), and provision of subsequent intervention services. Assessments must be conducted in a manner that is neither linguistically or culturally biased toward the child or family. Services must be provided within the child's community as defined by the family and often involve the child's home, day care setting and community based clinics. Services may be provided directly to the parent while the infant is still in a neonatal intensive care nursery. All aspects of the early intervention must recognize the role of parents and family members in a child's program.

The comprehensive nature of the assessments mandated by PL 99-457 has important implications for audiologists and speech-language pathologists. The ASHA (1991c) Committee on Infant Hearing has developed guidelines for the audiological assessment of infants and toddlers. The target population for audiologic evaluation includes (a) any child who fails a newborn hearing screening, (b) any child suspected by parent, primary caregiver, educator, or physician as having a hearing loss, (c) any child who exhibits abnormal auditory behavior or delayed speech and language development, and (d) any child not previously screening but who identified as at high risk for hearing loss (p. 39). Rossetti (1991a, b) and others speak about the possibility of hearing loss in high-risk infants (low birth weight and extremely premature infants) due to medications and the high noise levels of neonatal intensive care units (NICUs).

Speech-language pathologists must evaluate infant-caregiver interaction, in addition to the traditional areas of speech and language, as many of these children may have decreased language stimulation because of extensive stays in the NICUs. Communication specialists must also focus their assessments and intervention on the family, function with other team members, and plan for any transitions to other services as needed. Crais and Leonard (1990) suggest that these areas should be primary goals of professional training programs and continuing education.

INDIVIDUALS WITH LANGUAGE-LEARNING DISORDERS

Individuals with learning disabilities have been referred to by a variety of labels through the years, including "childhood dysphasia," "minimal brain dysfunction," and "dyslexia" (Wallach & Liebergott, 1984). Indeed,we now know that many children who were first treated for speech and language disorders later were found to have learning disabilities (Aram & Nation, 1980; Maxwell & Wallach, 1984). In 1982, ASHA began to use the term **language learning disorder (LLD)** (ASHA, 1982b) and adopted the 1981 National Joint Committee for Learning Disabilities (NJCLD) definition of a

learning disability (ASHA, 1982a). The NJCLD (1991) definition clearly identifies language as an underlying component of a specific learning disability for most children:

A disorder in one or more of the basic psychological processes involved in understanding or in using language, spoken or written, which may manifest itself in an imperfect ability to listen, think, speak, read, write, spell, or do mathematical calculations. (p. 18)

The prevalence of children considered to be learning disabled has increased since the implementation of PL 94-142. In 1983–84 there were 1.8 million children whose primary classification was learning disabled as compared to 800,000 children in 1976–77 (Hyman, 1985). These children generally receive services through their school district under the provisions of PL 94-142. The label has important implications for services, because children labeled "learning disabled," rather than the ASHA-recommended "language learning disordered," may be overlooked for language intervention (Cornett & Chabon, 1986; Wallach & Liebergott, 1984). Because of the importance of language for an individual with LLD, speech-language pathologists are encouraged to take an increasingly greater part in the educational programming for these children (Cornett & Chabon, 1986).

School-age children with LLD typically have academic difficulties, often first identified as a problem with reading decoding and/or comprehension (Cornett & Chabon, 1986). Word-finding difficulties, where a child has the vocabulary knowledge but often is unable to produce the word, are common, particularly with children who have reading difficulties (cf. German & Simon, 1991). Catts (1991) portrays the decoding problem as one of poor metaphonological awareness, although other speech-language pathologists have identified metalinguistic deficits, in general, as factors in comprehension difficulties (Wallach & Miller, 1988). Young children may demonstrate difficulties in recognizing the metapragmatics of the classroom (Wilkinson & Milosky, 1987). Older children show problems with deriving inferences from reading passages and often fail to recognize figurative language (Wallach & Miller, 1988). In addition to the specific language difficulties noted, children with LLD may have central auditory processing disorders that limit their ability to function in the classroom (Chermak & Musiek, 1992).

As can be seen in the above description, LLD is primarily a problem of academic performance and will be most significant in a child's classroom. Language assessment and intervention practices must include classroom information and procedures, in addition to direct individual pull-out services. The classroom model is most commonly called "collaborative consultation" and may incorporate observation, team conferences, and clinician facilitation through modeling or direct teaching. Silliman and Wilkinson (1991) describe this approach in detail, and the clinical forums in the July, 1990 and October, 1992 issues of *Language, Speech and Hearing Services in Schools* and the November, 1993 issue of *Topics in Language* provide extensive information on designing and implementing collaborative consultation.

PERSONS WITH MENTAL RETARDATION AND DEVELOPMENTAL DISABILITIES

As with individuals with LLD, persons with mental retardation have been referred to by a variety of labels over the years. As recently as the 1950s individuals with varying degrees of mental retardation were referred to as morons, idiots, imbeciles, and cretins (Mac-Millan, 1977). Institutionalization was a common practice; education and training were thought unnecessary, and communication intervention was thought to be inappropriate. The 1970s heralded the beginning of significant changes in practice that are still occurring. Again, PL 94-142 was the catalyst for much of this change, as it ensured the educational rights of all individuals with handicaps.

Mental retardation is defined as "significant subaverage general intellectual functioning existing concurrently with deficits in adaptive behavior, and manifested during the developmental period" (Grossman, 1983, p. 1).

Degrees of deficit range from mild (IQ range 52–68) to moderate (IQ range 36–51) to severe (IQ range 20–35) to profound (IQ below 20). Prevalence of mental retardation in the United States ranges from 1 to 3% of the general population, or more than 2.5 million individuals. The majority of these persons (about 89%) are considered mildly mentally retarded (Owens, 1993). The term "developmental disability" is often used instead of mental retardation, and many professionals are encouraging us to refer to this group as "cognitively challenged."

Initial communication intervention with the mentally retarded began by the 1970s and grew out of the application of behavior modification principles (cf., Bricker & Bricker, 1970). As a result of this focus, emphasis was placed on linguistic form and content; however, intervention has evolved to encompass use of language, or pragmatics, as well (McLean, McLean, Brady, & Etter, 1991). Current trends in intervention encourage the incorporation of the individual's natural environment (home, school, work setting) and naturally occurring communication partners including caregivers, teachers, peers, and work supervisors. This trend is often called functionalism (Mire & Chisholm, 1990; Owens, 1993).

Speech-language pathologists begin working with individuals with mental retardation as soon as they are identified through early intervention programs. Some individuals, such as those born with Downs syndrome, are identified at birth. Other persons are identified as toddlers when developmental milestones are not reached within normal limits. Often the speech-language pathologist is the first professional, other than the child's physician, to assess the child. The speech-language pathologist's role, which begins under mandate of PL 99-457, continues through school age (21 years for individuals who are handicapped) under mandate of PL 94-142. After these individuals "age out," speech-language pathologists may continue to provide direct and consultative services to these individuals in sheltered workshops, day-treatment centers, and other work settings.

Audiologists also serve very important professional roles for individuals with mental retardation. When early speech-language and cognitive milestones are not met, a hearing loss is often the first suspected disorder. Assessment of hearing status of these persons is very challenging. In addition, many syndromes associated with mental retardation, such as Down and Treacher-Collins' syndromes and mental retardation caused by cytomegalovirus (CMV) have accompanying sensorineural or fluctuating conductive hearing losses. Amplification, for example, a hearing aid, may be recommended for children with Down syndrome who have chronic fluctuating conductive hearing loss (Northern & Downs, 1991).

Speech-language pathologists and audiologists working with persons with mental retardation continue to be challenged. The impact of early intervention, as mandated by PL 99-457, has barely begun. Early intervention is expected to change the educational and vocational outcomes of these individuals which, in turn, will alter our clinical approaches and expectations.

PERSONS WITH TRAUMATIC BRAIN INJURIES

One population that has received increased attention from speech-language pathologists is survivors of traumatic brain injury (TBI). Approximately 500,000 individuals sustain a head injury each year, and of these, 30,000 to 50,000 sustain severe injuries (Kalsbeek, McLauren, Harris, & Miller, 1981). TBI is the leading cause of death for those under 35 years of age (Kraus et al., 1984) and the third leading cause of death in the United States (Turnkey, 1983). Overall, the most common causes of TBI are motor vehicle accidents and falls. Recreational accidents rank high as a cause of TBI for school children with assaults as a major cause for young adults (Beukelman & Yorkston, 1991).

An individual who suffers a brain injury may display a wide spectrum of physical, behavioral, emotional, cognitive, and communicative difficulties due to the possible diffuse pathophysiology of the injury. Of particular interest to the speech-language pathologist are the highly related cognitive and language disabilities. Difficulties are likely to occur in attention, concentration, visual processing, language, memory, reasoning, problem solving and executive functions (Sohlberg & Mateer, 1989). Other difficulties that fall within the purview of the speech-language pathologist include motor speech disorders and dysphagia (Lazarus, 1991; Yorkston & Beukelman 1991). In addition, audiologists may assess both peripheral and central auditory functioning as sequelae of TBI. Many of these problems are manifest long after the original injury and impair successful return to school, work, and community activities. Finally, TBI has numerous negative effects on the individual's family and social network.

In general, interdisciplinary approaches to rehabilitation for individuals with TBI are the most effective. Team members include but are not limited to the speech-language pathologist, audiologist, neurologist, physician, physiatrist, neuropsychologist, physical therapist, occupational therapist, special educator, clinical psychologist, rehabilitation nurse, and vocational counselor. In 1987 ASHA's Subcommittee on Cognition and Language (ASHA, 1987b) proposed that the specific roles of the speech-language pathologist include assessment of cognitive–communicative impairments and a wide variety of treatment components such as determining client candidacy for therapy; planning and implementation of individual and group therapy; counseling patients, families, and professionals; recommending and training in augmentative devices; preparing reports; and research.

INDIVIDUALS WITH DEMENTIA

Dementia involves a decline in cognitive function and memory from previously attained intellectual levels and is sustained over a period of months or years. The decline is manifest in at least three of five areas of mental activity: (a) language; (b) memory; (c) visuospatial skills; (d) emotion or personality; and (e) cognition such as abstraction, calculation, and judgment (Cummings & Benson, 1983). Dementia in its many forms is estimated to affect about 4 million individuals, the majority being elderly (Cross & Gurland, 1985). The most common form of dementia is Alzheimer's disease and may affect as many as 10.3% of those over 65 years (Evans, Funkstein, & Albert, 1989). Although studies differ on the prevalence of dementia in the elderly population, two constants emerge. First, the number of individuals with dementia rises with increasing age. Perhaps as many as 47% of those older than age 85 have Alzheimer's disease (Evans et al.,9 1989). Second, the prevalence of dementia is higher for those residing in nursing care facilities than for those in the community. Katzman (1986) estimated that 65% of patients in a large geriatric nursing home in the New York City area had dementia. Autopsy studies confirmed that 55% showed pathologic evidence for Alzheimer's disease.

The changes in communication abilities for those with dementia have stimulated much interest from the field of communication disorders (e.g., Bayles & Kasniak, 1987; Grimes, 1991; Kempler, 1991; Lubinski, 1991; Ripich & Terrell, 1988; Weinstein, 1991). Numerous studies have been done to delineate the cognitive, language, motor speech, and auditory changes that occur with dementia as well as differential diagnosis of dementia from aphasia or changes associated with normal aging. The major language difficulties involve word knowledge and pragmatics, the use of contextually appropriate language (Kempler, 1991). Auditory changes may parallel the changes associated with aging, but also include changes in central auditory processing (Grimes, 1991). Such research has led to new roles for speech-language pathologists in the interdisciplinary diagnosis of dementia, including documentation of communication changes with disease progression, individual and environmental intervention approaches, counseling family members, and education of professional staff. Audiologists are challenged in their comprehensive assessment of hearing abilities in individuals with dementia. Speech-language pathologists and audiologists working in long-term care facilities, home health care, or even acute care hospitals need academic and clinical experiences with this population to provide effective and innovative service. Considering the rapidly multiplying number of elderly living well into their 80s and 90s, such professionals are likely to encounter increasingly complex cases, such as those with dementia.

UNDERSERVED POPULATIONS

One of the most socially important issues faced by speech-language pathologists and audiologists is whether we truly are reaching the wide variety of the individuals who need our service. In 1985 ASHA convened a National Colloquium on Underserved Populations and identified six populations for whom service may be a "luxury and not a service." These populations included (a) linguistic minorities such as Hispanics, Asians, and those with social dialects; (b) the economically disadvantaged; (c) the institutionalized in prisons and psychiatric settings; (d) those residing in remote/rural areas including Appalachia and Micronesia; (e) American Indians; and (f) those residing in developing regions (ASHA, 1985).

Linguistic Minority Populations

The influx of immigrants from Asia and Latin America in the last two decades underscores the need for communication disorders professionals to become highly sensitive to the special cultural and language issues of clients from linguistic minority. From 1980 to 1990 there was a 107% increase in the number of Asian or Pacific Islanders in the United States and a 53% increase in individuals of Hispanic origin (U.S. Bureau of the Census, 1990). These percentages translate to over 5 million Asians and 19 million Hispanics. In addition, there are about 80,000 Black immigrants to the United States each year from the Caribbean, South America, Africa, and Central America (Cole, 1989). When the number of legal and undocumented immigrants is added to those of other racial/ethnic minorities who may have different social dialects, the actual population of those who constitute a linguistic minority increases. This growth is expected to continue well into the next century with the number of minorities expected to increase to at least 79 million by the year 2080. By the year 2000 about one third of the school-age population will be Black, Hispanic, Asian, or American Indian (Cole, 1989).

Cole (1989) described eight multicultural imperatives that potentially affect audiology and speech-language pathology service delivery to this population. They include: (a) there will be more minorities with communication disorders; (b) more minority children are born at-risk; (c) there are different etiologies and prevalences of communication disorders among these populations; (d) the heterogeneity among these groups contributes to difficulty in establishing norms; (e) these populations have different cultural views on health and disorders; (f) there is more potential for cultural conflict in clinical settings; (g) there may be different service delivery preferences among minority groups; and (h) linguistic minority populations cannot be categorized automatically into racial/ethnic minority groups.

To help audiologists and speech-language pathologists understand and meet the unique needs of linguistic minority clients, the Educational Standards Board of ASHA has mandated that, as of January 1, 1993, accredited graduate programs in speech-language pathology and audiology must offer course content pertaining to culturally diverse groups (ASHA, 1992b). There is also an effort to increase the number of minority professionals in the profession. Some college and university programs offer specialized multicultural-based programs. (For more indepth reading on the topic of multicultural issues see Chapter 22 by Kayser.)

Economically Disadvantaged Populations

The ASHA Colloquium on Underserved Populations (ASHA, 1985) raised the issue of the economically disadvantaged as a target population for inclusion in professional academic coursework, clinical experiences, and research

and for increased service availability and delivery. In 1990, the economically disadvantaged population consisted of individuals whose annual income was below $7,223 and $13,359 for a four-person family (*Statistical Abstracts of the United States*, 1992). In 1990, this represented about 33 million individuals or 13.5% of the United States population. Many of those in the economically disadvantaged cohort are also part of the linguistic minority population. For example, in 1990, Hispanics constituted 28.1% of those below the poverty level and Blacks about 31.9%. Cole (1989) states that economically disadvantaged populations are at greater risk for handicapping conditions related to environmental, teratogenic, nutritional, and traumatic factors (p. 68). Professional preparation should emphasize the differences in health care agenda held by middle class professionals and clients from poverty groups. In addition, recruitment and retention of individuals from economically disadvantaged populations into our professions are priorities in helping to access communication services to this underserved group. Changes in health care reform and financing need to ensure that the economically disadvantaged will have full and equal access to quality communication services.

Institutionalized Populations

The number of individuals residing in "institutional settings" in the United States is staggering. Institutional settings include prisons, nursing homes and other long-term care facilities, and psychiatric settings. In 1990 there were 1.1 million prisoners in correctional institutions, the majority of whom were males between 18 and 34 years of age. There were nearly 1.8 million individuals residing in 25,646 nursing facilities. In contrast, there were 228,000 inpatients in nearly 5,000 mental hospitals across the United States (*Statistical Abstracts of the United States*, 1992). Several authors (e.g., Lubinski, 1981, 1991; Nuru, 1985) propose that the psychosocial and physical nature of such settings create barriers to communication opportunities for residents. Although the communication characteristics of individuals residing in long-term care nursing facilities has been somewhat delineated (e.g., Mueller & Peters, 1981), less attention has been paid to the communication characteristics and needs of those living in correctional facilities or mental hospitals. What is known from the few studies available is that the incidence of communication and hearing impairments among adult male and female prisoners is sigificantly higher than the general population (e.g., Belenchia & Crowe, 1983; Wagner, Gray, & Potter, 1983). In 1973, ASHA published a task force report on Speech Pathology and Audiology Service Needs in Prisons and concluded that such services were "critically needed" in the setting. This population appears to continue to be a neglected and hence underserved population. A comprehensive approach to rehabilitation is a necessary component to reducing recidivism rates and successful return to the community.

Remote/Rural Populations

In 1990, about 25% of the United States population resided in rural areas. Rural populations tend to reside in small towns which have a dearth of professional resources. According to ASHA's Ad Hoc Committee on Services to Remote/Rural Populations (ASHA, 1991e) such areas include the Appalachian region of West Virginia, Kentucky, and Tennessee; Alaska; Hawaii; and the U.S. Territories including Puerto Rico; the U.S. Virgin Islands; American Samoa; and the Pacific Trust of Guam. Rural areas of other states also qualify as underserved. The populations of these areas overlap with other underserved populations such as American Indians and linguistic minorities. There is a higher prevalence of speech, language, and hearing disorders with a paucity of communication disorders professionals serving this category. The REACH model was developed by this committee to improve service delivery in remote/rural areas. REACH stands for remote, rural education, access, consultation, and habilitation. It focuses on six target areas:

data, grant funding, training programs, continuing education, professional resource development, and consumer resources.

Although service delivery in rural/remote areas can consist of traditional clinic- or school-based service, more creativity and flexibility are needed to meet the needs of clients in these areas. Olmstead and Bergeron (1993) describe two programs: an itinerant, consulting approach and a staff team approach. Both approaches rely heavily on inter- and transdisciplinary teamwork and cultural sensitivity. Olmstead stated that "We work hard not to be perceived as team members who 'blow in . . . blow off . . . and blow out'" (p. 44). She adds that teamwork in a rural/remote setting can be challenging in itself.

Native Americans

In 1990, there were about 2 million individuals classified as American Indian, Eskimo, or Aleut residing in the United States (*Statistical Abstracts of the United States*, 1992). About 1 million Native Americans reside on or near a reservation and the remaining 1 million reside in urban areas. The 1 million Native Americans who live on reservations receive health services from the Indian Health Service (IHS). In addition to serious health problems such as tuberculosis, alcoholism, diabetes mellitus, gastrointestinal disorders, head trauma, and cancer, otitis media ranks as one of the most prevalent diseases among this population. The IHS offers audiologic services usually on a part-time outreach basis by otolaryngologists, audiologists, and audiometric technicians. Hearing aids are dispensed to children and offered at cost to adults (Stewart, 1992).

It is estimated that the incidence of communication disorders among this population is between 5 and 15 times higher than in the general population (Friedlander, 1993; Toubbeh, 1982). Unfortunately, speech-language services are considered nonmedical and are not offered routinely through the IHS (Stewart, 1992). Toubbeh (1982) states that, "amelioration of these and other disorders is further complicated by cultural and linguistic factors, lack of indigenous manpower and inefficient intervention strategies. The multiplicity of federal agencies which purport to serve Native Americans today further aggravates an already complex and disparate situation" (p. 396). Thus, comprehensive speech-language and hearing services to this population appear to be in short supply and complicated by cultural diversity within the Native American population, their living environment, and medical conditions.

INDIVIDUALS WITH DYSPHAGIA

One area of assessment and treatment that has grown exponentially in recent years is the field of working with individuals who have dysphagia (a swallowing disorder). Dysphagia may be a sequela of neurological dysfunction such as stroke or progressive neurological diseases or of head and neck cancers. Although dysphagia may occur without a concomitant speech or language disorder, it is highly likely that these problems will co-occur. Martin and Corlew (1990) found that 87% of patients identified with dysphagia also had speech, voice, language, or cognitive difficulties.

In 1986, ASHA published a position paper describing the role of the speech-language pathologist with this population and followed this in 1990 with a description of the knowledge and skills needed by speech-language pathologists to provide service to persons with swallowing problems (ASHA, 1986, 1990). Among the specific roles delineated are the ability to: (a) identify individuals at-risk for dysphagia; (b) conduct clinical oral–pharyngeal and respiratory examinations with a detailed history; (c) conduct instrumental/structural physiologic examination with related professionals; (d) determine patient management strategies; (e) provide treatment with related professionals; (f) provide education and counseling to appropriate others; (g) manage and/or participate in an interdisciplinary team; (h) maintain quality control and risk management; and (i) provide discharge planning and follow-up care.

In 1992, again to meet the technological advances occurring in dysphagia assessment, ASHA published a position and guideline on instrumental diagnostic procedures for swallowing. Specific instrumental procedures with which a speech-language pathologist may be involved in include videofluorography, ultrasonography, fiberoptic endoscopy, scintigraphy, electromyography, and manometry. These procedures *require* the speech language pathologist to obtain education and training *beyond* that necessary for ASHA certification (ASHA, 1992a, p. 25).

SPECIAL SETTINGS

NURSING HOMES

As stated previously, about 2 million individuals reside in nursing homes and related care facilities (National Center for Health Statistics, 1989). Unfortunately, although the prevalence of speech, language, and hearing problems among this population is high, there is a dearth of communication services to individuals in this setting. The lack of service is particularly noticeable for individuals with hearing impairment. In a 1979 study of the availability of communication services in nursing homes in 29 states, Chapey, Lubinski, Salzburg, and Chapey (1979) found that only 30% of institutional respondents had a full- or part-time speech-language pathologist and only 14% received full- or part-time services from an audiologist. In a more recent survey of nursing homes in New York State, Lubinski and Weinstein (1988) found that although 70% of the nursing homes had a speech-language pathologist, less than one third employed an audiologist. To determine why there is such a dearth of audiological services in nursing homes, a follow-up survey in New York State queried both administrators and audiologists about this question (Lubinski, Stecker, Weinstein, & Volin, 1993). Contributing factors identified by both administrators and audiologists included an emphasis on an office-based diagnostic role for audiologists, misperception of suitable candidates for hearing testing, lack of on-site testing facilities, inadequate funding, and limited interaction between staff and audiologists.

Recent federal legislation, the Omnibus Budget Reconciliation Act of 1987, mandates that all persons in a nursing home setting receiving Medicare and Medicaid assistance have a comprehensive assessment of their needs. Part of the Resident Assessment Instrument (Morris et al., 1990) focuses specifically on communication. It is expected that with full implementation of this instrument in long-term care facilities across the country, there will be an increase in referrals for both audiological and speech-language pathology services. In addition, use of this tool should promote more interaction between facility staff and communication disorders professionals (Lubinski & Frattali, 1993).

HOME HEALTH CARE

Although the vast majority of elderly individuals (95%) reside in the community, many of these individuals and also some younger community-based chronically ill or disabled persons require regular assistance with activities of daily living (ADLs) and instrumental activities of daily living (IADLs) such as bathing, dressing, eating, transferring, walking, using the toilet, preparing meals, shopping, managing money, doing housework, and getting outside (National Center for Health Statistics, 1989). Rowland and Lyons (1991) state that about 5.5 million elderly individuals are functionally disabled and require some form of daily assistance. Of these, about 1.6 million are severely disabled and require long-term care in the community.

A relatively new approach to providing assistance with ADLs and IADLs, as well as health, rehabilitation, and social services to the community-based elderly and disabled, is home health care. With most assistance provided through informal caregivers such as family and friends, care given by paid help constitutes formal home health care. The first formal home health care program began in 1796 at the Boston Dispensary. Through the 19th century, various types of home health care programs surfaced across the United States, usually in larger metropolitan areas such as Buffalo, New York, Boston, Philadelphia, and Los Angeles. Rural home health care was established in Kentucky at the beginning of the 20th century. Gradually the focus of such programs included services other than direct nursing health care. Rice (1992) states that, "the current philosophy of home health care is to provide cost-effective and quality health care in a setting that is often more conducive to health restoration and patient contentment than a hospital setting" (p. 12). Such services focus on a prevention role to maintain the health of the individual and forestall further disabilities, dependence, and relocation to an institutional setting as well as providing supportive and therapeutic services (Lubinski, 1981; May 1993). The growth of such services is partly related to improved medical technology that allows individuals with special treatment needs such as intravenous chemotherapy, renal dialysis, and ventilator-dependent infusion services to be treated at home (May 1993). For a detailed history of home healthcare, see May (1993) and Rice (1992).

In 1990, there were at least 5,753 home health care agencies providing services to 5.8 million individuals (May, 1993). This number is probably an underestimation because it does not include services offered through health maintenance organizations that may contract for such services. In the 1970s home health care became more available, especially as Medicare began to limit hospital stays. In 1987, Medicare accounted for 78% of the revenue sources for home health care with Medicaid and private insurers accounting for small percentages. Two thirds of this population are severely physically disabled and one third are designated as having only cognitive impairment. Over half of the *entire* population has a cognitive disorder—indicating the complex nature of their problems. Most of those served through home health care are female, of a minority race, over age 85, and poor (Rowland & Lyons, 1991).

Although nursing care is the most prevalent service offered by home health care programs, rehabilitation also constitutes an important aspect of service delivery. Rehabilitation includes occupational therapy, physical therapy, and speech therapy. About 7% of all home health care patients receive speech therapy (May, 1993). Lubinski and Chapey (1980) surveyed 596 home health care programs in the eight states having the largest populations of elderly persons. At that time, 58% of the responding agencies offered speech and language services. The bulk of the relatively small caseloads consisted of individuals with neurological disorders. Audiology services were available in only 10% of the respondents' programs. The vast majority of home health care programs employed speech-language pathologists and audiologists part-time. Results of the study indicated that communication disorders specialists encountered numerous problems in providing service through home health care. These included (a) travel time and parking difficulties, (b) shortage of referrals from physicians, (c) inadequate funding, (d) lack of family involvement and follow through, (e) unsafe neighborhoods, (f) paperwork overload, and (g) competition from other agencies for referrals.

In 1987 the ASHA Task Force on Home Care (ASHA, 1987a) defined the role of speech-language pathology and audiology services in home health care. These roles included assessment, treatment, family involvement, record keeping, discharge planning, public education, referral to other professionals, research, and quality control. The task force commented specifically that professionals working in this type of setting need specialized academic and clinical experiences. For example, employment in home health care incorporates a team approach, and therefore, the practitioner needs familiarity with the roles and duties of other allied health care professionals. Other needed skills included knowledge of reimbursement issues, infection control, family intervention, drugs and medications, self-advocacy, and marketing.

As the United States grapples in 1994 with a change in its national health care program, speech-language pathologists and audiologists should be critical of how effectively rehabilitation programs are included in home health care funding. To date, financing for home health care programs is limited throughout most of the nation; and despite its objective of maintaining individuals in the community, full implementation has not occurred.

PRIVATE PRACTICE

One professional practice context that has experienced substantial growth in the number of practitioners is private practice. A professional in private practice is self-employed and has total control over ethical, professional, administrative, and financial aspects of the practice. According to 1990 statistics compiled by ASHA, 28.3% of speech-language pathologists and 35.8% of audiologists engage in either full- or part-time private practice. More than 60% of all private practitioners work part-time; 30% of speech-language pathologists and 57.5% of audiologists work full-time in this professional context (Keogh, 1991). Private practitioners offer their services to a wide range of settings including educational, hospital, long-term care, and nonresidential health care facilities as well as industry and research settings. The vast majority of private practitioners are females, have about 7 years of experience before starting a private practice, have at least a master's degree, and earn about one third more than the median salary for all other settings (Keogh, 1991). Private practitioners spend 71% of their professional time in direct clinical service as compared to about 59% spent by professionals in other settings (Shewan & Wisniewski, 1987).

The increase in popularity of private practice as a professional context has raised a number of important issues. In 1991, ASHA's Committee on Private Practice identified six major issues affecting private practice in our professions: education, legislation, marketing, reimbursement, interprofessional relationships, and recruitment. Although these issues are relevant to other settings, they have particular importance for the private practitioner, whose salary and professional identity are totally dependent on provision of and reimbursement of direct clinical services.

In 1988, Feldman stated that the educational preparation for private practice needed specific attention in minimum competencies, business management, and marketing. Considering the expanding knowledge base in communication disorders, increased and in-depth preparation in these areas may need to be taken through continuing education or doctoral level programs. The issue of doctoral level entry in audiology has roots in the rise in audiology private practice. (See Chapter 28 by Loavenbruck.)

To assist individuals interested in establishing a private practice, ASHA's Committee on Private Practice in Audiology and/or Speech-Language Pathology (American Speech-Language-Hearing Association, 1991b) developed an extensive list of considerations that help in deciding if private practice is for you. These considerations begin with the critical need for a careful analysis before establishing the practice, review of legal aspects, specialized services and dispensing of professional products, needed business management skills and practices, and strategies for buying or selling a private practice.

Review of these considerations indicates that today's private practitioner is not simply the "kitchen table" speech-language pathologist who "does a little extra therapy on the side." Individuals who choose private practice must be totally aware of business, marketing, ethics, and professional practice issues if they are to be successful. In addition to high level clinical skills, private practitioners must have personal qualities that will enhance professional activities such as a strong self-image, ability to handle stress, ability to go without income for awhile, strong family support, and a need for challenge and autonomy. Among the numerous articles in our professional literature in the past few years that have described and promoted private practice, Feldman's (1988)

comments summarize the challenge of private practice. "Given the necessary professional credentials, the will and incentive to engage in it, and the courage to accept the risks of failure as well as the joys of success, the opportunity (through private practice) is there. Accept the challenge and go for the gold. It will be good for you and the profession" (p. 30).

For a listing of relatively current readings on private practice, business, marketing, and other related issues, see the following two publications: *Considerations for Establishing a Private Practice in Audiology and/or Speech-Language Pathology* (ASHA, 1991b) and *Business, Marketing, Ethics, and Professionalism in Audiology: An Updated Annotated Bibliography* (ASHA, 1991a).

SUMMARY

The demography of our client populations and the variety of settings in which we provide services as audiologists and speech-language pathologists are rapidly changing. Our clientele crosses the age span, encompasses a variety of ethnic, economic, and cultural groups, and includes individuals with nontraditional problems such as head trauma, language learning disabilities, and dysphagia. Not only do we serve individuals and their families in schools, hospitals, and community agencies, but also in nursing homes, home health care, and private practice. The scope of new populations presented in this chapter is only the tip of the iceberg. Technological advance in both audiology and speech-language pathology will continue to expand our clientele. Each of these client groups and settings creates new avenues for service delivery but also requires the development or updating of new clinical and professional skills. Expanding frontiers necessitate continual self-evaluation as individual professionals and as professions devoted to improving the lives of our clients.

DISCUSSION QUESTIONS

1. What clinical groups or settings initially attracted you to the profession of speech-language pathology? How have these groups and settings changed?
2. Why and how should audiologists and speech-language pathologists update their professional skills to meet the changing demographic portrait of our clientele?
3. Describe some nontraditional clientele with whom we work who were not detailed in this chapter. Why does this population require the services of an audiologist or speech-language pathologist?
4. What might attract you to work in a nursing home, home health care, or private practice?
5. Imagine yourself as a practicing speech-language pathologist or audiologist 25 years from now. With what clientele and in what clinical settings do you think speech-language pathologists and audiologists will be working?

REFERENCES

American Speech-Language-Hearing Association. (1982a). Learning disabilities: Issues on definition. *Asha, 24,* 945–947.

American Speech-Language-Hearing Association. (1982b). Position statement on language learning disorders. *Asha, 24,* 937–944.

American Speech-Language-Hearing Association. (1985). 1985 national colloquium on underserved populations report. *Asha, 27,* 31–35.

American Speech-Language-Hearing Association. Ad Hoc Committee on Dysphagia. (1986). Ad Hoc Committee on Dysphagia report. *Asha, 29,* 57–58.

American Speech-Language-Hearing Association. (1987a). The delivery of speech-language and audiology services in home care. *Asha, 29,* 49–52.

American Speech-Language-Hearing Association. (1987b). The role of speech-language pathologists in the habilitation and rehabilitation of cognitively impaired individuals: A report of the subcommittee on language and cognition. *Asha, 29,* 53–55.

American Speech-Language-Hearing Association. (1988). Provision of audiology and speech-language pathology services to older persons in nursing homes. *Asha, 30,* 72–74.

American Speech-Language-Hearing Association. (1989). Communication based services for infants, toddlers, and their families. *Asha, 31,* 32–34.

American Speech-Language-Hearing Association. (1990). Skills needed by speech-language pathologists providing services to dysphagic patients/clients. *Asha, 32*(Suppl. 2), 7–12.

American Speech-Language-Hearing Association. (1991a). Business, marketing, ethics, and professionalism in audiology: An updated annotated bibliography (1986–1989). *Asha, 33*(Suppl. 3), 39–45.

American Speech-Language-Hearing Association. (1991b). Considerations for establishing a private practice in audiology and/or speech-language pathology. *Asha, 33*(Suppl. 3), 10–21.

American Speech-Language-Hearing Association. (1991c). Guidelines for the audiologic assessment of children from birth through 36 months of age. *Asha, 33*(Suppl. 5), 37–43.

American Speech-Language-Hearing Association. (1991d). Private practice in audiology and/or speech-language pathology. *Asha, 33*(Suppl. 3), 10–21.

American Speech-Language-Hearing Association. (1991e). REACH: A model for service delivery and professional development within remote/rural regions of the United States and U.S. territories. *Asha, 33*(Suppl. 6), 5–14.

American Speech-Language-Hearing Association. (1991f). Report on private practice. *Asha, 33*(Suppl. 6), 1–4.

American Speech-Language-Hearing Association. (1992a). Instrumental diagnostic procedures for swallowing. *Asha, 34*(Suppl. 7), 25–33.

American Speech-Language-Hearing Association. (1992b). *Professional certification standards.* Rockville, MD: Author.

Aram, D., & Nation, J. (1980). Preschool language disorders and subsequent language and academic difficulties. *Journal of Communication Disorders, 13,* 159–170.

Bayles, K., & Kasniak, A. (1987). *Communication and cognition in normal aging and dementia.* Boston: College-Hill Press.

Bebout, J. (1989). The aging of America. *The Hearing Journal, 42,* 7–12.

Belenchia, T., & Crowe, T. (1983). Prevalence of speech and hearing disorders in a state penitentiary population. *Journal of Communication Disorders, 16,* 279–285.

Beukelman, D., & Yorkston, K. (1991). Traumatic brain injury changes the way we live. In D. Beukelman & K. Yorkston (Eds.), *Communication disorders following traumatic brain injury* (pp. 1–14). Austin, TX: Pro-Ed.

Bricker, W., & Bricker, D. (1970). A program of language training for the severely handicapped child. *Exceptional Children, 37*, 101–111.

Brock, D., Guralnick, J., & Brody, J. (1990). Demography and epidemiology of aging in the United States. In E. Schneider & J. Rose (Eds.), *Handbook of the biology of aging* (3rd ed, pp. 3–23). San Diego: Academic Press.

Catts, H. (1991). Facilitating phonological awareness: Role of speech-language pathologists. *Language, Speech, and Hearing Services in Schools, 22*, 196–203.

Chapey, R., Lubinski, R., Salzburg, A., & Chapey, G. (1979, Winter). Survey of speech, language and hearing services in nursing home settings. *Long Term Care and Health Services Administration Quarterly*, pp. 307–316.

Chermak, G., & Musiek, F. (1992). Managing central auditory processing disorders in children and youth. *American Journal of Audiology, 1*, 61–65.

Cole, L. (1989). E pluribus pluribus: Multicultural imperatives for the 1990's and beyond. *Asha, 31*, 65–70.

Cornett, B., & Chabon, S. (1986). Speech-language pathologists as language-learning disabilities specialists: Rites of passage. *Asha, 28*, 29–31.

Crais, E., & Leonard, C. (1990). PL 99-457: Are speech-language pathologists prepared for the challenge? *Asha, 32*, 57–62.

Cross, P., & Gurland, B. (1985). The epidemiology of dementing disorders: A report on work performed by and submitted to the U.S. Congress, Office of Technology Assessment. New York: Columbia University Center for Geriatrics, Gerontology and Long Term Care.

Cummings, J., & Benson, D. F. (1983). *Dementia: A clinical approach*. Boston: Butterworth.

Evans, D., Funkstein, H., & Albert, M. (1989). Prevalence of Alzheimer's disease in a community population of older persons: Higher than previously reported. *Journal of American Medical Association. 262*, 2551–2556.

Fein, D. (1983). Projection for speech and hearing impairments to 2050. *Asha, 25*, 31.

Feldman, A. (1988). Some observations about us and private practice. *Asha, 30*, 29–30.

Friedlander, R. (1993). BHSM comes to the flathead Indian reservation. *Asha, 35*, 28–29.

German, D., & Simon, E. (1991). Analysis of children's word-finding skills in discourse. *Journal of Speech and Hearing Research, 34*, 309–316.

Grimes, A. (1991). Auditory changes. In R. Lubinski (Ed.), *Dementia and communication* (pp. 47–69). Philadelphia: B.C. Decker.

Grossman, H. (1983). *Classification in mental retardation*. Washington, DC: American Association on Mental Deficiency.

Houle, G., & Hamilton, J. (1991). Public Law 99-457: A challenge to speech-language pathologists and audiologists. *Asha, 33*, 51–54.

Hyman, C. (1985). PL 94-142 in review. *Asha, 27*, 37.

Kalsbeek, W., McLauren, R., Harris, B., & Miller, J. (1981). The national head and spinal cord injury survey: Major findings. *Journal of Neurosurgery, 53*, S19–S31.

Katzman, R. (1986). The prevalence of malignancy of Alzheimer's disease. *Archives of Neurology, 33*, 217–218.

Kempler, D. (1991). Language changes in dementia of the Alzheimer type. In R. Lubinski (Ed.), *Dementia and communication* (pp. 98–114). Philadelphia: B.C. Decker.

Keough, K. (1991). A profile of ASHA members in private practice. *Asha, 33*, 64.

Koury, L., & Lubinski, R. (1991). Effective in-service training for staff working with communication-impaired persons. In R. Lubinski (Ed.), *Dementia and communciation* (pp. 279–289). Philadelphia: B.C. Decker.

Kraus, J., Black, M., Hessol, N., Ley, P., Rokaw, W., Sullivan, C., Bowers, S., Knowlton, S., & Marshall, L. (1984). Incidence of acute brain injury and serious impairment in defined populations. *American Journal of Epidemiology, 119*, 185–201.

Language, Speech, and Hearing Services in the Schools. (1990). Clinical forum. Vol. 21, 205–252.

Language,Speech, and Hearing Services in the Schools. (1992). Clinical forum. Vol. 23, 361–372.

Lazarus, C. (1991). Diagnosis and management of swallowing disorders in traumatic brain injury. In D. Beukelman & K. Yorkston (Eds.), *Communication disorders following traumatic brain injury* (pp. 367–418). Austin, TX: Pro-Ed.

Lubinski, R. (1981). Speech, language and audiology programs in home health care agencies and nursing homes. In D. Beasley & G.A. Davis (Eds.), *Aging, communication processes and disorders* (pp. 339–356). New York: Grune & Stratton.

Lubinski, R. (1991). Environmental considerations for elderly persons. In R. Lubinski (Ed.), *Dementia and communication* (pp. 257–278). Philadelphia: B.C. Decker.

Lubinski, R., & Chapey, R. (1980). Communication services in home health care agencies: Availability and scope. *Asha, 22*, 929–936.

Lubinski, R., & Frattali, C. (1993). Nursing home reform: The resident assessment instrument. *Asha, 35*, 59–62.

Lubinski, R., Morrison, E., & Rigrodsky, S. (1981). Perception of spoken communication by elderly chronically ill patients in an institutional setting. *Journal of Speech and Hearing Disorders, 46*, 405–412.

Lubinski, R., Stecker, N., Weinstein, B., & Volin, R. (1993). Hearing health services in nursing homes: Perceptions of administrators and audiologists. *Journal of Long Term Care Administrators, 21,* 27–33.

Lubinski, R., & Weinstein, B. (1988). Status of communication services in nursing homes in New York state. *Asha, 39,* 69–72.

MacMillan, D. (1977). *Mental retardation in school and society.* Boston: Little, Brown.

Martin, B., & Corlew, M. (1990). The incidence of communication disorders in dysphagic patients. *Journal of Speech and Hearing Disorders, 55,* 28–32.

Maxwell, W., & Wallach, G. (1984). The language learning disabilities connection: Symptoms of early language disability change over time. In G. Wallach & K. Butler (Eds.), *Language learning disabilities in school-age children* (pp. 15–34). Baltimore: Williams & Wilkins.

May, B. (1993). *Home health and rehabilitation.* Philadelphia: F. A. Davis.

McLean, J., McLean, L., Brady, N., & Etter, R. (1991). Communication profiles of two types of gesture using nonverbal persons with severe to profound mental retardation. *Journal of Speech and Hearing Research, 34,* 294–308.

Mire, S., & Chisholm, R. (1990). Functional communication goals for adolescents and adults who are severely and moderately mentally handicapped. *Language, Speech and Hearing Services in Schools, 21,* 57–58.

Morris, J., Hawes, C., Fries, B., Phillips, C., Mohr, V., Katz, S., Murphy, K., Drugovich, M., & Friedlob, A. (1990). Designing the national resident assessment instrument for nursing homes. *Gerontologist, 30,* 293–307.

Mueller, P., & Peters, T. (1981). Needs and services in geriatric speech-language pathology and audiology. *Asha, 23,* 627–632.

National Center for Health Statistics. (1988). Advance report of final natality statistics, 1986. *Monthly Vital Statistics Report, 37*(3).

National Center for Health Statistics. (1989). *Vital and health statistics: Long term care for functionally dependent elderly* (Series 14, No. 104). Washington, DC: U.S. Department of Health and Human Services.

National Institute on Aging. (1987). *Personnel for health needs of the elderly through the year 2020.* Washington, DC: Author.

National Joint Committee on Learning Disabilities. (1991). Learning disabilities: Issues on definition. *Asha, 33*(Suppl. 5), 18–20.

Northern, J., & Downs, M. (1991). *Hearing in children* (4th ed.). Baltimore: Williams & Wilkins.

Nuru, N. (1985). Institutionalized people: Can we do a better job? *Asha, 27,* 35–38.

O'Connell, P., & O'Connell, E. (1978, November). *Speech language pathology services in a skilled nursing facility.* Paper presented at the Annual Convention of the American Speech and Hearing Association, San Francisco.

Olmstead, P., & Bergeron, L. (1993). A rural/remote perspective: Alaska. *Asha, 35,* 43–45.

Owens, R. (1993). Mental retardation: Difference and delay. In D. Bernstein & E. Tiegerman (Eds.), *Language and communciation disorders in children* (3rd ed., pp. 366–430). New York: Merrill.

Rice, R. (1992). *Home health nursing practice.* St. Louis: Mosby Year Book.

Ripich, D., & Terrell, B. (1988). Patterns of discourse cohesion and coherence in Alzheimer's disease. *Journal of Speech and Hearing Disorders, 53,* 8–15.

Rossetti, L. (1991a, Oct. 3–4). *Addressing the needs of at-risk infants and toddlers.* Workshop at the Speech and Hearing Association of Western New York Convention, Buffalo.

Rossetti, L. (1991b). Communication assessment: Birth to 36 months. *Asha, 33,* 45–49.

Roush, J. (1991). Expanding the audiologist's role. *Asha, 33,* 47–49.

Rowland, D., & Lyons, B. (1991). The elderly population in need of home care. In D. Rowland & B. Lyons (Eds.), *Financing home care: Improving protection for disabled elderly people* (pp. 3–26). Baltimore: The John Hopkins University Press.

Schow, R., & Nerbonne, M. (1980). Hearing levels among elderly nursing home residents. *Journal of Speech and Hearing Disorders, 45,* 124–132.

Scott, C. (1988). Producing complex sentences. *Topics in Language Disorders, 8,* 44–62.

Shewan, C., & Wisniewski, A. (1987). Who is a private practitioner? *Asha, 29,* 59.

Silliman, E., & Wilkinson, L. (1991). *Communicating for learning: Classroom observation and collaboration.* Gaithersburg, MD: Aspen Publishers.

Sohlberg, M., & Mateer, C. (1989). *Introduction to cognitive rehabilitation.* New York: The Guilford Press.

Statistical Abstracts of the United States. (1992). Washington, DC: U.S. Department of Commerce.

Stewart, J. (1992). Native American populations. *Asha, 34,* 40–42.

Topics in Language Disorders. (1993). Collaborative consultation: A problem-solving approach, *14,* 1–90.

Toubbeh, J. (1982). Native Americans: A multi-dimensional challenge. *Asha, 24,* 395–398.

Turnkey, D. (1983). Trauma. *Scientific American, 249,* 28–35.

U.S. Bureau of the Census. (1990). Press Release CB 91-216.

Wagner, C., Gray, L., & Potter, R. (1983). Communicative disorders in a group of adult female offenders. *Journal of Communication Disorders, 16,* 269–277.

Wallach, G., & Liebergott, J. (1984). Who shall be called "learning disabled": Some new directions. In G. Wallach & K. Butler (Eds.), *Language learning disabilities in school-age children* (pp. 1–14). Baltimore: Williams & Wilkins.

Wallach, G., & Miller, L. (1988). *Language intervention and academic success.* Gaithersburg, MD: Aspen Publishers.

Weinstein, B. (1991). Auditory testing and rehabilitaiton of the hearing impaired. In R. Lubinski (Ed.), *Dementia and communication* (pp. 223–237). Philadelphia: B.C. Decker

Wilkinson, L., & Milosky, L. (1987). School-age children's metapragmatic knowledge of requests and responses in the classroom. *Topics in Language Disorders, 7,* 61–70.

Yorkston, K., & Beukelman, D. (1991). Motor speech disorders. In D. Beukelman & K. Yorkston (Eds.), *Communication disorders following traumatic brain injury* (pp. 251–316). Austin, TX, Pro-Ed.

CHAPTER 13

Professional Liability

■ REBECCA KOOPER, J.D., M.A. ■

SCOPE OF CHAPTER

The term professional liability is one that usually evokes fear in the hearts of professionals. Fortunately, those of you entering or practicing speech-language pathology or audiology have little reason for concern as these fields have seen relatively few legal actions. A low number of litigated cases is also seen in other health care professions such as occupational or physical therapy, fields in which there are usually long-term relationships between therapists and clients. Such relationships permit problems that arise to be worked out in a timely fashion. The number of legal complaints increases in fields where the professional generally spends little time with the client. In such situations, problems can magnify, frustration and dissatisfaction build, and resolutions ultimately are sought in a court of law.

All professionals, however, regardless of the relationships they have with their clients, must recognize that, at some point in their careers, mistakes may be made or someone may question their professional competence. A legal action that arises from such a situation is an action based on professional liability principles.

This chapter defines professional liability and discusses how it relates to speech-language pathologists and audiologists. The elements needed to prove a classic professional liability action are discussed. The duties owed clients are reviewed and suggestions for optimizing the therapeutic relationship are offered. An understanding of legal procedure and definitions is presented.

PROFESSIONAL LIABILITY

Professional liability results when a professional's conduct is negligent in the course of treating a client and such conduct results in some injury to the client. The basis for this principle is found in tort law. A tort is a branch of civil law that deals with private legal wrongs. A tort may be intentional, such as assault and battery, or unintentional, such as negligence. There are many types of torts, but the one that most relates to professional liability is negligence, which courts will remedy by awarding damages. Negligence law covers compensation of individuals who have been accidentally harmed by another. It is based on the principle that all members of society have a duty to exercise reasonable care so that their actions will not hurt another. If failure to exercise reasonable care causes injury to another party, a potential liability can arise. When one is found to be legally liable to another person due to negligence, it means that the individual is held legally responsible for the harm caused the other person. Carelessness is not an excuse if someone is injured. We are all responsible for providing reasonable care when interacting with others.

Professional liability falls within the area of negligence. It is used to refer to negligent acts of people engaged in professions in which highly technical or professional skills are used. Professionals, when acting in a professional capacity, have to provide more than the usual standard of reasonable care when treating a client. They must provide care within a standard accepted by other professionals in their field (Kooper & Sullivan, 1986).

Four elements must be proved for a complainant to prevail in a professional liability action (Prosser, 1971):

1. A legal relationship between the professional and client exists,
2. A duty owed to the client has been breached,
3. This breach was the proximate cause of the client's injury, and
4. Actual loss or damages were caused to the client as a result of the injury.

The first element, establishing a relationship between the professional and the client, is easy to prove. As soon as the professional sees the client in any professional capacity, a relationship is formed. Proving the other elements is more difficult and are discussed in more detail.

PROFESSIONAL'S LEGAL DUTY

Providing clients with treatment within acceptable standards of care is the legal duty owed all clients. Acceptable standards of care can be found in both statutory and common law. Statutory laws are those created by federal, state, or local legislative bodies. State laws requiring professionals to obtain a license to practice in that state are examples of statutory laws. Common laws are those created as a result of principles established through the resolution of previous legal actions. An example of common law is the court-ordered desegregation of schools in the 1950s. These orders were not a result of legislation, but resulted from the U.S. Supreme Court's interpretation of laws at that time. These orders became the ruling law as long as no other subsequent court ruling changed or modified the existing order or until the legislatures changed the rulings.

STANDARD OF CARE

Establishing what standard of care is owed a client varies. Statutory standards are easy to prove. Practicing without a license in a state where such license is required is a breach of that state's statutory standard. Speech-language pathologists and audiologists are required to understand their state's statutes and requirements regarding the scope of their practice. Ignorance of the law is never a defense. The scope of practice permitted in each state may vary and it is incumbent on the professional to know the governing laws. Other statutory standards of care are those found in the American Speech-Language-Hearing Association's (ASHA's) professional Code of Ethics as well as each state's licensure requirements. (See Chapters 4 and 6 by Battle and Seymour.)

It is more difficult to establish the required standard of care as it relates to a professional's decisions about client care. Factors to be considered are the use of standardized tests and procedures utilizing the current technology available in your area. Other standards will evolve from court decisions involving speech-language pathologists and audiologists.

Certain standards may seem obvious, but are worth stating. For example, speech-language pathologists and audiologists have a duty to properly evaluate, to properly treat and instruct, to refer, to provide alternatives, and to obtain informed consent (Trace, 1993).

PROPER EVALUATION

Both speech-language pathologists and audiologists need to use standardized tests and procedures when they exist. Whenever possible, objective tests should be used to supplement standard behavioral testing. Clinicians should refrain from modifying accepted procedures unless the use of the modification is well documented. Video- or audiorecording help document a client's level of performance when behavioral tests are used. All test results should be well documented. Results should be shared with the client and this session should also be noted in the client's records. Any equipment used during this procedure should be in good working order and calibrated according to requisite standards.

PROPER TREATMENT

The duty to properly treat clients includes the development of a treatment plan by speech-language pathologists and audiologists. Once a client's problems have been diagnosed, a treatment plan is developed, documented, and reviewed with the client. The limitations of the plan must also be discussed. Clients must not have unrealistic expectations about the prognoses. A clinician must be careful not to become overly enthusiastic about a treatment plan, even when a prognosis appears to be excellent. One must remember that not all clients respond well to treatment and a disappointed client can be fuel for legal action.

Speech-language pathologists and audiologists must inform clients about the limitations of their treatment. It should be understood that hearing aids do not "cure" a hearing loss, or that progress in treatment may be uneven or slow. Periodic reviews of a treatment plan should be conducted and documented. A decision to continue treatment should also be reviewed and documented.

Professionals also have a duty to counsel clients regarding alternative treatment plans. On diagnosing a significant hearing loss in a young child, the audiologist often must counsel the parents about educational options. For example, the debate about total communication versus oral methods continues to flourish. It is not the audiologist's job to enter into this debate. The audiologist is responsible for explaining the options, regardless of personal preference. Cochlear implants are now a viable alternative for some children with profound hearing loss. Again, the audiologist has a responsibility to review this alternative, regardless of personal opinions.

Some treatments are new and/or controversial. You may consider discussing them with your clients before they learn about innovations from other sources and wonder why the information was withheld. Clients should be encouraged to explore as many options as they can with you. An example of a new treatment approach is the use of specialized auditory training for children who are diagnosed with autism. Speech-language pathologists treating this population should study this new approach and present the information to the parents of the child. Together, they can decide if this technique should be tried and the professional best qualified to perform this procedure.

Included in an audiologist's proper treatment plan is the duty to recommend proper amplification, when appropriate, and to instruct the client in the use of amplification devices. How to use and care for a hearing aid must be carefully demonstrated. Giving clients written instructions is encouraged because many people need to review what the audiologist showed them when they get home. Copies of such instructions should be put into the client's file and the date given noted. Children acquiring hearing aids often have special needs. Parents of these children must have specific instruction on how to meet their needs. For example, special devices to keep the hearing aids correctly attached to the child may be necessary, and the hearing aid may need to have a child-proof battery compartment. The dangers of hearing aid battery ingestion also need to be reviewed with caregivers.

REFERRALS

It is most important for speech-language pathologists and audiologists to know when to refer clients to other professionals in the same or related fields. For example, clients with voice problems should be seen by an otolaryngologist. The referral as well as the physician's report should be kept in the client's file. Similarly, audiologists need to refer to otologists whenever there is a question about the medical condition of the ear. These reports should also be kept in the file. It may be wise to recommend a second opinion if there is any doubt about the evaluation or if it appears that the client is not convinced about the problem. Many clients are grateful when a second opinion is recommended, and they will readily return to the original clinician if the diagnosis is confirmed. This demonstrates to the client that the clinician is looking out for the individual's best interests and will be willing to work with other professionals to develop the optimal treatment regimen.

DEVELOPING A POSITIVE RELATIONSHIP

Practicing professional competency will prevent clients from filing claims. It is important to repeat that, unless major damage occurred as a result of a professional's inability to act competently, most legal actions are a result of a client's dissatisfaction with the relationship with the professional. The initiation of a lawsuit is often the final stage of a deteriorating client/clinician relationship. Developing a positive relationship with your clients is one of the most important ways to prevent liability actions from arising (Kooper & Sullivan, 1986).

Your relationship begins when your client calls for an appointment. From the very beginning, all contacts should be professional and cordial. Many times, it is the little routine tasks that could contribute to the deterioration of a relationship. A client's unreturned telephone calls, waiting for long periods of time for an appointment, short visits in which questions are left unanswered, and inadequate explanation of bills are examples of unnecessary problems.

Establishing rapport is extremely important. Clients like to feel that they are being treated as individuals, not as a speech problem or a hearing loss. They need to feel that you, as a professional, are listening to them and are responding to their needs. Developing good listening skills is critical. A clinician who hears what a client is saying can pick up dissatisfaction at an early stage and can deal with client frustration before it magnifies. If you have not established a good rapport, weaknesses in your treatment plan will become more important.

The most effective and professional way to work with clients is to spend time educating them about the problem for which treatment is sought. Good communication skills will help clients feel that you understand their problems and will do your best to minimize the problems. Discussing the treatment plan and providing clients with alternative treatment plans promotes empowerment. Offering reading materials to further educate clients also is beneficial toward creating a good working relationship in which all parties are contributing members. The extra time spent with a client often ensures a good relationship in which realistic outcomes are expected. Informed clients who are encouraged to participate with their treatment become willing and cooperative partners in a therapeutic plan.

COMPLAINTS

Despite good intentions, mistakes are sometime made, misunderstandings occur, professional relationships deteriorate, and a legal action is initiated. If the client is not interested in an award for damages, a complaint may be registered with ASHA's Ethical Practice Board (EPB). If a violation is found after an investigation, the EPB has the power to take such actions as to suspend or revoke the professional's Certificate of Clinical Competence. Another place for clients to register dissatisfaction is to file a complaint with the state's licensing board (in states with licensure), which has the power to suspend or revoke a license to practice speech-language pathology or audiology in that state. However, if the client wants financial compensation for an injury that occurred from the alleged negligence by a speech-language pathologist or audiologist, a legal action will be initiated in the state court system.

LEGAL PROCEDURE

A professional becomes part of a legal proceeding on receipt of a summons and/or complaint. The person who initiated the action will be referred to as the "plaintiff" and the professional will be referred to as the "defendant." The names of both parties will appear on the summons, with a complaint briefly outlining the grounds for the action. The complaint may be served with the summons or may follow soon after.

In the complaint, the elements necessary to prove a professional liability action must be supported by the facts of the case. These elements were described earlier in the chapter, but are worth repeating. The plaintiff must show (Prosser, 1971):

1. That a legal relationship existed between the professional and the client;
2. That the professional breached some duty owed the client;
3. That this breach was the proximate cause of the client's injury; and
4. That the client suffered some actual injury or loss as a result of the injury.

CONSULTING WITH AN ATTORNEY

On receipt of a summons naming you as a defendant in a professional liability case, contacting your attorney or your professional liability insurance company is your first step. A meeting with an attorney needs to take place soon after this initial contact because responses to complaints must be answered within a limited time. At the meeting with your attorney, a few rules should be kept in mind. First, and most important, is that your attorney must hear all the facts that pertain to the particular situation. Do not withhold information that you feel may not be helpful or, in fact, may be harmful. All communications with your attorney are confidential and are protected by law. Let your attorney make these judgments of relevancy and appropriateness. Your attorney is best equipped to decide what to do with all the facts. Withholding information that, in fact, the opposing parties may have will put you and your attorney at a disadvantage when the facts arise. If your attorney knows these facts ahead of time, your advocate will be best equipped to respond to the issues.

AFTER THE SUMMONS

After you have met with your attorney, he or she will write an answer to the complaint, either admitting, denying, or claiming ignorance of the allegations. Once the answer to this communication has been received by your client's attorney, pretrial procedures will begin. The purpose of pretrial discovery procedures is to ensure that each party is aware of all the facts and allegations involved in the case. These procedures include depositions, interrogatories, or the requisition of records. Depositions are testimonies taken down in writing, under oath. Interrogatories are written questions that are submitted to the parties. An issuance of a subpoena duces tecum requires parties to submit documents for examination by the opposition.

Another purpose of discovery is to encourage a settlement between parties. When a case is settled, neither party wins nor loses. There is no determination of liability. A settlement is a compromise that eliminates the need for a trial. This is often done to eliminate the high costs of court trials. Much time and money are saved if a case can be settled. Your attorney will give you the best advice during all stages of these proceedings (Kooper & Sullivan, 1986).

After a period of discovery, if a settlement has not been reached, then the parties will have a court date set. Besides the testimony of both parties, expert witnesses will testify to give an opinion on whether the defendant's actions met the standard of care recognized by other professionals in the field.

Expert witnesses are usually practicing speech-language pathologists or audiologists who are aware of the local facilities. These witnesses must demonstrate that they have the necessary credentials to practice speech-language pathology or audiology and that they are well versed with the accepted practices in the field, especially in the subspecialty in which the client needs treatment. The facts of the case are explained to this witness, who then gives an opinion regarding to what extent the defendant's actions were within accepted practice standards. The witness need not agree with the practice, only confirm or deny that the procedure meets acceptable standards.

After all the testimony has been presented, the jury decides, in most cases, whether negligence has occurred and, if deciding yes, what damages should be awarded. At any time before a jury reaches a verdict, the parties may settle the case.

LIABILITY INSURANCE

Most speech-language pathologists and audiologists obtain legal advice from the insurance carrier that provides their professional liability insurance. This type of insurance will provide an insured professional with counsel and will provide financial compensation if damages are awarded to the plaintiff, up to the limit of the policy. Professional liability insurance is offered by the American Speech-Language-Hearing Association for all speech-language pathologists and audiologists employed in a clinical or educational setting or self-employed in a private setting. (See Resources at the end of this chapter for ASHA's liability group carrier.)

STAYING OUT OF COURT

As was stated earlier, the professions of speech-language pathology and audiology are relatively free of professional liability cases.

Like other health care providers who develop long-term relationships with their clients, these relationships are the best insurance against a liability action. However, it is interesting to review complaints that have been made to professional licensing boards. A survey of professional boards indicates that most complaints were based on violations that occurred in private practice. The most frequent complaints were: practicing without a license, practicing beyond the scope permitted by law, and incorrect or inadequate treatment. Other complaints included injury from equipment or premises, conduct demonstrating moral unfitness, fraud, failure to refer, failure to obtain informed consent, failure to file a report, and inappropriate fees for services (Miller & Lubinski, 1986).

The following steps are recommended to ensure against a legal complaint:

1. Practice competently. Be aware of all current practice standards and adhere to them. Keep abreast by reading journals and attending conferences.
2. Evaluations should be based on standardized testing procedures.
3. Foster a good business relationship with your clients by returning all telephone calls promptly, keeping waiting time to a minimum, having convenient office hours, and sending bills with an adequate explanation.
4. Develop a treatment program with your client that is realistic and provides for accountability.
5. Educate your clients so that their participation in the treatment process is active and cooperative.
6. Document everything. Keep accurate records of every visit, including test procedures, treatment goals, and notes toward these goals. Document all communications with your client and family and other professionals including telephone calls, letters, and informal discussions.
7. Continually foster a relationship based on mutual respect and professional competence.

SUMMARY

Professional liability results when a professional's conduct is negligent during the course of treating a client and such conduct results in some injury to the client. Negligent conduct results when a professional's actions are not within the acceptable standard recognized by other professionals in the field. Norms for acceptable standards are found in both statutory and common law. Examples of acceptable standards of care are practicing with a license when such license is required by state law, properly evaluating clients, properly treating and instructing clients, referring clients to other professionals when appropriate, providing treatment alternatives, and obtaining informed consent.

The initiation of a professional liability claim is usually the final stage of a deteriorating client/ clinician relationship. Developing a positive relationship with clients is the best way for clinicians to protect themselves against legal actions.

DISCUSSION QUESTIONS

1. What is professional liability?
2. What are the four elements needed to prove a professional liability action?
3. What are some standards of care owed the client who requests services from a speech-language pathologist or audiologist?
4. Where can a disgruntled client file a complaint?
5. What are some recommended steps clinicians can take to reduce the risk of professional liability actions?

REFERENCES

Kooper, R., & Sullivan, C. (1986). Professional liability: management and prevention. In K. Butler (Ed.), *Prospering in private practice* (pp. 59–80). Rockville, MD: Aspen Publishers.

Miller, T., & Lubinski, R. (1986). Professional liability in speech-language pathology and audiology. *Asha, 28,* 45–47.

Prosser, W. (1971). *Handbook of the law of torts* (4th ed.). St. Paul: West Publishing Company.

Trace, R. (1993). Legal issues in audiology. *Advance, 3,* 11.

RESOURCES

Kramer, M., & Armbruster, J. (1982). *Forensic audiology.* Baltimore: University Park Press.

Albert H. Wohlers & Co., Administrators Group Insurance Plans (ASHA liability group carrier), 1500 Higgins Road, Park Ridge, Il 60068-5750.

■ CHAPTER 14 ■

Health Care Legislation: Implications for Financing and Service Delivery

■ CAROL FRATTALI, Ph.D. ■
■ BONNIE CURL, M.S. ■
■ MARLENE BEVAN, Ph.D. ■

SCOPE OF CHAPTER

Health care in the United States is facing dramatic change. The American Speech-Language-Hearing Association (ASHA) Task Force on Healthcare (1993d), in view of the need for reform, cites some startling statistics:

■ Health care expenditures currently account for 14% of the gross domestic product, and increase at a rate twice that of inflation (Levit, Lazenby, Letsch, & Cowan, 1991). Forecasts predict a ratio of 18% for the year 2000 (Reinhardt, 1993).

■ The United States pays more for health care than any other industrialized nation (Schieber & Poullier, 1991).

■ An estimated 37 million Americans are uninsured, creating a two-tiered system in which quality services are provided primarily to those who can afford them or are otherwise covered adequately by third-party payer sources.

- Only a small fraction of the U.S. health care dollar is spent on children. Children from birth to 18 years of age make up nearly 28% of the nation's population, yet accounted for less than 14% of health care expenditures in 1987 (Lewit & Monheit, 1992).
- Currently, nearly 18% of all children in the United States lack health insurance (Monheit & Cunningham, 1992).

To appreciate the need for reform, it is important that you acquire an historical perspective on the federal laws that helped to structure our health care system. How did the health care system evolve into its current state? What changes are on the horizon? And how will these changes affect the delivery and financing of speech-language pathology and audiology services? These questions are addressed in an effort to prepare you for what lies ahead in competitive and cost-conscious health care environment.

This chapter chronicles some of the important federal health care legislation that has shaped the current financing and service delivery systems. This legislation will be interpreted both generally and specifically from the view of the professions of speech-language pathology and audiology. A discussion follows on imminent health care reform. The chapter closes with implications for the practice of the professions.

AN INTRODUCTION TO HEALTH CARE LEGISLATION

Wilson and Neuhauser (1982) provide a succinct account of the legislative, as well as regulatory process. It is summarized here.

The activities of the federal government in health care are authorized by the passage of **laws**, or **statutes**, by Congress. Proposed legislation is called a **bill**. It is introduced in the Senate or House of Representatives by a congressional sponsor. It is assigned a number (e.g., S. 43, H.R. 36) and referred to the appropriate committee(s) for study. Public hearings often are held, after which the bill is either amended or entirely redrafted. Often, a bill is never reviewed by a committee and languishes until the end of the congressional session and, in essence, dies. If the bill is approved by the committee, it is placed on the legislative calendar for vote by the entire House or Senate. If passed, the bill is sent to the other chamber where the same process of committee referral, reporting, and floor debate take place. Another process that can take place is the introduction of identical or similar bills in each chamber. If the versions passed by each body vary, the differences are then settled by conference committee composed of members of both the House and Senate authorizing committees. If a referred bill is passed by both houses, it is sent to the president for approval. When signed by the president, the bill becomes a law, or statute.

The law is then numbered sequentially and by number of the Congress. Public Law (P.L.) 89-97, for example, means the 97th law passed by the 89th Congress. Much legislation is **authorizing legislation**, which establishes or continues programs and authorizes funding for them. **Appropriations legislation** actually appropriates or provides the funds.

Finally, many of the details of the various laws are left to be spelled out in **regulations**. Regulations are developed by the various departments and their administrative agencies of the executive branch (e.g., the Health Care Financing Administration of the U.S. Department of Health and Human Services). As these are developed, they are published in the *Federal Register*. Most often, they are published as proposed regulations, which are then revised after comments have been received from interested parties. These regulations are then incorporated in the *Code of Federal Regulations* and have the force of law. The glossary at the end of this chapter will familiarize you with some of the terminology used to describe the legislative and regulatory process.

SPECIFIC HEALTH CARE LEGISLATION

The following chronology summarizes some of the major federal health care legislation that has influenced the provision of speech-language pathology and audiology services. Much of the information that follows, particularly as it relates to the Social Security Act, comes from Wilson and Neuhauser (1982). For more detailed information about the following and related health care legislation, you are referred to Wilson and Neuhauser (1982), Downey, White, and Karr (1984), and back issues of ASHA's *Governmental Affairs Review* and *Federal Legislative Issues*.

SOCIAL SECURITY ACT (1935)

The Social Security Act of 1935 was a landmark piece of legislation, developed and passed during the Great Depression. It represented the first major entrance of the federal government into the area of social insurance and it greatly expanded federal grant-in-aid assistance to the states (Wilson & Neuhauser, 1982).

The Social Security Act formed the base for important federal programs in health care, including Medicare and Medicaid. In general, the act provides for the general welfare by establishing a system of federal benefits for the elderly and by enabling states to make more adequate provisions for aged persons, blind persons, dependent and disabled children, maternal and child welfare, public health, and the administration of unemployment compensation laws.

Over the years several amendments were made to the act, including:

Social Security Amendments of 1965

These amendments established Medicare (Title XVIII), the national program of health insurance for the aged. The amendments also created Medicaid (Title XIX), federally supported and state administered programs of health insurance for public assistance recipients (which was an expansion of existing medical assistance programs to groups other than the elderly). There were also a number of amendments to Title V that formed the core services of many community health centers.

These amendments created two parts to the Medicare program: Parts A and B. Part A,

hospital insurance benefits, provides basic protection against the costs of hospital and related posthospital services. It was financed by an increase in the Social Security earnings tax (payroll tax). Benefits included: inpatient hospital services, posthospital extended care services, posthospital home health services, and hospital outpatient diagnostic services. Speech-language pathology services could be provided as part of inpatient hospital, skilled nursing facility (as part of extended care benefits), and home health services.

Part B, supplemental medical insurance benefits, is a voluntary program financed from premium payments by enrollees and matching payments from general revenues. Benefits included: physicians' services and related services such as X-rays and laboratory tests, supplies and equipment, and home health services. It was not until 1972 that speech-language pathology services were added to Part B benefits.

It is important to recognize that, to date, neither "audiology" nor "audiologist" appears anywhere in Medicare law. Audiological services and audiologists, however, are recognized in Medicare regulations and guidelines and are reimbursed by Medicare Parts A and B under certain circumstances (Downey et al., 1984). In addition, the definition of audiologist is included with that for speech-language pathologist in the home health agency conditions of participation. Diagnostic audiology for the purpose of assisting a physician in making a medical diagnosis and determining the course of medical treatment is covered. In addition, aural rehabilitation, provided by either an audiologist employed in a hospital or by a physician, or by a speech-language pathologist is included as a Medicare benefit. The Medicare statute specifically excludes coverage for hearing aids and any examination related to hearing aids.

To understand the intricacies of speech-language pathology and audiology services under Medicare, you are referred to Downey et al., (1984) and are well advised to contact staff from the Health Care Financing Division of the American Speech-Language-Hearing Association (ASHA) to receive the most current information on Medicare, as well as Medicaid. Two other publications of interest, prepared by ASHA's Health Care Financing Division, are *The Medicare Handbook* (ASHA, 1993b) and *Guide to Medicare Rehabilitation Agencies for Speech-Language Pathologists* (ASHA, 1991).

Medicaid also extended eligibility to medically indigent persons not on welfare. Under this program, states are to provide at least some of each of five basic services: inpatient hospital services, outpatient hospital services, other laboratory and X-ray services, skilled nursing facility services, and physician's services. A range of additional services, including audiology and speech-language pathology services, also could be offered by the states. The federal share of the program's costs is 50% to 83%, according to the state's per capita income.

Social Security Amendments of 1967

These amendments added outpatient physical therapy services under Part B of the Medicare Program. They also eliminated the requirement that a physician certify the medical necessity of outpatient hospital services. Periodic certification after admission, however, remains.

Social Security Amendments of 1972

These amendments expanded Medicare to include health insurance for individuals with severe disabilities. Persons who have received cash benefits under the disability insurance provisions of the Social Security Act for at least 2 years would be eligible for health care benefits under Medicare. Thus, Medicare became the health insurance program for individuals who are 65 years and older, and individuals under 65 years who have a disability. **The amendments of 1972 also added coverage of speech-language pathology services as part of outpatient physical therapy services under Medicare.**

As a result of these amendments, regulations were promulgated (effective in 1976) specifying conditions of participation for clinics, rehabilitation agencies, and public health agencies as providers of outpatient speech-language pathology services under Medicare Part B. Now speech-language pathologists independently can obtain a Medicare provider number if they meet the requirements for recognition as a rehabilitation agency.

In addition, the Early and Periodic Screening, Diagnosis and Treatment (EPSDT) Program under Medicaid was established. This program provides for child health screening (including screening for speech, language, and hearing), hearing aids, augmentative and assistive communication devices and subsequent treatment for children of families receiving aid for dependent children.

Social Security Amendments of 1982

Concern over rapidly rising ancillary costs led to amendments that changed the way in which hospitals were reimbursed for costs by Medicare. The Tax Equity and Fiscal Responsibility Act (TEFRA) marked the beginning of a new era in Medicare reimbursement. For the first time, hospitals were paid according to fixed payment levels or discharge limits rather than what they reported as their actual costs. These TEFRA limits were applied to all routine operating costs, costs of special care units, and costs of inpatient ancillary services including speech-language pathology and audiology services. Further, the TEFRA limits capped the rate of increase of a hospital's Medicare reimbursement per discharge from one fiscal period to the next.

TEFRA offered strong incentive to providers to contain costs, although Medicare's Prospective Payment System (PPS) (described later) would offer stronger incentive. As TEFRA continued and rehabilitation services have remained under its limits, providers have become increasingly dissatisfied with the effect of the system (National Association of Rehabilitation Facilities, 1990). According to the National Association of Rehabilitation Facilities (NARF) (NARF, 1990), recent increases in TEFRA limits have not been sufficient to pay for the increasing costs of as many as half of all rehabilitation facilities, and leading providers, themselves, to propose changes to the way in which rehabilitation services are reimbursed.

TEFRA also added a new Medicare provider setting. Section 122 established coverage for hospice care. The act specifically covers speech-language pathology services for the terminally ill. Section 418.92, Title 42 of the *Code of Federal Regulations* (1990) states, "Physical therapy services, occupational therapy services, and speech-language pathology services must be available, and, when provided, offered in a manner consistent with accepted standards of practice."

Social Security Amendments of 1983

In reaction to predictions that the Medicare program would go bankrupt by the year 2000 without drastic cost controls, the payment methodology of fixed payment levels or cost limits begun under TEFRA was strengthened dramatically in 1983. The Social Security Amendments of 1983 created a new system, the Prospective Payment System (PPS), in which a flat payment was determined prior to treatment and based on a patient's principal diagnosis or diagnosis-related group (DRG).

PPS was considered to provide strong incentive for hospitals to provide efficient services. Hospitals could keep any savings realized under the Medicare DRGs. If the hospital's actual costs to treat a patient were less than the flat amount assigned to that particular DRG, the hospital kept the difference. However, if the hospital's actual costs exceeded the payment assigned, the hospital absorbed the loss.

Although such incentive reimbursement offered strong encouragement to providers for efficiency, it also raised concerns regarding a number of less positive effects. Health care professionals reported that PPS compromised quality of care. They alleged that patients were being discharged quicker and sicker. Others raised the concern that hospitals, struggling to survive in the health market, would learn to "game the system" and simply shift costs to other areas.

Inpatient rehabilitation units and rehabilitation hospitals were exempt from Medicare's PPS (as were pediatric, psychiatric, and long-term care hospitals), but remained subject to the TEFRA cost limits.

Although anecdotal, the fallout of PPS for inpatient speech-language pathology and audiology services has reportedly been late or reduced inpatient referrals, fewer inpatient sessions, downsizing of staff, or reluctance to contract for new services. At the same time, however, units and hospitals exempted from Medicare's PPS enjoyed unprecedented growth (Wilkerson, Batavia, & DeJong, 1992).

U.S. PUBLIC HEALTH SERVICE ACT (1944)

The Public Health Service Act of 1944 revised and brought together in one statute all existing legislation concerning the U.S. Public Health Service. It set forth provisions for the organization, staffing, and activities of the service. There have been many amendments to this act, including the Health Maintenance Organization Act.

The Health Maintenance Organization Act of 1973

This act amended the Public Health Service Act to provide assistance and encouragement for the establishment and expansion of health maintenance organizations. The act added a new title, XIII, Health Maintenance Organizations (HMOs), to the Public Health Service Act. The act required the provision of the following basic medical services for a set, periodic payment fixed under a community rating system: physician services, inpatient and outpatient services, medically necessary emergency health services, short-term outpatient evaluative and crisis intervention mental health services (not over 20 visits), medical treatment and referral services for alcohol and drug abuse, laboratory and X-ray services, home health services, and preventive services. Supplemental health services were also to be made available to enrolled members who wished to contract for them. They were: intermediate and long-term care, vision care, and dental and mental health services not included under basic services, plus provision of prescription drugs.

Numerous amendments designed to make the requirements under the act less stringent were made to the act over the years. In 1976, an additional provision in the amendments required that HMOs receiving reimbursement from Medicare or Medicaid must be federally qualified. The regulatory language resulting from these provisions also resulted in limitations on the provision of speech-language pathology and audiology services:

Federally qualified HMOs must provide or arrange for outpatient service and inpatient hospital services [which] shall include short-term rehabilitation and physical therapy, the provision of which the HMO determines can be expected to result in the significant improvement of a member's condition within a period of two months. (*Code of Federal Regulations,* Title 42, Section 110.102 [1990])

This language has reportedly had an apparently unintended effect on the length of treatment allowable for speech-language pathology services in HMOs. The regulatory language designates 2 months or 60 days as a **minimum** for rehabilitation services. However, it appears to be used by HMOs as a **maximum** limit, at least for speech-language pathology services. In a 1986 survey of HMOs (Cornett & Chabon, 1986), most reported limitations on speech-language pathology services to a maximum of 2 months or 60 days.

TECHNOLOGY-RELATED ASSISTANCE FOR INDIVIDUALS WITH DISABILITIES ACT OF 1988

The purpose of the act is to provide financial assistance to states for developing and implementing a consumer-responsive statewide program of technology-related assistance for individuals with disabilities. Such programs must be designed, in part, to increase the availability of and funding for the provision of assistive technology devices and services. ASHA worked to include a broad definition of "assistive device" in the act (ASHA, 1990). The term refers to any item, piece of equipment, or product system—whether acquired commercially off-the-shelf, modified, or customized—that is used to increase, maintain,

or improve functional capabilities of individuals with disabilities. The term "assistive technology service" refers to any service that directly assists an individual with a disability in the selection, acquisition, or use of an assistive technology device. It includes evaluation of needs, acquisition of devices, repairing/replacing devices, coordinating services, and training or technical assistance.

OMNIBUS BUDGET RECONCILIATION ACTS (OBRAs)

Although many important pieces of legislation for health care have been authorizing statutes, much has also resulted from budget reconciliation. Traditionally, the budget process involved setting dollar outlays for broad budget categories or "functions," such as health and education. Specific programmatic changes to achieve those outlays were left to authorizing and appropriating legislation.

However, in the 96th Congress, the "reconciliation" procedure of the Congressional Budget and Impoundment Control Act of 1974 was used for the first time to "instruct" the authorizing committees to cut spending in numerous health programs. Since then, reconciliation has become an integral part of the budget process (National Health Council, 1993). Provisions in the following reconciliation laws are of interest to speech-language pathologists and audiologists.

OMNIBUS BUDGET RECONCILIATION ACT OF 1980

A component in the new law had a notable impact for speech-language pathologists providing services to Medicare beneficiaries. ASHA lobbied for legislation that was incorporated into OBRA 1980 that amended Medicare to eliminate the physician prescription requirement for outpatient speech-language pathology services. **Effective January 1, 1981, speech-language pathologists could write their own plans of treatment for Medicare beneficiaries.**

In their 1979 reports on the Medicare Amendments legislation, the Senate Finance Committee and the House Ways and Means Committee stated that, "Since speech[-language] pathology involves highly specialized knowledge and training, physicians generally do not specify in detail the services needed when referring a patient for such services" [House Report 96-588 at p. 15; Senate Report 96-471 at p. 37].

Consolidated Omnibus Budget Reconciliation Act of 1985

Provisions in this act, which contained amendments to the Medicare and Medicaid programs, established the Physician Payment Review Commission. This commission was required to make recommendations to Congress regarding changes in the methodology for determining the rates of payment for Medicare Part B services. This legislation led to the implementation of the Resource-Based Relative Value Scale (RBRVS). The RBRVS is a rating of Medicare Part B services on the basis of relative resource inputs (work and other practice costs) to provide medical services. Use of the system has implications primarily for provision of audiology services (ASHA, 1992b). These implications are detailed in the OBRA '89 subsection below.

Omnibus Budget Reconciliation Act of 1986

Section 9305 of OBRA '86 required the development of a Uniform Needs Assessment Instrument (UNAI) to evaluate the functional capacity and health care needs of the individual to assist with functional incapacities. The legislation was a response to the increased anxiety and alarm expressed by health care consumers at the decreasing length of the average hospital stay. It was thought to be a safeguard to ensure the quality of care provided to Medicare beneficiaries (U.S. Department of Health and Human Services, 1992).

According to the law, the tool can be used by discharge planners, hospitals, nursing facilities, other health care providers, and fiscal intermediaries in evaluating an individual's need for posthospital extended-care services, home health services, and long-term

care services of a health-related or supportive nature. These services would include speech-language pathology and audiology services. To date, a tool has been developed, but not yet implemented, to determine posthospital needs. Use of such a tool is currently tangled in debate about its need. A recent report, submitted by former Secretary of Health and Human Services Louis Sullivan, indicates that Congress should investigate unnecessary duplication of effort and wasteful expenditures that the UNAI may induce (U.S. Department of Health and Human Services, 1992).

The tool, Form HCFA-32 (titled the Assessment of Needs for Continuing Care), addresses communication among those factors that may affect postdischarge care needs. A draft of the tool can be found in the "Report of the Secretary's Advisory Panel on the Development of Uniform Needs Assessment Instrument(s)" (U.S. Department of Health and Human Services, 1992).

In addition, OBRA '86 directs the Health Care Financing Administration (HCFA), the federal agency that administers Medicare, to proceed with research on a new system of Medicare Part B payment to physicians and other practitioners. It led to implementation of the RBRVS.

Omnibus Budget Reconciliation Act of 1987

OBRA '87, in response to the pervasiveness of substandard conditions in the nation's nursing homes, made sweeping reforms on the care provided by all nursing homes participating in the Medicare and Medicaid programs. This legislation mandates nursing facilities receiving Medicare and Medicaid reimbursement to provide each resident the necessary care and services to "attain or maintain the highest practicable physical, mental and psychosocial well-being, in accordance with the comprehensive assessment and plan of care" (Code of Federal Regulations, Title 42, Section 483.25 [1990]). The regulations resulting from this legislation further specify that the comprehensive assessment include an assessment of functional status, including the ability to use speech, language, or other functional communication systems (Lubinski & Frattali, 1993; White, 1989).

OBRA '87 holds great potential for improving access to quality care for nursing facility residents with communication disorders and related disorders, such as dysphagia and cognitive deficits. As a result of this legislation, the Resident Assessment Instrument (RAI) was developed (Morris et al., 1991). The RAI contains a minimum data set that requires information on communication/hearing. It was developed with input from the American Speech-Language-Hearing Association (Lubinski & Frattali, 1993).

Three years after the tool was put in place in the nation's nursing facilities, survey data collected by the research consortium involved in the development of the RAI documented a 31% increase in referrals to speech-language pathology (audiology data were not reported at the time) (Lubinski, personal communication, 1993).

OMNIBUS BUDGET RECONCILIATION ACT OF 1989

OBRA '89 established the Agency for Health Care Policy and Research (AHCPR). It is one of eight agencies of the U.S. Public Health Service within the Department of Health and Human Services and replaces the National Center for Health Services Research and Health Care Technology Assessment. AHCPR supports studies on the outcomes of health care services and procedures used to prevent, diagnose, treat, and manage illness and disability (Agency for Health Care Policy and Research, 1990b).

An arm of AHCPR, the Office of the Forum for Quality and Effectiveness in Health Care, is charged with coordinating the development of national practice guidelines (Agency for Health Care Policy and Research, 1990a). These multidisciplinary guidelines are intended for widespread use by providers as well as consumers as a yardstick for measuring the quality of care for certain medical conditions.

The professions of speech-language pathology and audiology have been well represented on expert panels charged with drafting guideline language (Goldberg, 1993). Three guidelines of interest to the professions address otitis media in children, poststroke rehabilitation, and Alzheimer's disease screening.

OBRA '89 also required Medicare to begin paying for charge-based Part B services by January 1992, based on a resource-based relative value scale (RBRVS) with geographic adjustments for differences in costs of practice. This legislation replaced the reasonable charge payment mechanism with a fee schedule based on national uniform relative values for all "physician services" including outpatient rehabilitation services. The system was to have been phased in over a 4-year period, beginning in 1992.

The RBRVS has caused concern among audiologists and, to a lesser extent, speech-language pathologists (ASHA, Task Force on Resource-Based Relative Value Scale, 1992b). The system, which is based on the Current Procedural Terminology (CPT) Codes, does not recognize the interpretation of audiologic tests. Thus, audiologists could not bill for interpretation of audiologic testing (White & Kander, 1992). The RBRVS system also equates independent practitioners with those employed by physicians. Consequently, the system would have a detrimental effect on audiologists and speech-language pathologists who bill directly for their services. Finally, there is a potential, under the system, for physicians to use noncertified assistants to perform screening, diagnostic, and therapeutic services normally provided by speech-language pathologists and audiologists and to bill for these services. This practice certainly could lower quality of care and potentially lower Medicare payment rates for speech-language pathology and audiology services. A review of audiology and speech-language pathology relative value units is provided by White and Kander (1992).

Finally, OBRA '89 improved the Medicaid EPSDT program so that proper treatment for disorders discovered during screening be provided (White, 1990).

Omnibus Budget
Reconciliation Act of 1990

OBRA '90 (Omnibus Budget and Reconciliation Act, 1990) includes Section 4005(b)(1) which states:

The Secretary of Health and Human Services shall develop a proposal to modify the current system under which [excluded] hospitals receive payment . . . or a proposal to replace such system with a system under which such payments would be made on the basis of nationally determined average standardized amounts.

Through this provision, Congress made clear its intent to develop a more appropriate payment system for rehabilitation under Medicare (Wilkerson et al., 1992). The 1990 OBRA legislation, as an interim measure, also provided some relief to hospitals in the form of partial payment for differences between the TEFRA cap and actual hospital costs (Wilkerson et al., 1992).

THE ROLE OF STATE GOVERNMENTS

Historically, the states have played an important role in shaping the structure, delivery, and reimbursement of health care services. One of the ways in which states affect change derives from their ability to receive a waiver from a federally prescribed system of implementing a program. Under such a waiver, states can enact systems that are more responsive to the specific needs of their residents while maintaining compliance with the overall goals of the federal program. This action often has an impact far beyond the individual states.

For example, New Jersey sought and received such a waiver from the Health Care Financing Administration (HCFA) for the administration of Medicare within the state. As a result of that waiver, the state developed and implemented an alternative payment program that utilized diagnosis-related groups (DRGs) for reimbursement of hospital costs. In its health care cost containment efforts, the Reagan administration used the New Jersey system as a prototype in developing the federal Prospective Payment System under Medicare.

States also affect the structuring and delivery of health care services as well as the reimbursement for those services through direct authority over a number of health care issues. Those issues include the licensing of health care professionals, insurance regulation, public health, indigent care, rate setting, and access to health care services within the state. For example, states have considerable latitude for the administration of the Medicaid program. In fact, considerable variation is found from state to state in coverage of audiology and speech-language pathology services by provider setting, procedures, and assistive technology.

You can expect that the role of states in national health care will increase over the next few years. In fact, it is believed that the states rather than the federal government will drive health care reform in this country. Interest in extending considerable latitude to the states in providing and managing health care services has been expressed by players on all fronts including Congress and the Administration.

THE FUTURE OF HEALTH CARE

Dramatic changes lie ahead for health care in the United States. The legislative and regulatory changes outlined in this chapter were implemented slowly and often in piecemeal fashion. In contrast, the sharply elevating costs of health care, changing population demographics, and health care inequities are moving the nation rapidly toward comprehensive change. You can anticipate sweeping change in the way health care services are delivered and financed during the next few years.

Reform proposals by Congress, the Administration, consumers, states, and others all include certain fundamental factors for health care reform. Universal concerns will most likely result in a national health care package that:

- Controls costs
- Enhances quality
- Expands access
- Encourages local responsibility
- Focuses on patient outcomes
- Increases accountability
- Emphasizes health promotion and disease prevention

Consistent with these fundamental principles, The ASHA Ad Hoc Committee on National Health Policy prepared a position on health care reform to be used in ASHA's advocacy and lobbying efforts (ASHA, 1993c). According to this position statement, any national health policy must adhere to the following 12 principles: Provide universal access to consumers; recognize individual needs; ensure quality of life; ensure consumer and professional representation for policy development and implementation; support consumer education; allow consumers to choose provider settings; cover comprehensive services; provide cost-effective services; ensure broad-based financing; support research; recognize the autonomy of the audiology and speech-language pathology professions; and provide access to necessary assistive and augmentative technology.

Similarly, the disability community, through the work of the Consortium for Citizens with Disabilities (1992), drafted a disability perspective on health care reform. The perspective included a number of key features. Health care reform must be: nondiscriminatory (e.g., ensure that all persons have access to needed services); comprehensive (e.g., include audiology and speech-language pathology among benefits); appropriate (e.g., ensure appropriate amount, scope, and duration of services, ensure the availability of trained personnel); equitable (e.g., limit out of pocket expenses); and efficient (e.g., reduce administrative complexity, maintain effective cost controls).

Beyond the fundamental principles articulated by a variety of players, you can expect to see specific elements in all health care reform efforts. A standard benefits package will be created to define exactly which services each individual is entitled to by law. Although current proposals include speech-language pathology and audiology services, they impose limitations on length of service based on expectations of functional gain. Reimbursement will be linked directly to evidence that services provided are beneficial and cost-efficient. Health care providers will be held accountable for the quality and cost-efficiency of their services.

Overriding all of these principles and anticipated key elements, the major thrust of health care reform will be "managed care." But what exactly is managed care? It can be a type of health maintenance organization (HMO), a preferred provider organization (PPO), or even simply a requirement for a second opinion. Whatever its formal structure, managed care involves a system with several common dimensions (Griffin & Fazen, 1993):

- Selected providers who furnish comprehensive services to members;
- Fees and rates that have been negotiated with the plan's providers to be lower than the normal price of services;
- Formal quality improvement and utilization review programs; and
- Financial incentives for members to use providers and procedures covered by the plan.

Several trends appear on the horizon for managed care (Griffin & Fazen, 1993). Its importance and scope will increase. There will be a move toward shared risk, or capitated arrangements instead of discounts from fees-for-service. As mergers and consolidation among managed care plans continue, there will be larger but fewer players. Severity-adjusted clinical outcomes and clinical protocols will be used increasingly in service and payment decision making. More specialty managed care organizations (e.g., dental, mental health, rehabilitation) will evolve to subcontract with managed care plans for a particular segment of health care. Responding to capitated rates, acute and rehabilitation hospitals will develop lower cost alternative settings for the patient who requires a long medical stay.

The professions of speech-language pathology and audiology, through the efforts of ASHA, are preparing now for this restructuring. ASHA's efforts include lobbying and advocacy activities (ASHA, 1993a); work with several national coalitions (e.g., National Rehabilitation Caucus, Consortium for Citizens with Disabilities); a special project to collect, summarize, and disseminate treatment efficacy data; a grant project to develop a functional outcome measure (ASHA, 1992a); and an Ad Hoc Committee on Managed Care established to develop professional educational products on managed care for ASHA members.

What will restructuring of health care delivery and financing mean for speech-language pathologists and audiologists? In its broadest sense, reform will require professionals to look beyond their own disciplines. Clinicians must begin to think along service lines, such as rehabilitative, neurological, and pediatric services (Hospital Management Review, 1993). Professional collaboration and the development of multispecialty networks and new alliances, case management, team approaches to care, critical paths (a coordinated work flow plan from start to finish with estimated time frames for completion [Hofmann, 1993]), and use of support personnel will become increasingly important. Speech-language pathologists and audiologists, for example, may need to form alliances with physicians, psychologists, optometrists, physical therapists, and occupational therapists, depending on which service lines could be developed for contract negotiations with the major purchasers of care.

Finally, clinicians must become sensitive to and expert in "quantifying their practice." Available efficacy research and related cost/benefit studies must be used to support the benefits of treatment. More efficacy research and cost/benefit analyses must be conducted, disseminated, and used by members of the professions. Outcome measurement, particularly functional status measures and patient satisfaction measures, must be refined and used on a continuing basis by all professionals. Patients must be oriented to contribute to that information, and consumers, in general, must be educated to understand what that information means.

SUMMARY

The health care legislation summarized in this chapter has led to the creation of a complex health care system that has fallen far short of meeting the needs of all Americans. The current system has imposed layers of bureaucracy and program limitations that have led to often arbitrary decisions about who will provide what services, to whom, and at what cost. Soon you will be competing in yet a new system, most definitely on the basis of the cost and quality of your services. Thus, you must learn to collect and use objective and convincing evidence that what you do makes a difference and is cost-effective.

Change is on the horizon. Consequently, there will be both obstacles and opportunities facing speech-language pathologists and audiologists. The professions will continue to prepare for the future of health care. You are, however, well advised that the true measure of your success in a reformed health care system will be the ability to compete individually by acting collaboratively and beyond the boundaries of your own discipline.

DISCUSSION QUESTIONS

1. Describe the legislative process.
2. Why is prospective payment called incentive reimbursement?
3. Select an important piece of legislation and describe its impact on the practice or reimbursement of speech-language pathology and audiology services.
4. Describe the role of state governments in health care reform.
5. In view of health care reform, how might you compete successfully on the basis of cost and quality?

REFERENCES

Agency for Health Care Policy and Research. (1990a, August). Clinical guideline development. *AHCPR Program Note*. Rockville, MD: U.S. Department of Health and Human Services.

Agency for Health Care Policy and Research. (1990b, March). Medical treatment effectiveness research. *AHCPR Program Note*. Rockville, MD: U.S. Department of Health and Human Services.

American Speech-Language-Hearing Association. (1990, March). *Federal legislative issues: Current issues of interest to speech-language pathologists, audiologists and persons with communication disorders* (ASHA Congressional Relations Division Report). Rockville, MD: Author.

American Speech-Language-Hearing Association. (1991). *Guide to medicare rehabilitation agencies for speech-language pathologists*. Rockville, MD: Author.

American Speech-Language-Hearing Association. (1992a). New ASHA project to develop a functional communication measure for adults. *Project Newsletter*. Rockville, MD: Author.

American Speech-Language-Hearing Association. (1992b). Strategies for responding to the Medicare resource-based relative value scale (RBRVS) (ASHA Task Force on Resource-Based Relative Value Scale Report). *Asha, 34*(4), 63–68.

American Speech-Language-Hearing Association. (1993a). Health care reform: ASHA takes action. *Asha, 35*(8), 23–24.

American Speech-Language-Hearing Association. (1993b). *The medicare handbook*. Rockville, MD: Author.

American Speech-Language-Hearing Association. (1993c). Ad Hoc Committee on National Health Policy. Position statement on national health policy. *Asha, 35*(8)(Suppl. 10), 1.

American Speech-Language-Hearing Association. (1993d). Report of the Task Force on Health Care. *Asha, 35*(8), 53–54.

Consortium for Citizens with Disabilities. (1992, November). Principles for health care reform from a disability perspective (Health Task Force Update). Washington, DC: Author.

Cornett, B., & Chabon, S. (1986, November). *Speech-language pathologists: Winners or losers in the health care revolution?* Paper presented at the meeting of the American Speech-Language- Hearing Association, Detroit, MI.

Downey, M., White, S., & Karr, S. (1984). *Health insurance manual for speech-language pathologists and audiologists*. Rockville, MD: Author.

Goldberg, B. (1993). Translating data into practice. *Asha, 35*(8), 45–47.

Griffin, K. M., & Fazen, M. (1993). A managed care strategy for practitioners. *Quality Improvement Digest*. Rockville, MD: American Speech-Language-Hearing Association.

Hofmann, P. A. (1993, July). Critical path method: An important tool for coordinating clinical care. *Journal of Quality Improvement, 19*, 235–246.

Hospital Management Review. (1993, August). Case management model stresses discipline integration. *Hospital Management Review, 12*, 3.

Levit, K. R., Lazenby, H. C., Letsch, S. W., & Cowan, C. A. (1991, Spring). National health care spending, 1989. *Health Affairs, 10*(1), 117–130.

Lewit, E. M., & Monheit, A. C. (1992, Winter). Expenditures on health care for children and pregnant women. *The Future of Children* (pp. 95–114). Rockville, MD: Agency for Health Care Policy and Research.

Lubinski, R., & Frattali, C. (1993). Nursing home reform: The Resident Assessment Instrument. *Asha, 35*(1), 59–62.

Monheit, A. C., & Cunningham, P. J. (1992, Winter). Children without health insurance. *The Future of Children* (pp. 154–170). Rockville, MD: Agency for Health Care Policy and Research.

Morris, J. N., Hawes, C., Murphy, K., Nonemaker, S., Phillips, C., Fries, B. E., & Mor, V. (1991). *Resident assessment instrument training manual and resource guide*. Natick, MA: Eliot Press.

National Association of Rehabilitation Facilities. (1990). ProPAC examines excluded facilities. *Medical Rehabilitation Review, 7*(51), 1–2.

National Health Council. (1993, July). *Congress and health*. New York, NY: National Health Council, Inc.

Office of the Federal Register. (1990). *Code of Federal Regulations*. Washington, DC: U.S. Government Printing Office.

Omnibus Budget and Reconciliation Act, Pub. L. No. 101-508, Section 4005(b)(1) (1990).

Reinhardt, U. E. (1993, April). *Health care in an age of constrained (though not shrinking) budgets*. Paper presented at the Fifth Annual National Managed Health Care Congress. Washington, DC.

Schieber, G. J., & Poullier, J. (1991, Spring). International health spending: Issues and trends. *Health Affairs, 10*(1), 106–115.

U.S. Department of Health and Human Services (1992, December). Report of the Secretary's Advisory Panel on the Development of Uniform Needs Assessment Instrument(s): Report to Congress. Washington, DC: Health Care Financing Administration.

White, S. (1989, April). Medicare and nursing home services. *Asha, 31*, 75, 59.

White, S. (1990, June/July). EPSDT: A program you should know. *Asha, 32*, 77–78.

White, S., & Kander, M. (1992, April). Medicare resource-based relative value scale (RBRVS) summary and guide. *Asha, 34*, 60–62.

Wilkerson, D. L., Batavia, A. J., & DeJong, G. (1992). Use of functional status measures for payment of medical rehabilitation services. *Archives of Physical Medicine and Rehabilitation, 73*, 111–120.

Wilson, F. A., & Neuhauser, D. (1982). *Health services in the United States* (2nd ed.). Cambridge, MA: Ballinger Publishing.

GLOSSARY OF LEGISLATIVE, REGULATORY, AND REIMBURSEMENT TERMS

Acts: Bills (or joint resolutions) that have been passed in both houses of Congress and become law. Also, measures introduced as "A Bill" are re-designated as "An Act" after passage in the house of origin, whether or not they finally become law.

appropriations: Legislation to provide the money required to fund governmental programs previously established by authorizing legislation.

appropriations legislation: Legislation that appropriates or provides the funds for established programs.

authorizing legislation: Legislation that establishes or continues programs and authorizes funding for them.

Bills: Measures proposing legislation to create a new act (or amend or repeal existing law). Must be passed by both houses and

signed by the President before finally becoming law (abbreviated as "H.R." in the House and "S." in the Senate).

capitation: A payment option in which charges are paid per capita or per enrollee for the range of health care services. Capitation rates are usually expressed in units of "per enrollee per month."

Code of Federal Regulations (CFR): A codification of the regulations of the various federal agencies, published in 50 titles according to subject matter. Generally revised on an annual basis to incorporate changes adopted during the previous year.

current procedural terminology (CPT) codes: A listing and five-digit coding of procedures and services performed by physicians and published by the American Medical Association. The purpose of CPT codes are to accurately communicate medical, surgical, and diagnostic services among physicians, patients, and third parties. Speech-language pathology and audiology services are among those listed.

diagnosis-related groups (DRGs): A system for classifying hospital inpatients into groups, codified by principal diagnosis, that are clinically coherent and homogeneous with respect to resource use. The Health Care Financing Administration bases its Medicare Part A hospital reimbursement levels on DRGs.

Federal Register: A daily publication that provides a uniform system for publishing presidential and federal agency documents. Divided into five major sections: Presidential Documents, Rules and Regulations, Proposed Rules, Notices, and Sunshine Act Meetings.

health maintenance organization (HMO): A comprehensive health service organization

Sources: Legi-Slate. (1988). *Glossary of congressional and regulatory terms.* Washington, DC: Author; Downey, M., White, S., & Karr, S. (1984). *Health insurance manual for speech-language pathologists and audiologists.* Rockville, MD: Author; Wilson, F. A., & Neuhauser, D. (1982). *Health services in the United States* (2nd ed.). Cambridge, MA: Ballinger Publishing; Griffin, K. M., & Fazen, M. (1993). A managed care strategy for practitioners. *Quality Improvement Digest.* Rockville, MD: American Speech-Language-Hearing Association.

that provides health care services to members (enrollees) in a geographic area through a panel of providers. Members pay a fixed, pre-paid amount of money, usually on a "per member per month" basis, without regard to the amount of actual services utilized.

laws: Acts passed by both houses of Congress and signed by the President, or passed over his or her veto.

legislation: A proposed or enacted law or group of laws. Also, the act or process of lawmaking.

managed care: A system of managing and financing health care delivery to ensure that services provided to managed care plan enrollees are necessary, efficiently provided, and appropriately priced.

preferred provider organization (PPO): A managed care plan that contracts with independent providers for negotiated discounted fees for services rendered to plan members. Patients have a financial incentive, such as reduced copayments or lower deductibles, to use the PPO's network of providers.

prospective payment: A payment methodology in which the rate of payment is determined before the provision of services.

Public Laws (P.L.): Laws resulting from passage of public bills, having national applicability.

rehabilitation agency: Per Medicare guidelines, a health provider that supplies speech-language pathology services, occupational therapy, and/or physical therapy and social or vocational adjustment services.

relative value scale: A listing of services and procedures that are given an index number reflecting the relative length and difficulty of the task. This index can then be multiplied by a fixed dollar amount to obtain an appropriate fee.

resource-based relative value scale: Rating of Medicare Part B services on the basis of relative resource inputs (work and other practice costs) to provide medical services. Specifi-cally refers to relative physician work values developed by the Harvard RBRVS study.

retrospective denial of payment: A procedure in which the payer reviews the appropriateness of the use of services after they have been provided and denies payment on the basis that they were medically unnecessary.

retrospective payment: A payment methodology in which payment is determined after services are provided, based on costs or charges incurred.

rules and regulations: Regulatory documents having general applicability and legal effect, most of which are keyed to and codified in the *Code of Federal Regulations* (CFR).

statutes: A compilation of all laws enacted by Congress. They are termed "Statutes-at-large" and numbered by volume and page number where the text of each law can be found (e.g., "93 Stat. 326").

third-party payer: Any organization, public or private, that pays or insures health and medical expenses on behalf of beneficiaries or recipients. The individual generally pays a premium for such coverage in all private and some public programs. The person receiving the service is the first party, the provider or supplier is referred to as the second party, and the organization paying for it is the third party.

RESOURCES FOR ADDITIONAL INFORMATION

Audiology and Speech-Language Pathology Services and the Mandate for Health Care Reform. American Speech-Language-Hearing Association. Rockville, MD, 1993.

Congress and Health: An Introduction to the Legislative Process and its Key Participants. National Health Council. New York, NY, 1993.

The Dance of Legislation. Eric Redman. Simon and Schuster. New York, NY, 1973.

Health Groups in Washington: A Directory. National Health Council. New York, NY, 1993.

Legi-Slate Glossary of Congressional and Regulatory Terms. Legi-Slate, Inc. Washington, DC, 1988.

A Managed Care Strategy for Practitioners. Griffin, K., & Fazen, M. *Quality Improvement Digest.* American Speech-Language-Hearing Association. Rockville, MD, Winter, 1993.

HOW TO OBTAIN A BILL, REPORT, OR PUBLIC LAW

A free copy of a House or Senate bill, committee report, or conference report may be obtained by sending a written request (reference the bill or report number) and self-addressed label to:

Senate Document Room (for Senate items)
SH-B04
Senate Hart Office Building
Washington, DC 20510

or

House Document Room (for House items)
H-226
Capitol
Washington, DC 20515

Requests for a free copy of a public law may be sent to either document room.

HOW TO BECOME ACTIVE IN HEALTH CARE ADVOCACY

If you are interested in becoming active in advocating for speech-language pathology and audiology services in health care, contact the Congressional Relations Division of the American Speech-Language-Hearing Association (ASHA) to become a part of a member grassroots network.

■ CHAPTER 15 ■

Service Delivery Issues in Health Care Settings

■ BECKY SUTHERLAND CORNETT, Ph.D. ■

SCOPE OF CHAPTER

The practice of audiology and speech-language pathology in health care settings is highly varied, according to the mission and objectives of specific facilities or programs. The persons served, clinical knowledge and skills needed, and job responsibilities are defined by the requirements of the work setting. As the roles of speech-language pathologists and audiologists expand, it is difficult to determine which members of our professions are "health care" professionals and which are "education" professionals. The traditional dichotomy between health and education in our professions is rapidly disappearing. For example, speech-language pathologists in schools are treating students with swallowing problems, traumatic brain injuries, and multiple disabilities. These professionals are also increasingly billing public and private third-party payers for services rendered to students.

Conversely, hospital-based speech-language pathologists are consulting with education teams to determine goals for Individualized Education Programs (IEPs) for persons with traumatic brain injuries. Professionals in private practice may often cross the traditional "boundaries" in the course of daily clinical work.

However, for the sake of order, I will use information from the American Speech-Language-Hearing Association (ASHA) to classify those who work in health care. According to the 1992 ASHA Omnibus Survey (ASHA, 1992a) approximately 70% of audiologists and 40% of speech-language pathologists currently work in diverse health care environments. These settings include hospitals, residential facilities, and nonresidential facilities. The category of hospitals is further subdivided into acute-care, rehabilitation, and specialty hospitals such as psychiatric, pediatric, cancer, or eye and ear centers. Residential facilties may include skilled nursing, intermediate, or extended care centers, mental retardation/developmental disabilities (MR/DD) residential treatment centers, transitional living facilities, and hospices. Examples of nonresidential facilities are home health agencies, physician's offices, speech-language pathology or audiology private practice offices, outpatient rehabilitation centers, and community speech and hearing clinics. (See Chapter 9 by Shewan on characteristics of ASHA members.)

Although it will not be possible to address service delivery issues in all situations, this chapter provides an overview of clinical practice and management issues applicable to audiology and speech-language pathology services in most health care settings. The chapter describes the various clinical roles of speech-language pathologists and audiologists and discusses the clinician's role in management and departmental operations. The chapter concludes with a presentation of health care trends related to the practice of speech-language pathology and audiology.

SPEECH-LANGUAGE PATHOLOGY AND AUDIOLOGY SERVICES IN HEALTH CARE SETTINGS

The clinical practice of speech-language pathology and audiology in health care settings presents unique challenges and rewards. During the past decade, the term "medical speech pathology" has been used by several authors (Golper, 1992; Miller & Groher, 1990) to designate the special skills and knowledge required of professionals who work in medical environments. The role of the medical speech-language pathologist varies with the specific place of employment. For example, one SLP may specialize in the evaluation and treatment of swallowing disorders, leading a dysphagia team in a large urban teaching hospital. Another SLP in the same facility may evaluate and treat persons who need augmentative or alternative communication (AAC) systems. Still another staff member may be the community integration specialist for the head injury team. Other SLPs in smaller hospitals or in clinics may be generalists, responsible for treating persons of all ages who present a wide variety of communication and related disorders. Figure 15–1 presents some of the clinical roles of medical speech-language pathologists. This list is not all-inclusive; there are many special populations, advanced procedures, and setting-specific activities that may not be included.

Audiologists who work in health care settings also have varied roles. The audiologist who works in the hospital newborn nursery and neonatal intensive care unit (NICU) identifies and provides early intervention for infants who are at-risk for communication disorders resulting from hearing impairments. Another audiologist may conduct comprehensive audiologic assessments and special tests, with yet another colleague specializing in hearing aid and assistive device assessments, selection, dispensing, fitting and orientation. Examples of the clinical roles of audiologists are presented in Figure 15–2.

In her discussion of speech-language pathology practice in medical settings, Golper (1992) stresses the importance of understanding the relationship between illness and communication: "clinicians . . . should have a basic understanding of the conditions that bring patients into the hospital and what is being done, medically or surgically, to manage them. Patients are not hospitalized because they have a communication problem" (p. ix). Miller and Groher (1990) agree that medical speech-language pathologists must view their services within the context of the overall medical management of the patient. Speech-language pathologists can serve the health care team by contributing to differential diagnosis and ongoing monitoring of medical conditions as well as in their traditional roles of rehabilitating persons with communication disorders. Miller and Groher (1990) offer this assessment:

CLINICAL ROLES OF MEDICAL SPEECH-LANGUAGE PATHOLOGISTS

Assessment and treatment of:

aphasia

dysarthria

apraxia

right-hemisphere dysfunction

cognitive-communicative disorders associated with brain injuries, or Alzheimer's or other dementias

dysphagia and other disorders of oral-pharyngeal function

speech, language, and swallowing disorders associated with cleft palate or other oral and oropharyngeal anomalies

organic and nonorganic vocal pathologies

fluency disorders

Providing preoperative counseling, postsurgical evaluation and selection of communication methods, and rehabilitation for persons who have undergone oral, velopharyngeal, or laryngeal surgery.

Augmentative and alternative communication system (AAC) assessment, selection, orientation, training, and follow-up.

Participation in the evaluation, selection, and use of voice prostheses ("talking trach" tubes, one-way speaking valves) in persons with a tracheostomy.

Counseling patients, families, and caregivers regarding communication and swallowing assessment and treatment, progress, prognosis, facilitating techniques, coping and adjustment strategies.

Consultation with other professionals and agencies regarding patient management issues related to communication and swallowing processes, disorders, interactions, and environments.

Providing in-service education to other professionals.

Figure 15–1. Examples of clinical roles of medical speech-language pathologists.

To obtain equal status in the medical setting it is imperative that speech/language pathologists demonstrate how their expertise can be used to solve the problems of establishing medical diagnoses and how their skills can assist physicians in managing patients after and, more importantly, during the hospital stay. It comes initially from an understanding of medical disciplines to which speech/language pathologists relate on a daily basis and how to establish a mutual environment of respect as diagnosticians and treatment providers. (p. 25)

Interestingly, the audiologist has always been viewed as a diagnostician, assisting in differential diagnosis and assisting in the medical man-

agement of patients. This role for audiologists has increased as some audiologists participate in neurophysiologic intraoperative monitoring, balance system assessment, electrical stimulation for cochlear implant selection and rehabilitation, and cerumen management. ASHA has published position statements and guidelines for these and other advanced procedures (see ASHA, 1992b).

Golper (1992) suggests that concurrence, cooperation, and coordination are the key words for practice in health care settings. That is, speech-language pathologists and audiologists see patients by referral in health

---

CLINICAL ROLES OF AUDIOLOGISTS IN HEALTH CARE SETTINGS

Evaluation and diagnosis of peripheral and central auditory nervous system dysfunctions.

Hearing aid and assistive device or system assessment, selection, dispensing, fitting, orientation, and monitoring.

Assessment and monitoring of the vestibular system.

Aural rehabilitation assessment and provision of aural rehabilitation services.

Special tests or procedures to assist in medical diagnosis and monitoring (e.g., neurophysiologic intraoperative monitoring, high-frequency ototoxicity tests).

Audiologic assessment of central auditory processing.

Participation in cochlear implant assessment, selection, placement, orientation, and follow-up.

Counseling patients, families, and caregivers regarding auditory and vestibular system assessment, treatment, progress, prognosis, facilitating techniques, and coping and adjustment strategies.

Consultation with other professionals and agencies regarding patient management issues related to auditory and vestibular system functions and disorders and communication interactions and environments.

Providing in-service education to other professionals.

Figure 15–2. Examples of clinical roles of audiologists in health care settings.

care settings, and so the *concurrence* of the physician and other members of health care teams is important. Speech-language pathologists and audiologists work in *cooperation* with other health professionals and also must *coordinate* service delivery with other activities, tests, and procedures during the patient's day. It is important that speech-language pathology and audiology services be viewed as integral to patient care. Therefore, it is incumbent on the professional to learn about the roles of other members of the health care team and to determine how speech-language pathology and audiology services can best serve the team and the patient. Health care teams may include many health professionals: physician, nurse, occupational, physical, and respiratory therapists, dietitian, psychologist, social worker, speech-language pathologist, audiologist, chaplain, vocational specialist, and others. Team approaches vary and may be multidisciplinary, interdisciplinary, or transdisciplinary. Readers are encouraged to investigate other

sources for information about members and functions of health care teams (Catlett & Halper, 1992; Cornett & Chabon, 1988; Frattali, 1993; Miller & Groher, 1990; Scholtes, 1991).

In their discussion of the principles of treatment and management in medical speech-language pathology, Miller and Groher (1990) stress the importance of functionally based care plans. The purpose of treatment is to assist the patient to achieve maximum functional communication and swallowing behaviors following discharge. We facilitate quality and efficiency of communication or swallowing patterns, promote compensatory communication skills when complete recovery does not seem realistic, and attempt to prevent complications and maladaptive behaviors that impede recovery. According to Miller and Groher, "if goals are realistic and attainable, then reaching the goals should make a difference in the patient's life" (p. 275).

Functional assessment and treatment philosophies are being increasingly emphasized as legislative, regulatory, and accrediting body requirements are enacted. Functional assessment tools evaluate an individual's ability to complete activities of daily living in his or her environment. A number of instruments have been developed to assess functional abilities, including communication and swallowing behaviors, and clinicians incorporate these assessments as part of regular clinical practice. See Chapter 24 by Frattali on functional assessment in this book; also Frattali (1992) and Lubinski and Frattali (1993) for detailed information about the status and use of functional assessments.

The development and use of treatment guidelines, clinical protocols, and care paths are also becoming integral to speech-language pathology and audiology services in health care settings. According to Johnston and Wilkerson (1992), treatment guidelines are "systematically developed statements based on scientific evidence and clinical experience that assist decisions about appropriate care for specific clinical circumstances" (p. 77). Treatment guidelines have been mandated by the Omnibus Budget Reconciliation Act of 1989, which created a new agency within the U.S. Public Health Service to develop practice guidelines, and to promote medical effectiveness research (see Chapter 14 by Frattali, Curl, and Bevan). A number of practice guidelines are currently being developed by teams of experts. The American Speech-Language-Hearing Association (ASHA) has also developed a number of guidelines for effective clinical practice in specific areas. A complete list of available guidelines, position statements and definitions is in the March reference issue of Asha magazine annually. They are also compiled in the current *ASHA Desk Reference*. Many are of particular interest to speech-language pathologists and audiologists in health care settings, among them the *Preferred Practice Patterns for the Professions of Speech-Language Pathology and Audiology*, approved in November, 1992, and published in March, 1993 (ASHA, 1993).

Clinical protocols and care paths are typically developed by individual facilities, programs, teams, or departments, and provide standard procedures for assessment, treatment, and management based on diagnosis or disorder. A care path is essentially a protocol illustrated as a "decision tree." A care path for dysphagia management developed by speech-language pathologists who work in a large university teaching hospital is illustrated in Figure 15–3.

Effective clinical practice also requires the timely, accurate, and complete documentation of services rendered. Medical information management is a rapidly developing area; some hospitals and other health care facilities are documenting most patient information electronically. Care paths and protocols are incorporated into the patient record; a laser pen is used to document care rendered. Other facilities still produce a paper record, and speech-language pathologists and audiologists contribute written assessment, treatment, and discharge reports. Some departments use dictation and transcription; other departments have standard forms to complete. Still others may have software programs that generate reports completed by individual clinicians using their own personal computers. Speech-language pathologists and audiologists should be thoroughly familiar with the content and format of medical or patient care records. Detailed presentations about medical records are found in Cornett and Chabon (1988) and Miller and Groher (1990), and explanations of medical terminology in Golper (1992).

The patient care record serves as a basis for planning and continuity of care, documents the course of care, facilitates communication among health professionals, and provides data for payment, quality improvement, utilization management, and research purposes. Cornett and Chabon (1988) summarize the importance of documentation in the following statement:

Our clinical records and reports are our primary vehicles of communication with other speech-language pathologists and audiologists, health and education professionals and administrators, government agencies, and third-party payers. Patient or client records with supporting reports should provide a complete written history of the course of our work with individual patients. The accuracy and thoroughness of our documentation is often the key to third-party payment for our services and can also influence administrative decisions about the effectiveness and efficiency of our work. (p. 91)

Readers are referred to the chapters in this book about health care financing, quality improvement, policies and procedures, and professional liability for additional information about documentation issues.

Discharge planning or continuing care planning is another very important clinical role for speech-language pathologists and audiologists. Lamprey and Berry (1989) define continuing care planning as "a patient-centered, multidisciplinary process designed to plan for the continuing care needs of a patient following discharge from the hospital" (p. 83). This definition can be expanded to include all treatment locations and programs. Continuing care planning is also needed for discharge from outpatient treatment. Planning begins at or before admission for treatment and includes all professionals involved, the patient, and the individual's family or caregivers. Some of the primary objectives of discharge planning for medical speech-language pathologists and audiologists are to: identify current and anticipated future communication and swallowing needs; prepare the patient and family for a change or termination of services; assist in the transition from one facility or program to another or to the home. Discharge or continuing care planning is an ongoing process; current treatment plans, objectives, and activities should be based on discharge goals and disposition. More information about discharge planning is found in Cornett and Chabon (1988), Lamprey and Berry (1989), and Miller and Groher (1990).

THE CLINICIAN'S ROLES IN MANAGEMENT

According to Shewan and Blake (1991), an average of 24.7 hours of the majority of hospital-based speech-language pathologists' and audiologists' work week is spent in direct patient contact; an additional 14.5 hours are spent completing administrative duties. These duties encompass a wide variety of tasks and may occur daily, weekly, monthly, or quarterly. Figure 15–4 lists a number of management tasks in which clinicians participate. The majority have been included under the heading "quality assessment and improvement." I have chosen to broaden the traditional definition of quality improvement activities to include numerous duties and responsibilities related to achieving and maintaining a quality speech-language pathology and audiology department or program.

Many of the activities listed in Figure 15–4 are discussed in other chapters in this book. They also correspond with the contents of the report "Major Issues Affecting the Delivery of Services in Hospital Settings," prepared by ASHA's Ad Hoc Committee on Hospital and Health Services (1990). The issues identified were: reimbursement, professional education, professional practice, quality assurance (now called quality improvement), productivity, and marketing. Clinicians, as well as supervisors and managers, have a role to play in each of these areas.

Issue 1: Reimbursement

Third-party payment and reimbursement patterns are evolving rapidly. Our health care system is poised for sweeping change. The professions of audiology and speech-language pathology will need to keep pace with the demands of the purchasers of our services, particularly in a managed care environment, by demonstrating the effectiveness and efficiency of our work with patients. Clinicians have a major contribution to make in this area. One of the strategies suggested by the Ad Hoc Committee on Hospital and Health Services (1990) to improve coverage of our services in health care plans is to "collect data on various communication disorders with regard to expected course of treatment,

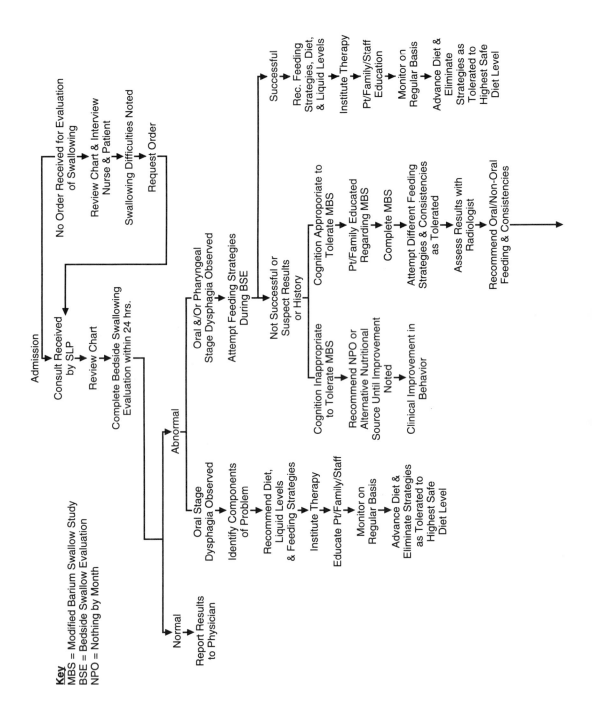

Key
MBS = Modified Barium Swallow Study
BSE = Bedside Swallow Evaluation
NPO = Nothing by Month

Admission

No Order Received for Evaluation of Swallowing

Review Chart & Interview Nurse & Patient

Swallowing Difficulties Noted

Request Order

Consult Received by SLP

Review Chart

Complete Bedside Swallowing Evaluation within 24 hrs.

Normal

Abnormal

Report Results to Physician

Oral &/Or Pharyngeal Stage Dysphagia Observed

Attempt Feeding Strategies During BSE

Not Successful or Suspect Results or History

Successful

Rec. Feeding Strategies, Diet, & Liquid Levels

Institute Therapy

Pt/Family/Staff Education

Monitor on Regular Basis

Advance Diet & Eliminate Strategies as Tolerated to Highest Safe Diet Level

Cognition Appropriate to Tolerate MBS

Pt/Family Educated Regarding MBS

Complete MBS

Attempt Different Feeding Strategies & Consistencies as Tolerated

Assess Results with Radiologist

Recommend Oral/Non-Oral Feeding & Consistencies

Cognition Inappropriate to Tolerate MBS

Recommend NPO or Alternative Nutritional Source Until Improvement Noted

Clinical Improvement in Behavior

Oral Stage Dysphagia Observed

Identify Components of Problem

Recommend Diet, Liquid Levels & Feeding Strategies

Institute Therapy

Educate Pt/Family/Staff

Monitor on Regular Basis

Advance Diet & Eliminate Strategies as Tolerated to Highest Safe Diet Level

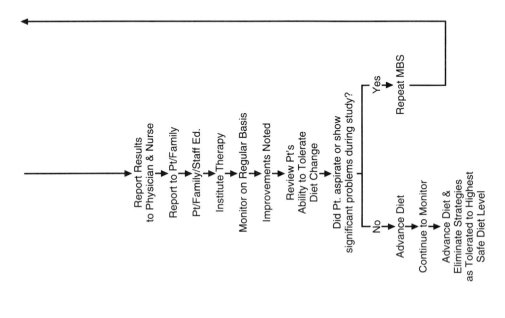

Report Results
to Physician & Nurse

Report to Pt/Family

Pt/Family/Staff Ed.

Institute Therapy

Monitor on Regular Basis

Improvements Noted

Review Pt's
Ability to Tolerate
Diet Change

Did Pt. aspirate or show
significant problems during study?

No

Advance Diet

Continue to Monitor

Advance Diet &
Eliminate Strategies
as Tolerated to Highest
Safe Diet Level

Yes

Repeat MBS

Figure 15–3. Example of a care path for dysphagia. (From *Care Path for Dysphagia* by J. Dickerson and M. Fitch, 1993. Unpublished document. Copyright 1993 The Ohio State University. Reprinted by permission.)

QUALITY ASSESSMENT AND IMPROVEMENT PROGRAM

Assist in development of clinical indicators

Monitor and evaluate services:

   self-assessment

   peer review

Participate in continuous improvement/total quality management teams

Develop and follow treatment guidelines, clinical protocols, and care paths

Comply with productivity requirements; provide suggestions for modifications to productivity-monitoring systems and departmental operations regarding efficiency of services

Participate in utilization management activities

Participate in risk management, safety, and infection control activities

Assist in development of policies, procedures, and suggest modifications to departmental operations

Provide timely, thorough, and accurate documentation of clinical services; suggest modifications to reporting systems;

Monitor third-party payment requirements for documentation and record-keeping; provide accurate billing data.

Know standards for accreditation; assist in monitoring compliance and maintaining accreditation.

CONTINUING EDUCATION, STAFF DEVELOPMENT, AND TEAM ISSUES

Participate in formal and informal professional education activities

Provide in-service education to colleagues and other health professionals

Participate in "clinical ladder" or clinical advancement programs to increase expertise in clinical area or develop departmental management role (clincal supervisor or manager)

Supervise support personnel

Participate in team management; monitor effectiveness of service delivery models; serve as team leader, coordinator or case manager as appropriate

---

Figure 15–4. The Clinician's Roles in management.

benefit of such treatment, and patient demographic information" (p. 67). As inpatient lengths-of-stay (LOS) decrease, clinicians are focusing primarily on functional assessment, improvement, and outcomes; and early continuing care planning.

The emphasis on efficiency and effectiveness is a primary component of health care reform, but there are many other service delivery and payment issues to consider. For more information, refer to Chapter 14 by Frattali, Curl, and Beven on health care legislation and Cornett and Chabon (1988); De Lew, Greenberg and Kinchen (1992); and Griffin and Fazen (1993).

Issue 2: Professional Education

Professional education begins with earning a graduate degree and continues throughout one's career. In health care settings, there are typically many opportunities for continuing professional education and staff development. These activities may be formal, such as presenting an inservice to nursing staff about communication strategies with persons who have aphasia or attending a seminar on neuropharmacology, or informal, such as reading a journal article or discussing a patient with another health professional. The Ad Hoc Committee on Hospital and Health Services reported that the scope of practice of speech-language pathologists and audiologists in hospitals and other health care settings has expanded with scientific, technological, and clinical advances (ASHA, 1990). As a result, many professionals may need to acquire additional competencies in specific areas of practice. ASHA offers membership in special interest divisions in areas such as dysphagia, neurophysiology, neurogenic speech and language disorders, and hearing and hearing disorders, but specialty certification is not currently available. It is incumbent on the professional to acquire the necessary knowledge base and skills to offer high quality services. Clinicians will be increasingly challenged to keep pace with advances in clinical practice in health care settings.

Issue 3: Professional Practice

Among the issues presented by the Ad Hoc Committee on Hospital and Health Services report (ASHA, 1990) in the area of professional practice is the growing use of alternative staffing models such as support personnel and multiskilled or cross-trained professionals; and "turf" issues associated with the services offered to patients by other health professionals such as occupational therapists and psychologists. The appropriate use of support personnel in both health and education settings has been debated by ASHA members for many years (see ASHA, 1981, 1988c; Freilinger, 1992; Slater & Shewan, 1992; Werven, 1992). The multiskilled health practitioner concept has evolved over the last

15 years and will continue to develop as health care administrators seek to redesign services to compete in a managed care environment (Cornett & Chabon, 1988). There will likely be increased demand for speech-language pathologists and audiologists to define their special skills and roles within the health care team, and to cooperate in efforts to streamline service delivery approaches. (See Chapter 26 by Frattali on professional autonomy and collaboration.)

Issue 4: Quality Improvement

The clinician's role in quality assessment and improvement in health care settings is more important than ever. Our understanding of quality has evolved from a "look for problems" approach under "quality assurance" programs to an approach based on continuous monitoring of service delivery and a focus on opportunities to improve care. We no longer wait until one aspect of our services has fallen below a "threshold" before we take action. As this chapter is written, the Joint Commission on Accreditation of Healthcare Organizations (JCAHO) is further revising the hospital standards for improving organizational performance. The 1994 JCAHO standards address nine dimensions of service delivery: appropriateness, availability, and continuity of care; effectiveness; efficacy; respect and caring for the patient; safety of patients and personnel; and timeliness of services. These dimensions are the essence of service delivery.

Quality assessment and improvement is no longer a "management" activity; it is the responsibility of all health care professionals. Speech-language pathologists and audiologists have the opportunity for professional self-assessment, peer review, and participation in work groups, councils, and task forces to assist in redesigning and refining processes of care throughout a health care facility or program. Readers are referred to Chapter 19 by Frattali on quality improvement for more information about trends and issues in this area.

Issue 5: Productivity

Speech-language pathology and audiology departments in health care settings are revenue-producing. That is, clinicians charge for services rendered. The productivity rating of each clinician, and the department's budget, is based on the number of "billable hours," or units of service produced. According to Coelho and Murphy (1988), productivity is:

the ratio of resources utilized (inputs) to services rendered (outputs). Resources include all of the expenses which contribute to the provision of the service (output). Inputs are generally defined as the paid productive staff hours and outputs as the hours of direct patient care (billable hours). (p. 45)

It is sometimes difficult to balance the clinical and administrative tasks assigned to clinicians each day. Sometimes clinicians may feel that managers are overemphasizing revenue and productivity issues, but in an increasingly competitive environment, managers and clinicians alike will be asked to offer quality services at the lowest cost. Larkins (1992) points out that the use of productivity data is important, not only for determining staffing and reimbursement patterns and for budget planning, but also to assess patient care variables such as average length of treatment, diagnostic groups, and treatment outcomes.

Issue 6: Marketing

Two major marketing issues were raised in the Ad Hoc Committee on Hospital and Health Services (1990) report: low visibility and utilization of speech-language pathology and audiology services in some health care settings and lack of awareness of the scope of practice of the professions. The American Speech-Language-Hearing Association has developed a series of marketing workshops and publications to assist professionals in increasing public and professional awareness of our services and programs, but a great deal must be done by each speech-language pathologist and audiologist to communicate the value of our professional services. Marketing is a very important part of professional practice in health care as hospitals and other facilities redesign, consolidate, and compete for a secure place in the service delivery system. See Chapter 20 by Loavenbruck in this book for more information about the role of marketing in the practice of speech-language pathology and audiology.

SUMMARY

This chapter has presented an overview of the many clinical roles and management issues in which speech-language pathologists and audiologists participate in health care settings. Unfortunately, I was not able to specifically discuss two growing practice settings: long-term care facilities and home care. As the population ages and as hospital inpatient stays shorten, there will likely be many more opportunities for practice in these environments. ASHA has published several statements and reports that describe the work of our professions in these areas (ASHA, 1988a, 1988b, 1991). See also Chapter 12 in this book by Lubinski and Masters titled "Special Populations and Special Settings."

It is difficult to predict the future of speech-language pathology and audiology in a rapidly changing health care system, but it is an exciting time for those just beginning practice. New clinicians will have the opportunity to shape new ways in delivering services and streamlining clinical management procedures and processes. Quality assessment and improvement concepts will continue to evolve and drive service delivery. Clinicians will participate in all levels of facilitating organizational change as the health professions "work smarter."

The issues discussed in this chapter related to reimbursement for services, professional education, professional practice, quality improvement, productivity, and marketing form the essence of service delivery in health care settings. Together they present many challenges to and opportunities for our professions' growth and development in the future. In a previous publication (Cornett & Chabon, 1988), I ended a chapter on quality of care with this statement: "Speech-language pathology and audiology are professions in transition. We are poised to enter a new era of accountability, assisted by technology but guided by our principles, ethics, and dedication to those we serve" (p. 193). This statement seems particularly appropriate today.

DISCUSSION QUESTIONS

1. Should ASHA offer specialty certification to speech-language pathologists and audiologists who work in health care settings? Why or why not?
2. What is "functional" assessment and treatment? Why is it imperative to focus on facilitating functional communication in health care settings?
3. As the nation's health care system undergoes reform, which of the issues delineated by ASHA's Ad Hoc Committee on Hospital and Health Services is most important to the future of speech-language pathologists and audiologists who work in health care settings? Why?
4. What are some similarities and differences between the activities, interests, and goals of speech-language pathologists and audiologists in health care settings? What impact might these differences have on our professions in the future?

REFERENCES

Ad Hoc Committee on Hospital and Health Services, American Speech-Language-Hearing Association. (1990). Major issues affecting the delivery of services in hospital settings. *Asha, 32*, 67–70.

American Speech-Language-Hearing Association. (1981). Employment and utilization of supportive personnel in audiology and speech-language pathology. *Asha, 23*, 165–169.

American Speech-Language-Hearing Association. (1988a). Provision of audiology and speech-lan-

guage pathology services to older persons in nursing homes. *Asha, 30*, 72–74.

American Speech-Language-Hearing Association. (1988b). The roles of speech-language pathologists and audiologists in working with older persons. *Asha, 30*, 80–84.

American Speech-Language-Hearing Association. (1988c). Utilization and employment of speech-language pathology supportive personnel with underserved populations. *Asha, 30*, 55–56.

American Speech-Language-Hearing Association. (1991). Guidelines for the delivery of speech-language pathology and audiology services in home care. *Asha 33*(Suppl. 5), 29–34.

American Speech-Language-Hearing Association. (1992a). *1992 omnibus survey results*. Rockville, MD: ASHA Research Division.

American Speech-Language-Hearing Association. (1992b). *Asha, 34*(3)(Suppl.).

American Speech-Language-Hearing Association. (1993, March). *Preferred practice patterns for the professions of speech-language pathology. Asha, 35*(Suppl. 11).

Catlett, C., & Halper, A. (1992, Summer). Team approaches: Working together to improve quality. *Quality Improvement Digest*. Rockville, MD: American Speech-Language-Hearing Association.

Coelho, C., & Murphy, K. (1988). Monitoring productivity in a hospital-based speech-language pathology and audiology program. *Asha, 30*, 45–48.

Cornett, B., & Chabon, S. (1988). *The clinical practice of speech-language pathology*. Columbus, OH: Merrill.

De Lew, N., Greenberg, G., & Kitchen, K. (1992, Fall). A layman's guide to the U.S. health care system. *Health Care Financing Review, 14*, 151–169.

Frattali, C. (1992). Functional assessment of communication: merging public policy with clinical views. *Aphasiology, 6*, 63–83.

Frattali, C. (1993). *Professional collaboration: A team approach to health care*. Clinical Series No. 11. Rockville, MD.: National Student Speech-Language-Hearing Association.

Freilinger, J. (1992). Support personnel. *Asha, 34*(11), 51–53.

Golper, L. (1992). *Sourcebook for medical speech pathology*. San Diego: Singular Publishing Group.

Griffin, K., & Fazen, M. (1993, Winter). A managed care strategy for practitioners. *Quality Improvement Digest*. Rockville, MD: American Speech-Language-Hearing Association.

Johnston, M., & Wilkerson, D. (1992). Program evaluation and quality improvement systems in brain injury rehabilitation. *Journal of Head Trauma Rehabilitation, 7*, 68–82.

Lamprey, J., & Berry, N. (1989). *Guide to utilization management*. Westborough, MA: InterQual.

Larkins, P. (1992, Fall). Measuring productivity: Finding the right quality quotient. *Quality Improvement Digest*. Rockville, MD: American Speech-Language-Hearing Association.

Lubinski, R., & Frattali, C. (1993). Nursing home reform: The resident assessment instrument. *Asha, 35*, 59–62.

Miller, R., & Groher, M. (1990). *Medical speech pathology*. Rockville, MD: Aspen.

Scholtes, P. (1991). *The team handbook*. Madison, WI: Joiner.

Shewan, C., & Blake, A. (1991). Speech-language pathologists and audiologists in hospitals. *Asha, 33*, 60.

Slater, S., & Shewan, C. (1992). Support personnel in the professions. *Asha, 34*, 28.

Werven, G. (1992). Training support personnel to provide services to persons with head injury. *Asha, 34*, 72–74.

■ CHAPTER 16 ■

Federal Legislation Affecting School Settings

■ JUDITH B. MONTGOMERY, Ph.D. ■

SCOPE OF CHAPTER

Until the mid-1970s, many parents of children with special needs or handicapping conditions, including communication disorders, faced incredible barriers to the education of their children. Their children were excluded from public schools, or if enrolled, they found segregated programs, limited services, and poorly prepared staff members. Some were charged fees for what was provided free to other students. Sometimes children were institutionalized or were declared wards of the state when it was the only avenue to receive daytime care or activity programs. Picture a 5-year-old boy with a repaired cleft palate, mild hearing loss, and nasalized speech patterns denied entry into kindergarten because he "isn't like the other students."

This chapter reviews the history of special education in the United States from the early 1950s to the present. Federal legislation is described in detail, with an emphasis on the development of services for communicatively disabled children, birth to age 22.

THE BACKGROUND OF SCHOOL SPECIAL EDUCATION LEGISLATION

Laws evolve from the perceived or real social needs of a population only when there are strong demands for change from several directions that converge on lawmakers. In the case of special education, including services for children with communication disorders, the overpowering demands for change evolved from the civil rights movement of the 1950s and '60s through the then new phenomenon of organized groups of parents of disabled children.

Earlier actions that pointed the way to this critical legislative juncture were:

1. Compulsory education laws in place in every state by 1918
2. Child labor laws enacted in 1938
3. The first standardized intelligence tests in the 1920s
4. The emergence of new professional fields such as speech-language pathology, audiology, and psychiatry/psychology, providing a body of knowledge that applied to atypical children
5. Medical advances in treatment of previously misunderstood disorders, such as cerebral palsy and cleft palate
6. Educational and technological advances in designing prostheses, providing transportation, and assisting ambulation and communication.

By the early 1970s these forces had coalesced into a nationwide commitment to educate all the children in this country in our public schools, if at all possible. The spirit of this commitment needed to be established in law to assure nationwide compliance. Despite the grassroots momentum, fueled by the passage of civil rights legislation, it still took 4 years of debate in the U. S. Congress to finally pass Public Law 94-142 (P.L. 94-142) in 1975. Although there were only seven dissenting votes in each house of Congress (Gallagher, Trohanis, & Clifford, 1989), there were protracted battles to convert the idea of a free appropriate education for all children in this country into specific language for an acceptable combined Senate and House bill. Many compromises were made, and hotly contested items were accepted by one group only if equally controversial items were agreed to by the other side.

Although there were no real opponents to the education of children, there were significant financial restraints to such all-encom-

passing legislation. Parents wanted to rectify every condition they had faced for years, fearing there would never be another chance to take the giant leap forward for disabled youth. Educators and medical personnel (most of them parents themselves) could not imagine strongly entrenched systems changing so radically without tremendous disruption and backlash. They advised more cautious steps. No one really knew how many children with disabilities were in need of services, what kind, and for how long.

Court cases in the 1950s centered on the segregation of African-Americans in educational institutions. In each case, the court found that the refusal to admit African-Americans into previously white schools, public buildings, public transportation, and colleges was based solely on race. When five school cases went to the Supreme Court in 1954 in the landmark case known as Brown v. the Board of Education (347 U.S.483, 1954) segregated schools were declared inherently unequal. The "separate but equal" schooling position was struck down. The success of civil rights groups was viewed by disabled rights advocates as a strong affirmation of the rights of all Americans. But it would be almost 20 years before this energy culminated in P.L. 93-112, the Rehabilitation Act (Section 504) in 1973, and the several more years before special education was legislated in every state with P.L. 94-142 in 1975.

In the meantime, efforts toward public awareness of persons with special needs were strengthened by several new institutions. In 1961, President John F. Kennedy called a Presidential Panel on Mental Retardation, and in 1965 P.L. 89-10, the Elementary and Secondary Education Act, was passed to provide states with funds to evaluate and educate some students with special needs, including children classified as gifted. In the next year, the Bureau for the Education of the Handicapped (BEH) was created and model demonstration programs for working with children with disabilities were funded with P.L. 90-247, the Handicapped Children's Early Education Act.

Section 504 of P.L. 93-112 was the next critical step toward mandating programs for school children with communication disorders. This act guarantees that people with disabilities may not be discriminated against because of their disability. Although not directed specifically at schools, it protects the person with disability for life and encompasses the right to vote, to be educated, to be employed, and to access all environments open to the general public. We continue to invoke this law today to ensure that school buildings, restrooms, public recreation activities, and so on are accessible for all persons. As we will discuss later, violations of Section 504 of the Rehabilitation Act can be charged by parents as easily as failure to live up to the better known P.L. 94-142. Section 504 is essentially a civil rights statement, with P.L. 94-142 specifically defining and authorizing education programs.

P.L. 94-142 LANDMARK LEGISLATION

In 1975, The Education of the Handicapped Act (EHA) was enacted as the 142nd piece of legislation in the 94th Congress and signed by President Gerald Ford. This is referred to as P.L. 94-142. There are five general purposes to this monumental act:

1. To ensure to all children with handicapping conditions a free appropriate education and all related services necessary to benefit from it;
2. To guarantee protection of student and parent rights through legal due process;
3. To provide funds for state and local agencies to carry out the prescribed programs;
4. To monitor and evaluate the programs designed;
5. To establish the individualized education program (IEP) as the written record of commitment to meet a student's goals as determined by parents and professionals.

Special education is defined by the EHA as education designed to meet the needs of a child who is handicapped at no cost to parents. This includes classroom instruction, home instruction, and instruction in hospitals and institutions. Children must be evaluated and found to have one of the handicapping conditions listed in Figure 16–1. The figure is an excerpt from P.L. 94-142 Rules and Regulations taken from the *Federal Register*, Volume 42, No. 163, August 23, 1977. The last two sections were added in 1992.

P.L. 99-142 defines the scope of services for communicatively handicapped children within the public schools as listed by Dublinske and Healy (1978) in Figure 16–2.

Six major principles are reflected in the law. The first four are rights, and the last two are protections. In the early years of implementation, each one initially constituted a new and

---

Handicapping Conditions
from P.L. 94-142 (EHA) 1975

Now re-named:

Special Education Disabilities
Categories from P.L. 101-476 (IDEA)
1991

1. Deaf
2. Deaf-blind
3. Hard of Hearing
4. Mentally retarded
5. Multi-handicapped
6. Orthopedically impaired
7. Other health impaired
8. Seriously emotionally disturbed
9. Specific learning disability
10. Speech impaired
11. Visually handicapped
12. Traumatic brain injury*
13. Autism*
*added in 1991

Figure 16–1. Handicapping conditions with services mandated by federal legislation.

Speech and Language Services include:

1. Identification of children with speech or language disorders

2. Diagnosis and appraisal of specific speech or language disorders

3. Referral for medical or other professional attention necessary to the habilitation of speech or language disorders

4. Provisions of speech and language services for the habilitation or prevention of communicative disorders

5. Counseling and guidance of parents, children, and teachers regarding speech and language disorders

Audiology services include:

1. Identification of children with hearing loss

2. Determination of the range, nature, and degree of hearing loss, including referral for medical or other professional attention for the habilitation of hearing

3. Provision of habilitative activities such as language habilitation, auditory training, speechreading, hearing evaluation, and speech conversation

4. Creation and administration of programs for prevention of hearing loss

5. Counseling and guidance of pupils, parents, and teachers regarding hearing loss

6. Determination of the child's need for group and individual amplification, selection and fitting of an appropriate aid, and evaluating the effectiveness of amplfication

Figure 16–2. Scope of services in schools for children with communication disabilities. (From "P.L. 94-142: Questions and Answers for the Speech-Language Pathologist and Audiologist" by S. Dublinske and W. Healey, 1978. *Asha, 20,* 188–205. Copyright 1978 by American Speech-Language-Hearing Association. Reprinted by permission.)

demanding change in the existing educational systems in the United States. Each one has been challenged in the courts and has been upheld.

1. **Zero Reject:** Every school-age child (5–22 years) must be served with no cost to the family. The state must have a program for identifying the eligible population.
2. **Testing, Evaluation, and Placement:** Prescribed methods for nonbiased evaluation and appropriate placement must be followed.
3. **Individualized and Appropriate Education:** Programs must be individualized to meet the specific needs of each child. This section is probably the most crucial to implement for school principals, special education directors, and teachers. The visible record of this effort on behalf of each child is the IEP.
4. **Least Restrictive Environment:** Now referred to as LRE, this section requires that children who are disabled be educated in the company of their nondisabled peers to the greatest extent possible. Not every child will be placed in a regular classroom.
5. **Procedural Due Process:** The right of parents to protest the actions of state or local agencies is derived from the United States Constitution. Parents may call on these legal procedures, carefully spelled out in the law, and question activities they may regard as discriminatory, inappropriate, or unfair.
6. **Parent Participation and Shared Decision Making:** Parents, legal guardians, or appointed surrogates must be involved at each stage of the special education process. They must be notified of every change before it is proposed or discussed, and they must be actively involved in writing the IEP, providing goals, and objectives of their own for the child.

The Individualized Education Program (IEP)

The IEP is surprisingly universal in procedure, but has great variability in written format. Most plans are 3 to 5 pages long, and include goals and objectives for the child from all the professionals involved in a child's program. In some instances, IEPs can be 20–25 pages long. The intent, of course, is to write a succinct description of the child's needs and treatment plan for the following school year. It must be developed at a face-to-face meeting of the IEP team and must be based on a nonbiased assessment previously approved by the parent.

The IEP team is composed of the parent, the professional(s) who did the assessment (e.g., speech language pathologist or audiologist), and an administrator. Sometimes the child is involved if all parties agree it is advantageous. If there are many educators or specialists involved there can be 10–12 people attending. For a student with only a speech disorder, three people can participate in the IEP—the parent, speech-language pathologist, and the administrator. If other assessments were completed and need to be reported, even if the student is not found to be eligible for services in that area, several other educators or psychologists may attend. Parents often remark that the IEP process is intimidating. This was not the intent, however, and it can be made less formal in local settings. Figure 16–3 lists the people who should attend an IEP team meeting for a specific child with a communication disability that substantially impedes learning. In this case, it is a 9-year-old child with a severe sensorineural hearing loss. The speech-language pathologist needs to report all of the assessment data, listen to the parents' concerns and ideas, suggest goals and objectives to remediate the problems, write these into an IEP with appropriate measurement instruments or methods, and get the agreement of the parent to provide such services. An audiologist may write an IEP for a child with a hearing loss; though, a speech-language pathologist often writes the curriculum-related goals. The report can be reviewed on request at any time during the year, by personnel or parents. It should be a practical, easy-to-read written statement on what and how educational instruction and related services are to be delivered to a child. Legally, the form must always contain the following:

- **Present Level of Performance.** The IEP must state the child's current level of performance in areas of need. This lays the foundation for its content and design.
- **Annual Long-Term Goals.** The IEP must contain at least one goal clearly stating what the speech-language pathologist will strive to accomplish in 1 year.
- **Short-term Objectives.** These are a series of intermediate steps to be taken to achieve one or more of the goals. They must be written with a measurable end point such as a test, an observation, an accomplished activity, or a skill. This is how progress is determined each year.
- **Designated Instruction and Services.** Services that are needed to help a child reach the student's goals are written into this section. These are also called related services.

Student: Male
Age: 9 years, 5 months
Diagnosis: Severe hearing loss
Home language: Vietnamese

Student
Parents
Grandparents
Language interpreter
Audiologist
Speech-language pathologist
Classroom teacher
Classroom aide
School principal
School psychologist
Resource teacher
School nurse
Signing aide for elementary school
District director of special education
Program specialist for program for hearing
   impaired students
Advocate from local deaf community
Youth minister from student's church

*This list reflects the participants of an actual IEP meeting. More or fewer participants may be included on the team when the most appropriate program is selected for and with the student.

Figure 16–3. IEP team participants*.

Examples of related services are occupational therapy, physical therapy, counseling, a signing aide, speech-language pathology services, transportation, audiology, and home instruction.

- **Placement.** This is the setting where a child is to be educated, ideally the least restrictive place that will meet the youngster's goals and objectives. PL 94-142 assumes it will be the regular classroom in the home school. If it is not the regular classroom, a justification must be written for an alternative placement such as a special day class, a resource class, or a nonpublic school. The date this will begin and the duration must also be written. In the case of severe speech and language disorders, children may be placed in self-contained classrooms with other severely communication delayed children. This type of class may appeal to the parent and the directional team in some instances. It must still be carefully justified as it is more restrictive than a regular classroom with typical language-intact peers.

The Speech-Language Pathologist and Procedural Forms

The written IEP is the final step in a carefully constructed referral, assessment, reporting, and program decision process. Each time a student is referred for assessment, the clinician must go through every step to address the above mandatory points on the IEP. There are many forms, permission slips, and documentation steps on the way to the IEP meeting. The number and types of forms are determined by the individual districts as well as the individual state plans. The federal government does not produce or prescribe any of these forms, only the content and the timeline for each step. There is wide variability in actual paperwork, but always the same steps in the same order. Figure 16–4 shows these steps. The timelines are important in ensuring that agencies or schools do not fall far behind in meeting with parents, reporting results, and offering

1. Screening, identification → Referral
2. Informed consent for evaluation signed by parents
3. Formation of multidisciplinary evaluation team
4. Comprehensive assessment
5. Report of assessment team → Recommendations
6. IEP meeting → development of IEP
7. Parental consent to program and placement
8. Implementation of IEP
9. Annual review
10. Three-year reevaluation

Figure 16–4. Steps in the IEP process.

programs. Individual speech-language pathologists typically see 125 children a year for assessments and have an equal number of IEP meetings (Montgomery, 1989). Maintaining this assessment and compliance schedule, plus therapy and intervention for 55–60 children per month, can be decidedly challenging for the school-based clinician.

Although procedural forms vary from school district to school district, they must all contain the same statements, assurances, and information for parents and professionals. Following are five examples of forms important to speech-language pathologists. Figure 16–5 is a typical IEP front page or cover page with all the necessary information for officially recording the placement decisions and related services. Speech and language services are written in the category of designated instructional (or related) services.

The second form is a sample of typical language articulation goals and objectives (Figure 16–6). There are usually two to four such goals per IEP. The third form (Figure 16–7) shows an innovative combination of all the assessment procedures and written report for a child who requires speech-language services. This is used by interdisciplinary teams in schools. The fourth form (Figure 16–8) displays the parents' rights assessment procedure referred to in the middle section of the previous assessment procedure. This form must be given to the parent every time the parents and professionals meet to decide on

any change in a student's program. Look at it carefully and you will see a delineation of the procedural safeguards and rights of the parent described earlier as one of the five major principles of the EHA.

The final form (Figure 16–9) is an IEP for unduplicated, or speech-language-only services, meaning the child has a voice, articulation, language, or fluency disorder that does not require other interventions. Note the format with the goal and two objectives statements arranged to reduce the amount of writing needed. Typically, one objective is for the first 6 months and the second objective for the second 6 months of the annual goal. Linguistically appropriate goals address the need to modify the intervention when students speak a language other than English. On the IEP sample shown in this chapter, the parent must sign three times—once to agree to the IEP, once to agree with the child's placement, and the third time to note attendance at the actual meeting. In this format, the parent could agree to a portion of the IEP, such as the goals and objectives, but not the place suggested for carrying them out. In some cases, the signature of parents indicates only that they attended the meeting. In some cases, continuation meetings are needed, to finally arrive at the level and type of service everyone agrees is best for the child.

THE RELATIONSHIP BETWEEN FEDERAL AND STATE LAWS

It is important to recall here that this discussion has focused on federal legislation, not state laws. Although public education is guaranteed at the federal level through the United States Constitution, it is carried out by individual states. Thus, there is great variability. We do not have a national school system. In the same way, the EHA is a federal law and operates as a contract between the federal government and the states. In this contract the states agree to follow certain procedures and regulations in exchange for federal funds. To qualify for these funds the states must sub-

PAGE _____ OF _____

INDIVIDUALIZED EDUCATION PROGRAM, DISCHARGE AND TRANSFER   Initial ☐   Review ☐   3 Yr. Re-Eval ☐

Recommendations

	Projected Date of Initiation	Anticipated Duration
☐ Resource Specialist Program		
☐ Special Class		
☐ Regular Class		
☐ Home/Hospital		
☐ Non-Public School		

Designated Instruction	Initiation Date	Duration	Sessions/ Week	Minutes/ Week

☐ Transportation   ☐ Extended yr. no. days _____

☐ P.E. (type) _____   ☐ Integration-extent _____

☐ Voc. Ed. (type) _____

☐ Inclusion of Linguistically Appropriate Goals and Objectives

☐ Other _____

Placement Options Considered but Rejected as Inappropriate:

_____

_____

_____

Rationale for Placement Outside School of Residence & Regular Class:

_____

_____

_____

Projected Date of Review: _____

Differential Standards for Graduation: _____

_____

_____

Reason for Delay In Initiation of Services: _____

_____

Student Name _____

Address _____

Name of Parent/Guardian _____

Phone No.   Home: _____   Work: _____

Birthdate _____   Age _____   Sex _____

Primary Language Student _____   Home _____

District: Reside _____   Attend _____

School _____   Grade _____

Date of Last 3 Year Re-Evaluation _____

I agree with the Individualized Education Program:

_____   Date _____
Parent/Guardian Signature

I give my permission for placement

_____   Date _____
Parent/Guardian Signature

Signature of those in attendance:

_____   _____   Date _____
Name   Administrator
                  Title

_____   _____   Date _____
Name   Teacher
                  Title

_____   _____   Date _____
Name   Parent/Guardian*
                  Title

_____   _____   Date _____
Name   Title

_____   _____   Date _____
Name   Title

_____   _____   Date _____
Name   Title

_____   _____   Date _____
Name   Title

_____   _____   Date _____
Name   Title

_____   _____   Date _____
Name   Title

*I acknowledge receipt of a copy of *Parents' Rights and Appeals Procedures* (as printed on the reverse side of this form.)

Distribution: White - File; Yellow - Teacher; Pink - Parent

Figure 16-5. Sample IEP cover page.

These statements were selected to reflect a variety of formats in use in schools.

Goal: To improve expressive communication skills.

Objectives: 1. Sharon will orally describe three characteristics of one main character from her current literature text, in 4 out of 5 stories (80%) read to her.

2. Sharon will use appropriate pronouns in responses to questions about the work of the students in her assigned science group 60% of the time in a 3-minute discussion.

Goal: To increase vocabulary.

Objectives: 1. Zachary will name (or write) five items in a category from the social studies unit when provided a Major heading three out of four times.

2. By November 15, Zachary will complete one assigned integrated language arts book of 10 pages or more.

3. Millie will use context clues to identify the meaning of a new vocabulary word in her science or health book with two or fewer clues from teacher or peers.

Goal: To increase comprehension in reading and written work.

Objectives: By April, Jorge will identify the main idea and supporting details of a given short story from the seventh grade core literature as measured by a completed story map in his portfolio.

Goal: To carry over the correct production of "r" in sentences.

Objectives: Twan will use the correct production of "r" in a conversation with a peer of his choice using 4 words containing "r" from his mathematics book.

By June, Twan will use the correct production of "r" in his math class each day when asking or answering the oral quiz questions.

Figure 16–6. Sample IEP goals and objectives.

mit annual plans, include assurances that timelines and due process are followed, monitor their own programs, set guidelines and eligibility criteria within the 13 federal definitions, account for the funds being used, and undergo a review every 3 years.

The state makes a portion of these federal funds available to each school district through its own accounting system. Districts receive both state and federal money for their programs for children with disabilities. This is necessary because the federal government never fully funded P.L. 94-142. In fact, less than 10% of the funds to operate these programs now come from the federal government (Montgomery, 1992). Most of the funds must be raised by the states to meet the federal requirements. The excessive paperwork often lamented by school-based speech-language pathologists and others is created not by federal requirements but by state laws. The paperwork serves to demonstrate compliance with the national policy and justify the need for extra funding from the state's treasury.

Education has become big business in many states, a significant call on the state budget, and, consequently, a highly political issue.

STATE ELIGIBILITY CRITERIA

As noted above, states must determine how they are going to meet the mandates of the EHA within program structures that are meaningful to their educational units or districts. One of the first concerns must be "who is eligible for service?" The federal definitions are useful up to a point. They do not describe in measurable detail such phrases as "so severe that the child is impaired" or "significantly subaverage general intellectual functioning." This is left to the states to define operationally. Each state has done this by developing eligibility statements that define the 13 categories in Figure 16–1 through test scores, standard deviations, formulas for discrepancies between ability and achievement, and percentages that indicate disability versus delay within normal limits. Thus, a stu-

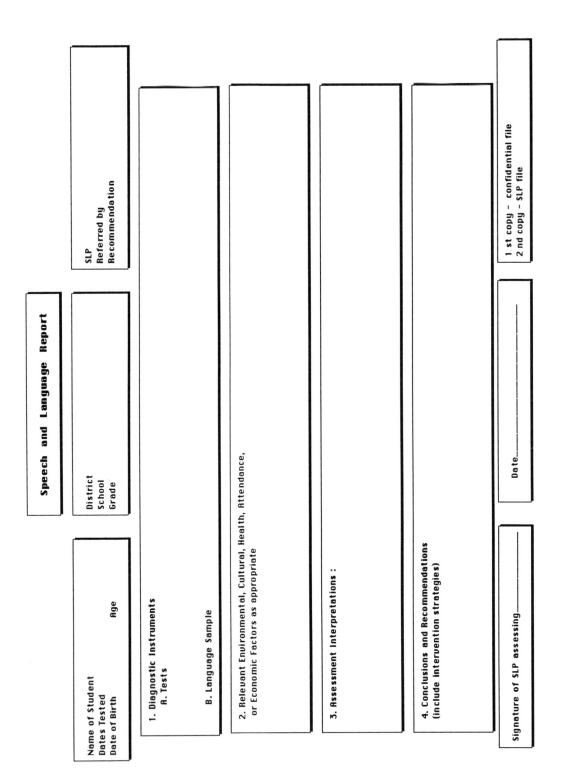

Figure 16–7. Sample speech and language report.

FREE APPROPRIATE PUBLIC EDUCATION

All handicapped children have the right to a free and appropriate public education.

All handicapped children have the right to placement in the least restrictive learning environment which offers maximum interaction with nonhandicapped peers.

If no appropriate public program is available, a program in a state-approved nonpublic school may be offered as an alternative.

All individuals shall receive a full explanation of all procedural safeguards and rights regarding their child's education.

RECORDS

The confidentiality of your child's records shall be maintained.

You may examine all records concerning your child within five days of your request.

You may request copies of records. (The district may charge a reasonable fee for copying them unless you cannot afford such fees.)

You may challenge the content of records in accordance with federal and state laws.

ASSESSMENT

You may request an educational assessment for your child.

You must give your written permission for any assessment before it may be conducted, and you may revoke that consent at any time.

You shall be given, in writing, a proposed assessment plan within 15 calendar days of the referral for assessment. A copy of the Parent's Rights shall be included with the assessment plan. The assessment plan shall explain each type of assessment instrument to be used, the purpose of the instrument, the professional personnel responsible for administering the instrument, and the facts which make an assessment necessary or desirable.

You shall have at least 15 calendar days from your receipt of the proposed assessment plan to arrive at a decision. Assessment may begin immediately upon district's receipt of your consent.

You shall be fully informed of the assessment results and may obtain, upon request, a copy of the findings of the assessment.

You have the right to obtain, at public expense, an independent educational assessment if you disagree with the assessment conducted by the district. However, the district may initiate a due process hearing to show that its assessment is appropriate. If the decision resulting from the hearing is that the district's assessment is appropriate, the parent still has the right to an independent assessment, but not at public expense.

INDIVIDUALIZED EDUCATION PROGRAM

You will be notified before an Individualized Education Program team meeting is held to discuss the assessment, the educational recommendations, and the reasons for these recommendations. You will be invited to participate in the development of your child's Individualized Education Program (IEP).

An IEP shall be developed within 50 calendar days, not counting days in July and August, from the date of receipt of the parent's written consent for assessment, unless the parent agrees in writing to an extension.

Your child's program placement will be based upon the goals and objectives as stated in his/her IEP.

The IEP team meeting shall be arranged at times and places mutually agreeable to you and the district.

INDIVIDUALIZED EDUCATION PROGRAM (cont.)

You are entitled to receive written notice of the proposed meeting.

A copy of the IEP shall be provided in the primary language at the request of the parent.

You have the right to present information to the IEP team in person or through a representative and the right to participate in eligibility recommendations and program planning.

You have the right to request a review by the IEP team.

Your child's IEP and placement will be reviewed at least once each year by the IEP team and you will be invited to participate.

A meeting of the IEP team requested by a parent to review the IEP shall be held within 30 days, not counting days in July and August, from the date of receipt of your written request.

Your child shall not be required to participate in all or part of any special education program unless you are first informed in writing of the facts which make participation in the program necessary or desirable.

Your voluntary written consent is necessary before any program placement or special education services may begin. You may consent to all or part of the proposed IEP.

You may withdraw your consent at any time after consultation with a member of the IEP team, and after submitting written notification to an administrator.

PROCEDURES FOR RESOLVING DIFFERENCES

Either the parent or the district may request a due process hearing in the event of a disagreement regarding a proposal or a refusal to initiate or change the identification, assessment, educational placement of a child, or the provision of a free, appropriate public education. The due process hearing procedures include the right to a mediation conference, the right to examine pupil records, and the right to a fair and impartial administrative hearing at the state level.

All requests for a due process hearing shall be submitted to the Superintendent of Public Instruction with a copy provided to the other party at the same time.

The district will advise the parent of free or low-cost legal services and other relevant services available within the geographic area.

The parent and the public education agency may meet informally to resolve the issue or issues.

The parent has the right to be accompanied and advised by counsel and by individuals with special knowledge or training relating to the problems of handicapped children.

The parent has the right to present evidence, written arguments and oral arguments.

Any party to the hearing has the right to prohibit the introduction of any evidence at the hearing that has not been disclosed to the other party at least five days before the hearing.

The parent has the right to a written or electronic verbatim record of the hearing.

Any party to the hearing has the right to written findings of fact and the final administrative decision.

Either party has the right to appeal the final administrative decision to a court of competent jurisdiction.

A court may award reasonable attorneys' fees to the parent who is the prevailing party.

During the hearing proceedings, the pupil shall remain in his or her present placement, unless the district and parent agree otherwise.

Any individual may file a written complaint with the State Department of Education with a copy to the district alleging a violation of federal or state law involving special education and related services.

Figure 16–8. Parents rights and appeals procedures.

□ Language   □ Articulation   □ Voice   □ Fluency

Student Name _____ File No. _____ IEP Date _____

DOB ____ Age ____ Sex: **M F** School _____ Grade ____

Parent/Guardian _____ Phone: **H** (   ) _____ **W** (   ) _____

Address _____

IEP Meeting
Status: ____ Initial ____ Annual ____ 3 Year Review Date Last Review ____

Present Performance Level _____

Goal: _____

Objective 1 _____

  Evaluation   Initiation   Completion
  Criteria: _____   Date _____   Date _____

Objective 1 _____

  Evaluation   Initiation   Completion
  Criteria: _____   Date _____   Date _____

Education Program:
Speech-Language—Unduplicated Service   Percent Participation in Reg. Ed. ____

Service Delivery: ____ In class: ____ Group: ____ Combination _____

Session/Time/WK ____ / ____   Special Adaptations _____

Inclusion of Linguistically Appropriate Goals _____

  I agree with the IEP as explained to me: I give permission for placement:

  _____ _____   _____ _____
  Parent/Guardian Signature   Date   Parent/Guardian Signature Date

IEP Developed by

  Name   Role   Name   Role

  _____ _____   _____ _____

  _____ _____   _____ _____

Figure 16–9. Example of an IEP for unduplicated speech-language pathology services.

dent could qualify for services as a communicatively disabled child in one state, move to another state and not be eligible to get assistance from the speech-language pathologist or audiologist in the schools. The child's disorder, of course, is the same, but the responsibility of the schools to provide free intervention do change based on varying state criteria.

The term "speech impaired" from the EHA categories is a case in point. As defined by 34 CFR section 300.5 (b) (10) of the EHA, speech impaired is a communication disorder such as stuttering, impaired articulation, a language impairment, or a voice impairment that adversely affects a child's educational performance. Does a child who stutters, but whose report card has all As, have a speech impairment? Some states interpreted the definition literally and said no services could be provided in such a case, because the child's academic performance was not affected. Others used the judgment of the speech-language pathologist who stated that a fluency disorder exists whether or not the child maintains educational achievement from year to year. This was resolved in 1980, when the Federal Office of Special Education, after careful consultation with the American Speech-Language-Hearing Association, declared that,

"the determination of a child's status as a handicapped child cannot be conditioned on a requirement that there must be concurrent deficiency in academic performance. Therefore, a child with a speech impairment established through appropriate appraisal procedures that does not affect his/her academic achievement can still be identified as an eligible handicapped child under EHA." (Education of the Handicapped Law Report, January, 1990, p. 15)

There is still considerable variance among states in determining what constitutes a speech and/or language handicapping condition (Neidecker, 1987). This continues to be an issue for school-based professionals who must follow these guidelines, yet recognize that their colleagues in private practices or health care settings appear to make other

determinations. It is important for the school-based speech-language pathologist to remember that such state-determined criteria identify only the children who will be considered disabled for reasons of the yearly child count for federal funds and the number of service personnel needed in the field. Setting limits of this type is within the realm of any employer. It does not alter the clinician's professional judgment of a communication disorder. Any agency that receives federal funds must abide by all federal regulations. The child may indeed require therapeutic services in another setting that does not include educational goals or time during the youngster's school day to remediate the problem. Finally, keep in mind that the IEP team can always decide jointly that there is overwhelming evidence of a communication disorder despite standardized tests results or state criteria. The professional judgment of the entire team, including the parent, is paramount under EHA.

Hearing loss is a more readily agreed-on condition in children. The audiologist can objectively measure the existence of a hearing loss. Its effect on educational performance must be determined by the entire IEP team.

STUDENT LEGAL RECORDS

Student records are particularly sensitive for disabled students, because they are subject to more tests, evaluations, reports, and observations than typical children. The Family Education Rights and Privacy Act (FERPA) requires educational agencies to provide parents access to their child's educational records and prohibits record dissemination to third parties without written permission from the parents. When students are 18 years old they have the same rights as their parents. Both EHA and FERPA spell out the confidentiality and accessibility of disabled students' records and note that translators must be provided, if necessary for the parents to meaningfully review their child's records.

A clinician's daily records are not considered educational records if kept in the sole possession of the clinician. As soon as these are made available to other specialists or educators, however, they are considered educational records and subject to the FERPA rules. Parents who disagree with the content of official school records can have the materials they find offensive removed. School districts can request a hearing to retain the records if the action is considered unwarranted or irresponsible.

APPRECIATING THE DUE PROCESS PROTECTION

Due process rights assure that no changes can be made in a disabled child's educational program without prior notice to the parents. It provides a mechanism for the resolution of disagreements between schools and parents. The procedural safeguards (see Figure 16–8) list all of these steps for the parent. Specifically, parents are entitled to the following procedures which must be set up by the local school district:

1. A written notice before any action is taken or recommended for their child
2. A right to examine all official records of the child
3. A chance to voice any complaints relating to services for their child
4. An impartial hearing before a hearing officer or a judge to settle a dispute
5. An adequate appeals procedure if they are not satisfied

There are three types of legal procedures:

Fair Hearing—is requested in situations that involve differences of opinion between the parent and the public education agency on what is *educationally appropriate* for a particular child.

Compliance Complaint—is used in situations that involve an alleged *violation* by the school *of state or federal law or regulation* governing special education.

"504" Complaint—is used against agencies receiving federal funds who have *violated civil rights* by discriminating on the basis of a handicapping condition of a child.

During the hearing or complaint procedures, the child remains in the placement in question. The process can take weeks or months to reach settlement, often with lengthy appeals. If the school is found to be at fault, it must rectify the situation immediately and pay the parents' attorney fees as well as its own. Clinicians are involved in the legal procedures when the students they serve are subjects of any type of special education litigation.

BROADENING THE LEGISLATION: P.L. 99-457

In October, 1986, the Education of the Handicapped Amendments, in the form of P.L. 99-457 were signed into law by President Ronald Reagan. The law made three important changes and many long-term alterations to the service delivery to children with special needs. It (a) established a new program that provided funds for planning and development of programs for disabled infants and toddlers age birth through 2 years; (b) increased federal financial support for states to provide programs and services for children with handicaps ages 3 through 5; and (c) reauthorized the discretionary programs of the EHA, including personnel training, programs for children with severe disabilities, and research and demonstration projects and materials. A critical change was also made to Part B of the EHA to ensure the use of qualified personnel to provide special education and related services. Specifically, all service providers in the schools must meet the highest requirement in the state for that discipline. In many states, that means that speech-language pathologists must meet the academic criteria for licensing (a master's degree) to provide the same services in schools as all state agencies. This was a protection to assure parents that specialists in schools were as well educated and prepared to work with children as other professionals who worked in other state or private agencies.

By the 1991–92 school year, all states accepting federal funds for disabled preschoolers had to guarantee a full range of services for 3- to 5-year-olds. The intent of the 1986 amendments was to reduce or eliminate the number of children who needed continuing special education placements in later years. Early intervention, according to the drafters of this legislation and much of the literature in the field, should make a difference and reduce the overall number of students needing remediation during their school years.

The resources of special education were also extended to preschool children "at-risk" due to personal factors, cultural factors, and traumatic life events. Into these categories would fall substance abuse, infants with Aquired Immunodeficiency Syndrome (AIDS), depression, child abuse, chronic illness, and so on.

Families are a key element of P.L. 99-457. Educators must design individualized family service plans (IFSP). These are comprehensive plans to target the family, the agencies, the community, and the child with special needs.

Interagency agreements were mandated in this new legislation, requiring the utilization of existing resources, programs, and agencies outside the realm of education. Thus, preschoolers and infants may be seen in community programs after assessments are com-pleted by school personnel or interagency assessments planned.

This law has many ramifications for the speech-language pathologist and audiologist. Disabled infants and toddlers are defined in P.L. 99-457 as individuals from birth through age 2 (actually 2 years, 11 months) who need early intervention services because they (a) are experiencing developmental delays as measured by appropriate diagnostic instruments and procedures in one or more of the following areas: cognitive development, physical development, language and speech development, psycho-social development, or self-help skills; or (b) have a diagnosed physical or mental condition that has a high probability of resulting in developmental delay. At-risk infants are determined by a state as facing substantial developmental delays if early intervention services are not provided.

Communication plays a major role in the development of infants, toddlers, and preschoolers. The law recognizes this by listing speech and language development in the body of the act, as well as listing speech-language pathology and audiology as two of the ten professions that must be made available to serve these children and infants. Many of the programs piloted during the first 2 years following enactment of the new law were based on speech, language, and hearing services then available in schools, as well as expanding such services in Head Start and public and private preschools.

Preschool and infant services were a relatively new undertaking for many school boards, and partnership with private or medical agencies was relatively uncharted territory. The new service delivery models for P.L. 99-457—home-based instruction, parent education, working within existing preschools, arena assessment, at-risk students—will require significant adjustments and policy changes by schools and state education agencies. Speech-language pathologists and audiologists will continue to be key providers of services for infants and toddlers. (See Chapter 17 by Montgomery for a discussion of these new service delivery models.)

TECHNOLOGY AND P.L. 100-407

The U.S. Department of Education Office of Special Education and Rehabilitation Services has been charged with the implementation of the most recent federal legislation to assist disabled students in schools and beyond. In 1988, Congress passed P.L. 100-407, the Technology-Related Assistance for Individuals with Disabilities Act. The funds helped states develop comprehensive programs of statewide technology-related services and set up resource centers to serve children and adults with disabilities. Grants from the Office of Education encourage effective partnerships between the public and private sector and consumers of such products, themselves. A substantial portion of this act was fueled by both the speech-language pathologists who promote and the consumers who use augmentative and alternative communication (AAC). Speech-language pathologists have served as staff members and consultants for the newly awarded state grants in technology.

REAUTHORIZATION OF THE LAW INTO IDEA

In 1991, refinements and additions to P.L. 94-142 were proposed, and some were passed. All laws are reviewed on a regular timetable, and some include automatic sunset provisions if they are not reauthorized by a specific congressional review and vote. A sunset provision provides that an act expires in a given period without special action. The overarching change in the law was the replacement of the term handicap with disability. The new law was renamed Individuals with Disabilities Education Act, or IDEA. Thus, P.L. 94-142, called EHA, was now embodied in the new IDEA legislation. There was a strong movement to expand the number of categories of disabilities. Four were proposed and two were finally voted in. IDEA has 13 disability conditions, an increase from the original 11, with the addition of traumatic brain injury and autism. Lobby groups continue to collect data to persuade their congresspersons to add attention deficit disorder and dyslexia. These conditions exist in school-age children, but could not be defined sufficiently to meet the criteria for a disabling condition. Students with either condition may receive modified programs under Section 504 of the Rehabilitation Act discussed earlier. Severe emotional disorders are in-cluded in IDEA; however, the identification and treatment of these disorders vary widely, as state and local criteria place more restrictions than the federal definition.

Nationwide discussion of the least restrictive environment raised the awareness of many school communities and of individual parents and parent groups. Educators and parents wanted to change special education to fit more closely with core curriculum and the delivery of support services in the general education classroom. A new term arose—inclusion or inclusive schooling—that was not actually used in the law, but in many people's opinion, more accurately represented the concept of blending special and general education (Regular Education Initiative, 1993). Inclusion referred to the provision of all modifications needed to educate children in their neighborhood school and the classroom they would have attended if they were not disabled. Speech-language and hearing services were already provided in the classroom for large numbers of students, but many schools also continued traditional programs of pull-out services. As general education reforms and restructuring took on greater political and economic implications, inclusion became the next step in the development of least restrictive environment. Collaboration and consultation became the implementation guideposts for the reauthorized federal law for individuals with disabilities. (See Chapter 17 by Montgomery for a more complete discussion of the new service models.)

SUMMARY

Providing services to children who are communicatively disabled in the public schools requires a thorough knowledge of the highly complex legislation that makes such programs possible. The four major federal laws discussed in this chapter (P.L. 94-142, P.L. 93-112, P.L. 99-457, and P.L. 100-407) plus the background of Supreme Court civil rights decisions set the stage for a free appropriate education for all children in our schools. To make education appropriate for children with communication disorders, speech-language pathologists and audiologists must know how to legally refer, assess, identify, treat, and measure student progress in schools. These children need to be served in the mainstream as much as possible, with every effort made to remediate their disability and enable them to succeed in school. The comprehensive legislation discussed in this chapter enables the highest qualified personnel in the professions of speech-language pathology and audiology to provide critical assessment and intervention for school-age children with communication disorders. Professionals entering this work setting are rigorously challenged to carry out the spirit and the letter of the Individual with Disabilities Education Act (IDEA).

DISCUSSION QUESTIONS

1. What role does civil rights legislation play in the development of special education law?
2. What are the five general purposes of P.L. 94-142?
3. Explain the critical elements of an IEP found in every state's forms.
4. P.L. 99-457 was significant for speech-language pathologists and audiologists for two reasons. Name them.
5. Why do you think assistive technology was mandated by federal law?

REFERENCES

Dublinske, S., & Healey, W. (1978). P.L. 94-142: Questions and answers for the speech-language pathologist and audiologist. *Asha 20* (3),188–205.

Education of the Handicapped Law Report (16 EHLR 82). Washington, DC: U.S. Goverment Printing Office.

Federal Register. (1977). Educational for All Handicapped Children Act, P.L. 94-142 Regulations, 42(163), Sec. 121a. 303. Vol. No. 163 42, Washington, DC: U.S. Government Printing Office.

Federal Register. (1986). Education of the Handicapped Act Amendments of 1986, Part H for Infants and Toddlers with Disabilities, and the Preschool Grant Program (now IDEA), P.L. 99-457.

Gallager, J. J., Trohanis, P. L., & Clifford, R. M. (Eds.). (1989). *Policy implementation and PL 99-457.* Baltimore: Paul H. Brookes.

Handicapped students and special education (7th ed.). (1990). Rosemont, MN: Data Research, Inc.

Montgomery, J. (1989). *Special education annual report.* (Available from Fountain Valley School District, 17210 Oak Street, Fountain Valley, CA.)

Montgomery, J. (1992). *Special education annual report.* (Available from Fountain Valley School District, 17210 Oak Street, Fountain Valley, CA.)

Neidecker, E. (1987). *School programs in speech-language.* Englewood Cliffs, NJ: Prentice-Hall.

Regular Education Initiative: Expanding Horizons (1993). (Available from Illinois State Board of Education, Springfield, IL 62777.)

RESOURCES

Cornett, B., & Chabon, S. (1988). *The clinical practice of speech-language pathology,* Columbus, OH: Merrill.

Hardman, M., Drew, C., & Egan, M. (1987). *Human exceptionality, society, school, and family.* Boston: Allyn & Bacon.

Meyer, E., & Skritic, T. (1988). *Exceptional children and youth: An introduction* (3rd ed.). Denver: Love.

■ CHAPTER 17 ■

Service Delivery Issues for Schools

■ JUDITH B. MONTGOMERY, Ph.D. ■

SCOPE OF CHAPTER

School-based speech-language pathologists (SLPs) and audiologists provide a wide variety of screening, assessment, and intervention services to children with all types of communication disorders. Each state defines its own eligibility criteria to identify communication disorders. The models of service delivery vary from state to state, district to district, and school to school. Programs are designed and managed by individual SLPs and audiologists to meet the demands of their schools and the needs of their students and communities. In this chapter, both traditional and new service delivery models are discussed, including specializations, observation, curriculum-based programs, and preschool programs, with an emphasis on collaborative consultation as a skill and responsibility of the SLP. The role of the educational audiologist is also discussed as a collaborative team member to assist children with hearing loss.

A REVIEW OF SCHOOL SERVICES

More speech-language pathologists provide services in the schools than in any other work setting. Education is mandatory through at least age 16 in this country by state laws. Therefore, all children are mandated to attend school and comprehensive screening for communication disorders takes place there. Once screened, children who are eligible may receive services without cost from the school district. Schools must employ large numbers of speech-language pathologists and audiologists to conduct a comprehensive program of screening, evaluation, and intervention services for children from birth through age 22 (IDEA, 1990). Public Law 94-142, now reauthorized and renamed IDEA, requires that these services be provided by professionals who meet the highest qualifications set by each state.

Each state, however, determines which children qualify for services. State eligibility criteria differ from state to state. The criteria may also differ from definitions of specific communication disorders found in the professional literature. Thus, one student may have a language disorder according to a particular set of norms, but the discrepancy is not great enough to have an adverse educational impact; another student may not have a communication disorder from the school's viewpoint, but the youngster could still benefit from therapy provided in a private practice setting, for example. This causes confusion for parents who request services for children who do not "qualify as disabled" in state guidelines.

There is considerably less confusion for children with a hearing loss. In education programs, hearing loss is considered a medical condition and the child, once identified, receives related services. States differ in the availability of various services for children with hearing loss. Thus, some states may offer separate residential schools for children who are deaf; whereas, others have highly developed integrated programs in the public schools for children with mild, moderate, or profound hearing losses. The important decisions about use of manual, total, or oral communication are made by the parents and the educational team. Often these decisions are influenced more by the expertise of the local professionals and programs available to the child, than the best match for the child's skills or degree of hearing loss. For example, parents may want a fully inclusive educational setting for their child with hearing impairment, but resources for audio-looped classrooms or trained signing interpreters may be limited or relatively undeveloped. Identified children in such a community may have routinely attended a day school for hearing impaired students. Parents will feel pressure if educators suggest the "best" services are at the day school. In some parts of the United States, there are large well-defined deaf communities, and deaf individuals will take strong issue with the concept of deafness as a disability. Some deaf parents will argue that their child knows another language (i.e., manual sign) so perhaps it is the rest of the people at school who cannot communicate with their child in sign language who are disabled. Making valid educational and communication decisions for children with hearing loss can require many resources and our best thinking.

It is important to recognize the role that schools play in providing no-cost services to children with communication disorders. Although they must meet the needs of every child, the form of intervention may not resemble that found in other settings. The service is provided during the school day, with state-qualified clinicians, often with groups of peers, and in the context of the academic program for the child's chronological-age grade level. Teams of professionals from several disciplines, including psychology, remedial reading, special education, and nursing may work together with the speech-language pathologist or audiologist in the schools. It is a unique practice setting that is attractive to many professionals and assures access to services for all children.

RESPONSIBILITIES FOR SCHOOL-BASED SERVICES

Every school district in the country must provide speech, language, and hearing services for the children in its boundary area, including those who attend private schools (IDEA, 1990). SLPs may be school district employees, private practitioners under contract, or available to a school district through an interagency agreement. Audiologists may be employees in very large urban school districts, but typically they provide contracted services to school districts through a regional joint agreement with an agency or private practice. Typically, speech-language pathologists provide therapy several times a week, although audiologists need to be available in a different form of scheduling for identification of hearing loss, fitting or maintenance of hearing aids, support for instruction, and yearly status updates. Aural rehabilitation services may be provided by audiologists, speech-language pathologists, and, in some schools, itinerant teachers who work with children who experience hearing loss. Although specific job descriptions vary among educational audiologists, it is widely agreed that five activities take up most of the workday: (a) manager of the screening program, (b) audiological evaluator and manager, (c) amplification manager, (d) referral source, liaison, team member, (e) advocate for the child with a hearing impairment (Lenich, 1993).

SLPs evaluate and treat between 25 and 100 children per year, with an average caseload of 55 to 70 children with communication disorders (ASHA Omnibus Survey, 1993). The caseload size can vary greatly in both urban and rural areas during a school year as new students enter and staffing units are not adjusted upwards. SLP staffing units are typically calculated and set for 1 year, leaving little flexibility if there are significant increases in student populations. Many clinicians report they plan eleven 30-minute group or individual treatment sessions a day. Audiologists may evaluate between 100 to 300 children per year. Practitioners in both professions write extensive reports on each child evaluated and treated, meet with families, and coordinate each child's program with all the other professionals involved at the school or in health care settings.

The SLP may use a different title in the school setting. Terms such as speech-language specialist; communication disorders specialist; and language, speech, and hearing specialist are used. Educational systems often cannot recognize the term "pathologist" in its state teacher credentialing structure, and speech-language pathologists are most often hired as direct-service providers and covered in teacher unions, associations, or bargaining units. They may be labeled pupil personnel staff or support staff to differentiate their tasks from classroom teachers. Sometimes this terminology confuses parents who perceive school-based clinicians as less qualified or otherwise different from hospital-based clinicians or private practitioners. Most school-based clinicians, however, have the same educational background as their health care-based cohorts. Furthermore, they must meet additional education-related criteria to work in the schools, usually resulting in a state teaching credential. They can do this in addition to or instead of the state license. In some cases, schools hire clinicians who have not completed their master's degree, leading to variations in the amount and breadth of professional education of school based practitioners. SLPs who do not have a master's degree cannot provide treatment for children who receive services through third-party payers such as Medicaid and private health insurance companies. Audiologists must have a master's degree to practice audiology. In 43 states, they must also have a state license and, in some cases, a type of educational credential or certificate to receive salary advancement in districts with such requirements.

Paraprofessionals or instructional aides assist some SLPs and audiologists who work in schools. They usually assist with scheduling, clerical tasks, parent contacts, and homework follow-up. In some cases, they are trained by SLPs and audiologists to oversee testing or therapy sessions, collect data, and work with students on computerized or similar programmable intervention tasks. They must be supervised directly by the SLP or audiologist and cannot work independently. Aides are employees of the school district and their educational level and previous training are determined by the district's personnel standards. In some situations, SLPs can place a request for a person with special training or skills to assist in a communication disorders program; but realistically, the shortage of such personnel often defeats the purpose. Audiologists often utilize technicians or aides to assist them in reaching the hundreds of children with hearing loss. In many culturally diverse areas of the country, SLP aides are assigned to provide language interpretation and translation for students who have limited English skills and may need to have therapy provided in their first language.

TRADITIONAL MODELS OF SERVICE DELIVERY

School-based programs to speech, language, and hearing services have three main components: screening, assessment, and therapy.

Each of these components will be discussed from a traditional school services viewpoint.

SCREENING

Traditionally, school-based speech-language pathologists screen all children in one or more grade levels to determine the need for assessment to identify communication disorders. This is usually a 3- to 5-minute screening with of a set of uniform questions or activities designed to enable children to display their speech and language skills to the observant clinician. Often all kindergarten or first grade classes are "screened" in this way. In some areas, third grade students are routinely screened, taking articulation maturation norms into account. Children who "fail" a screening are referred for additional testing.

Screening is not used in all school settings; consequently, many districts use a teacher referral process that concentrates on the same grade levels as screening. Educators are instructed to refer children who appear to have speech and language delays. If the teachers are carefully trained by the SLP, they may become fairly astute observers of communication behaviors. Most teachers are encouraged to err in the direction of overreferral to be sure not to miss children who may benefit from evaluation and services from the SLP. Many districts use a combination of screening and teacher referral. Middle and high schools typically screen student records to locate children who need services or rely on teachers' recommendations.

Students' hearing is screened in the schools by school nurses, contracted health services, or SLPs. Audiologists do not typically do pure-tone threshold screenings in schools. Each state has a mandated schedule for this routine testing in the health and safety code of its education policy. A typical schedule might mandate the hearing screening of all students at three frequencies in kindergarten and Grades 3, 5, 8, and 11. School nurses are more likely to conduct hearing screenings, because SLPs are the only professionals who can assess and treat speech and language disorders. Children who fail the screening and a follow-up pure-tone

threshold test conducted by the school nurse are referred to their parents for medical follow-up and then for an audiological evaluation, if needed. If parents do not or cannot take their children to a physician, the school will refer the child through the education system's health care network services for audiological and medical services. If identified with a hearing loss, the child is eligible for special education services including yearly audiological evaluation and appropriate educational modifications.

ASSESSMENT

Assessment is a complex issue for school-based SLPs. Assessment tools must be appropriate to the communication problem, age level of the child, and linguistic cultural background of the child, also yielding data that will be acceptable by the state and school district. Some schools require that assessment results be reported in percentiles, IQ deviation scores, or standard scores. Thus, SLPs may be required to select tests that provide such data rather than more clinically useful and intervention-focused information. Although most tests in use today meet a wide range of psychometric and statistical criteria, some extremely helpful assessment tools such as language samples cannot be used easily for state eligibility formulas. Further complicating the assessment issue in the schools is the use of norms developed on white, middle-class children that yield inappropriate results for minorities or children of a lower socioeconomic group.

School-based SLPs assess students for speech, language, and hearing disorders within the parameters of academic expectancies of other children of similar age and ability. Assessment results must show evidence of the adverse impact of a communication problem on a child's educational performance for the youngster to be served in the schools. For instance, a straight-A student with a reverse swallowing pattern and a tongue thrust without an articulation disorder would not be found eligible for services in most states. A student who scored below the 18th percentile on an expressive language test but was getting

Bs in all classes would not reflect an adverse educational impact. Other student factors such as positive self-esteem and the ability to make friends and feel comfortable communicating orally or in writing in one's classes are also components of educational performance. Thus, high achieving students who are disfluent or who have articulation problems are eligible for services from the speech-language pathologist because their communication disorder affects their ability to make social and/or emotional progress expected of their age (Hoskins, 1990).

Assessment results are often shared with other team members working in the school setting, because children may need several remedial services to benefit from their educational program. SLPs often integrate their report with the findings of the other team members to create a total picture of the child's functioning level. For example, in one case, the SLP identified a child with a severe delay in receptive and expressive language. When this information was integrated with the findings of the psychologist and learning disabilities teacher, a comprehensive program could be designed. The team approach to assessment is vital in the school setting to provide a complete and appropriate approach to the child, teachers, and parents.

Some school districts have their own audiology sound suites or test booths for assessments. Most do not. When an educational audiologist joins the school team to assist a child with a diagnosed hearing loss, the child may be tested at an audiology office, hospital, or similar outside agency. Ideally, the audiologist will also observe the child in the classroom. The evaluation results are shared with the parents and other team members as soon as possible after assessment so that educational interventions can be undertaken. Complete and frequent audiological assessments are essential for school-age children. Hearing conditions can change rapidly, especially in children under the age of 5. When children are known to have recurrent otitis media, a common childhood condition characterized by a fluid build-up in the middle ear, weekly assessment may be needed. Children who have hearing aids or use amplification need reassessments yearly or any time the teacher or parent notices a difference in the child's attention or learning skills.

THERAPY

The SLP determines the number of therapy sessions per week and the length of each session. The school day is typically 4 to 6 hours in length, depending on the age of the child. Kindergarten may only be 2½ to 3 hours. A 30-minute speech session in kindergarten may comprise 20% of the entire school day for that child. The SLP tries to match the child with other children with similar needs or age or both. Group sessions can be an effective therapeutic tool. Homogeneous groups have the advantage of allowing clear focus on a specific target area. Heterogeneous groups with diverse communication problems may also be highly effective. Children may correctly model target behaviors for each other. These sessions must be carefully planned so that each child is working on personal objectives and moving toward specific self-goals. In both homogeneous and heterogeneous groups, there are opportunities for realistic interaction and peer reinforcement. Such interaction parallels much of the everyday classroom interaction.

Individuals or groups must meet during school hours, and thus children attending therapy must miss academic class time (pull-out model of service delivery). In some cases, children may attend therapy sessions before or after school, but they cannot miss their recess or lunch period to have speech remediation sessions. Missed class time is a long-standing issue for school-based clinicians. For some children, this can be very disruptive and further delay their academic growth. For others, 30 to 90 minutes less of instruction each week does not diminish their learning program. Therapy scheduling should be monitored carefully for each child. SLPs must be sensitive to the overall educational program, yet clearly establish the importance of their own programs. This clash with academic time has led to the new service delivery models which are explained later in this chapter.

School-based SLPs must develop an individualized education program (IEP) for each child identified with a communication disorder. The plan format varies from district to district but essentially includes the same components across programs. The child's level of functioning at the time the plan is written is stated in each area assessed. The overall goal for improvement is stated, followed by the specific objective, with prognosis for measurable gains in month or year increments set. The tests to be used to show change and/or the strategies to be used to meet the goal may be added, but the list is not exhaustive and other approaches can be used at any time without returning to the IEP to change the wording. If the goal is changed, however, or new or expanded objectives are written, the IEP must be updated during the year. The IEP is basically a 1-year treatment plan for the child that the clinician, educational staff, and parent sign. If objectives are met, the next skill to be learned is listed, until the child is released as corrected or significantly improved. Some children do not meet their objectives and the team must discuss the problem, change the expectancies, or search for additional barriers to learning that were not previously identified. The IEP frames the intervention for one, complete year but may begin and end in any school month and overlap from one school year to the next. A sample of an IEP is included in Chapter 16. Samples of speech and language goals and objectives can also be reviewed in Figure 16–6.

INTERVENTION FOR CULTURALLY DIVERSE STUDENTS

Many schools today have children with diverse linguistic and cultural backgrounds. For example, in 1993 a moderately sized school district in southern California had a total of 6,000 students who spoke 54 different languages. The Los Angeles school district reported 122 languages among its student population in the same year. SLPs and audiologists need to be aware of the profound effect of culture, first language, and the number of years of formal schooling on the communication skills of children. What may appear as a communication disorder may actually be an effect of the child's first language. It could also be an effect of the context in which the child learned English or of the child's cultural background. School-based clinicians see a larger number of culturally diverse children and a wider range of cultures than seen in most other work settings because of the requirement that all children must attend school. Translators and interpreters need to be used extensively in the assessment process if the SLP does not speak the child's language. Background information must be carefully gathered to understand a particular child's pattern for the acquisition of English. It is imperative that children not be labeled as disabled, needing special education, and/or communication disordered if they are still in the process of learning English. This learning task is challenging for many children, and they need the best possible language models around them to learn their second language in an enriching, accepting, and natural environment. Many times it is the SLP who identifies the effects of second language acquisition and helps other educators and parents to support the children as they acquire language in the natural contexts of school.

THE DESIGN OF A SCHOOL-BASED PROGRAM

In addition to meeting the needs of the general caseload, the school-based SLP may specialize in a particular aspect of communication. School-based professionals often become specialists in areas that reflect the students they serve such as: augmentative and alternative communication (AAC), fluency, alternative assessments for second language learners, apraxia, preschool intervention, or voice disorders. Figure 17–1 shows all the programs in one school district that are operated by speech-language pathologists. Programs are arranged into three groups: assessment, therapy, and

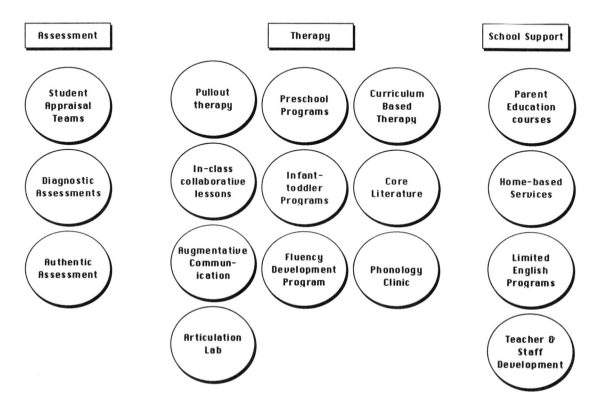

Figure 17–1. School-based services for children with communication disorders.

school support services. There are 12 SLPs in this district, and each SLP has 55 cases, including those in the practitioner's specialty area. Some students are transported from one site to another to take advantage of a clinic or center once or twice a week. In other cases, the specialty SLP drives from one school to another, serving the students who have special needs or working with the SLP assigned to each school.

Audiologists also have designed unique programs to fit the needs of students, equipment, distance, age levels, and the number of students in each location. They will often plan their schedule around frequent visits to children aged birth to 5 years, as small children develop and change rapidly. Twice a week visits to a preschool are not uncommon. If district students are in a variety of neigh-

borhood schools, travel can be excessive, and the audiologist may visit a school only when called there. If students with hearing loss are grouped in one school or at three to four sites chosen for age groupings, the audiologist may visit each site once every 2 weeks to assist the teacher, do routine maintenance, and submit regular reports. Schools that house large numbers of disabled children, particularly children with cognitive delays or multiple disabilities, need to schedule considerable time for the audiological testing to be complete and accurate, with the results conveyed to all the staff members. An audiologist may schedule this type of school for a weekly visit for the same day each week, or on varying days each week to accommodate the instructional program.

COLLABORATION IN GOAL SETTING AND GOAL WRITING

In Figure 16–6, samples of both traditional and curriculum goals and objectives are listed. These goals were written for individual children who met eligibility criteria for services in the schools. Although SLPs have typically developed such goals and objectives to independently address the communication needs of a student, collaboration has changed this approach in some schools. Shared goals are fast becoming the product of team assessment and team intervention. Teamwork is one of the most effective means for regular and special educators to work together and measure progress of children who receive services from more than one support staff member. The SLP can prepare the communication aspect of a goal, while the teacher can decide the best way for the child to reach an academic goal.

Here are some ways that student goals can become shared ventures for the child, the clinician, and the other school staff members.

1. Several special educators will meet and plan their actions together, resulting in two or three joint goals rather than a series of goals from each specialist.
2. For some children, setting one common goal is most effective. All the team members responsible for the child's program contribute to the writing of this statement and rotate the responsibility for monitoring it throughout the year.
3. Educators may write goals and objectives in their own areas of expertise (e.g., speech and language, resource, adaptive physical education); however, the titles of other adults or peers are written into the section listing "persons responsible" or "carried out by." In this way, the goal is designed by the expert, although the implementation may occur in other settings and be measured by various team members or peers.
4. Goals having two objectives may be written for a child. One objective might be carried out at home (parent responsibility) and the other objective carried out at school (teacher responsibility).
5. Parents and educators can write goals and objectives together, with a single method of monitoring progress. A check sheet, folder, or communication board can be carried back and forth by the child and used in school and at home. In some cases, separate monitoring systems are needed in each setting, and these are compared on a regular basis.
6. Teams can write embedded skill goals, in which all objectives lead to a single goal such as improved expressive communication written by the SLP. (Occupational therapy and physical therapy would have embedded motor goals, with the teacher having embedded cause-and-effect cognition goals, and the vision therapist having embedded left-to-right sequencing goals.)
7. The student's school day can be viewed through life domains (e.g., homeroom, hallways, bus stop, scouts, and cafeteria) and objectives written by the team to be carried out with the help of non-special-education personnel in each setting.

NEW MODELS OF SERVICE DELIVERY

School speech, language, and hearing programs are changing rapidly as the general education reform movement takes shape throughout the 1990s. Many schools are asking all their staff members, including the SLP, to form site-based teams that tackle tough school issues such as dropout rates, crime and violence, illiteracy, poor math scores, few female students in science and technology courses, and other system-wide issues (Boyer, 1983). The separation of general education and special education has led to some inequalities over the past 20 years, and many students do not have access to the core curriculum if they are identified for special education (Reid, 1990; Will, 1987). To some extent, this affects speech and language students, too, as they must miss important curriculum concepts when they are removed from class for our services. To reduce this fragmentation and lack of coordination, schools are providing more intervention services in the classroom.

The reform and restructure movement in special education is a global issue because of two factors: limited resources in all countries and the recognition of human rights for all persons (Rouse, 1993). Throughout the world, governments are attempting to educate more students with less available money or, in the case of third world countries, attempting to circumvent the educational problems that western industrialized nations experienced in segregating persons with disabilities. Persons with communication disorders in all countries are more likely to be educated with same-age peers than ever before (Stubbs, 1993). Education agencies everywhere are seeking new models of service delivery.

SLPs are joining with their educational colleagues to help ensure that children receive the core curriculum, even when they must receive additional remedial services. Some children with communication disorders may have greater academic and organizational problems because of their language learning disabilities and, thus, need services that bridge the gap between pullout or individual therapy and language performance in their classroom. Terms like consultation/collaboration, collaborative consultation, literature-based therapy, inclusive education, and meaning-based instruction are used to refer to these new models. There are some similarities among these programs, although they vary greatly in format, design, and expectations.

There are many compelling justifications for these new models. SLPs, often wrestling with the highest caseload in all of special education, have among the most pressing needs to be successful with children who require services. In some cases, SLPs may work without professional peers. They may miss the energy of many minds analyzing a problem or forming alternative solutions. These solo professionals often do their own assessment, determine eligibility for services using their state's criteria, design the method of intervention, carry out therapy, and measure the rate of change of the student. The SLP, alone, must determine if the student's progress is sufficient to continue the current intervention or if another approach is necessary. Again, the SLP alone must recognize and record the student's steps toward improved communicative competence, and many times these early steps are not reflected in the classroom. Although the SLP and the child may be working diligently on a series of objectives that will lead to an improvement in reading, for example, the teacher may not see the connection with everyday classroom activities. The child may also feel responsible for another "class" called speech with a separate set of drills, new vocabulary, and unrelated homework. This "parallel" curriculum is unnecessary in the new models, as content from the classroom serves as the content for therapy; or even more effectively, therapy occurs in the classroom with the assistance and modeling of children who are not disabled. Field-based investigators (Eger, 1990; Fischer & Boncher, 1989; Montgomery, 1990a; Moore-Brown, 1989) suggest that SLPs are embracing new curriculum-based models for four reasons:

1. The classroom is the most natural context for the use of language. Children communicate there all day, everyday. Any other setting is artificial or contrived compared to the classroom.
2. Carryover and generalization are the most difficult parts of therapy. The more therapy taking place in the classroom, the greater the opportunity for the acquisition and maintenance of new skills.
3. We have a changing population of children in our schools today: greater needs, more cultural diversity, and more children at risk for academic failure. We cannot serve all children; but if SLPs are present in the classroom, more children will benefit from the activities designed for the targeted students (Hoffman, 1990).
4. When SLPs work in the school setting, their employers are educators, not other SLPs or health care administrators. Educators mea-

sure the success of speech and language programs by the SLP's ability to enhance the academic success of identified students. It is not enough to say that a child has improved on a language or speech test; children must be able to use that new skill to become more effective learners in the classroom (Simon, 1991). This is expected of each educational team member. Considering that SLPs in other settings become members of their hospital or university teams, school-based clinicians must do the same to maintain credibility in the educational system.

Observing target students in the classroom is a critical strategy for SLPs and audiologists (Reid, 1990; Simon, 1991). Selecting the appropriate assessment tools, or providing meaningful interventions is much easier if the students' behaviors in the classroom can be observed and noted beforehand. What may appear to a teacher as a child's poor concentration skills may actually be rooted in a word retrieval problem that can be assessed by the SLP. Observation in the classroom requires time and the trust of other educators. Demanding daily schedules make it difficult to designate time for watching children learn in their classroom environment. Nonetheless, it is one of the most powerful tools and is uniquely accessible to the SLP in the schools (Simon, 1991). Observation in the classroom also results in valuable information about teaching styles and teacher expectations for students, as well as a firsthand glimpse of how typical students use their communication skills.

Some of the consultation/collaboration programs in use today for speech, language, and hearing services in the schools are outlined below. Each program or model is unique to the skills of the clinician, the needs of the child, the degree of organization of core curriculum in a school, and the political and social environment of each community. The models also have several elements in common. All of the programs described here provide service in the natural environment of the classroom, reduce the amount of time the child spends out of class, blend objectives and content of the speech/language remediation with the class, and utilize peer rewards and reinforcement. These programs have been in operation for more than 5 years, have special application in schools with culturally diverse children, and the author has worked closely in the implementation of each of them.

SAMPLES OF NEW MODELS

ARTICULATION AND LANGUAGE THERAPY IN THE CLASSROOM.

Each child is scheduled for 90 minutes of therapy a week, which is provided in the classroom. For example, the SLP clusters students with a variety of language learning disorders and articulation carryover goals into a sixth grade science class. The SLP coteaches with the teacher three times a week—alternately teaching the lesson, doing guided practice, working with target children in a small group, demonstrating semantic organizers, mind mapping, and predicting to assist special needs children to learn the material and practice their target phonemes in the regular class.

TEAM TEACHING/REMEDIATION

In this program the SLP and resource teacher alternate in assisting in the regular classroom. The SLP goes into the regular tenth grade U.S. History class one or two times a week for 42 minutes (length of high school period). The SLP has three children with special needs in the classroom, and the resource specialist has four students. The resource specialist alternates with the SLP by going into the classroom every other week. These specialists outline the lecture on the chalkboard behind the teacher who conducts class. All important points are underlined, new vocabulary spelled correctly, and the sequence of main ideas maintained. Items for the weekly quizzes are starred by the teacher. The entire class may use the outline; however, it is specifically designed for the seven identified students.

Each youth is scheduled for 80 minutes of therapy a week provided in the classroom. Goals and objectives are written to reflect skills in sequencing, written language, main idea grasp, and categorization using the history class content.

THREE-WEEK PULLOUT, ONE-WEEK IN-CLASS MODEL

The SLP meets with caseload students during 3 weeks each month. The fourth week, each child's classroom is observed. This provides an opportunity to answer questions, assist cooperative learning groups, correct papers for the whole class (an excellent method to find out how target children function compared to the rest of the class), conduct language enrichment activities for the core literature, and remind children of their target sounds, or easy speech, or use of full sentences. All children scheduled for speech and language services in the classroom are credited with the time the SLP spends in their classroom (i.e., four children in a class the SLP visits for 30 minutes are each seen for 30 minutes that day).

CORE LITERATURE APPROACH

Students are scheduled to receive 60 minutes of therapy a week, in class and in pullout sessions. The SLP meets with the primary teacher and determines what core literature books are being taught that year. They share their goals for the children in the SLP's caseload and decide that the children will not iss any of the introduction activities (also called "into" or "bonding" activities by general educators) for the core literature in the classroom. On those days the SLP will be in the room as an assistant and take two mixed groups of students who are identified and nonidentified. The SLP will use the core literature book for all content for a student with multiple articulation disorders and use the book and the workbook pages for the students with severe orientation, conceptual, and reading disorders. At least three of the

activities conducted in the pullout therapy program will be used in the classroom the following week assuring the identified students' success in front of their peers. The teacher's aide will assist with the in-class practice if the SLP is unable to attend the class meeting due to unusual travel conditions or a meeting at another site.

TEACHER-PROVIDED CONTENT FOR PULLOUT SESSIONS

In this program, students are scheduled for 60 minutes a week of therapy which utilizes either the math curriculum or the SLP's selected content for their goals. The SLP meets weekly with the classroom teachers for five students who are in eighth grade math classes that meet at different times of the day. The teacher gives the SLP the lesson to be taught the following week, and the SLP preteaches the new vocabulary, the sequence words, the operational terms, and the question statements in all the word problems.

STORYTELLING WITH SEMANTIC ORGANIZERS

The SLP has three schools and visits one class a week to present a lesson on storytelling. She selects a folk tale or similar high-interest/high-action, 5-minute story and tells it to the whole class. The students are all encouraged to practice good listening habits, oral comprehension skills, auditory memory techniques, and visualization strategies. The SLP coteaches the remainder of the session using quick draws, journal writing, semantic organizers, dictation, or similar facilitating approaches to reinforce the story for all students. The ensuing discussion enables the SLP to tap each identified child's target behavior in a group setting. Frequently, the practitioner combines two or more classes to increase the number of speech/language students in the group. All students in the storytelling group are counted for therapy minutes for the whole session (typically 40 minutes).

PRESCHOOL/PARENT COLLABORATION MODEL

The SLP enrolls 10 preschool children in a program to remediate severe language delays. The children attend with a parent or care provider for one, 60-minute session per week in the group. The SLP conducts the session with parents switching as facilitators for their children for 15 minutes, then as observers, then as facilitators again. The preschoolers attend a Head Start preschool or a typical local preschool the remainder of the week, and the SLP works with them and the preschool teacher another 30 minutes per week in the company of their peers who are nondisabled. The students receive 90 minutes of therapy a week and the parents and teachers are collaborators with the SLP for all interventions.

Each of these models has been successful for the SLP with one or multiple schools in a large geographic area that includes considerable driving time and distance. In each case, the SLP became a critical member of the school team, learned the core curriculum of the grade level or subject area involved, wrote meaningful, easy-to-read and measurable goals, and enjoyed a productive, satisfying year (Bardzik, 1990; Christensen & Luckett, 1990; Welsh, 1990). Student outcomes in these new models have met or exceeded released-as-corrected rates for students in the traditional service delivery models (11% vs. 12%) for four years (Montgomery, 1986, 1987, 1988, 1989). Additional comparative data are needed on this topic from other field-based practitioners in schools including other culturally diverse rural and urban settings.

RECURRING SERVICE DELIVERY ISSUES

School-based SLPs and audiologists frequently list other service delivery issues that affect the scope and effectiveness of their programs. One issue is meeting the needs of children with severe or multiple disabilities, cognitive delays, and traumatic brain injury.

A second issue is development of working relationships with educators, colleagues in other work settings, and parents. These issues change from one school site to another as administrators, school board policy, and community expectations shape our service delivery programs.

STUDENTS WITH SEVERE AND MULTIPLE DISABILITIES

Due to the increasing emphasis on providing education for all children in a least restrictive environment, there are more severely disabled children in the mainstream of education than ever before. These children may have significant cognitive delays, medically fragile conditions, physical limitations, and vision or hearing disorders. Children with mulitiple impairments may have a combination of two or more disabling conditions, plus a culturally diverse background or inadequate medical or emotional support at home. Communication problems can arise from any one or several of these factors, and the SLP and audiologist must assess the child carefully, using appropriate tools and the team approach. The SLP needs to determine the most effective method to deliver services, weigh traditional models with alternative ones, experiment with shared goals as described earlier, and blend therapy with liberal doses of observation in the child's other settings. Successful programs for children with cognitive delays require a commitment to functionally based goals and objectives, close contact with other professionals serving the child, and meaningful reinforcement systems for the child and the family. The SLP and audiologist often work closely together when students with multiple impairments also have hearing loss. This can be easily overlooked if a child has several other more visible needs.

Communication is vital to students with multiple disabilities and the SLP often sets up augmentative and alternative communication (AAC) systems for the nonspeaking child, as mentioned in the section on program design. Teachers, parents, and peers often raise their level of expectation for children who begin to communicate with others. Designing communication boards, selecting a lexicon, teaching symbols, or matching communication methods with emergent literacy are commonly coordinated by SLPs. Students who are physically disabled but have academic skills should have access to the core curriculum, and the SLP often initially builds that bridge for the teacher and the child. Team planning is essential for effective AAC use, student self-esteem, and the development of pragmatics and educational skills.

TRAUMATIC BRAIN INJURY

Children who have experienced traumatic brain injury may or may not have concomitant physical disabilities. Ideally, these students should return to their general education classrooms with appropriate support systems in place for them to be successful. Memory, speech, language, and cognitive skills are often compromised after head injury, as are emotional stability and orientation. Difficulties can occur many times in a busy school day and the SLP can assist as a member of the support team. Collaborative consultation can be a useful tool in these cases, as teachers need a source of information for dealing with the returning student's possible erratic academic performance and behaviors. Again, the team needs to review alternative therapy models to respond appropriately to the immediate needs of a traumatically brain injured child in the natural contexts of school, peers, and family life.

WORKING WITH EDUCATORS, PROFESSIONAL PEERS, AND PARENTS

A recurrent professional issue discussed throughout this chapter is the importance of good working relationships with educators, professionals in other work settings, and parents/care providers. This is true of traditional and new service delivery models; it is true in rural and urban schools; it is true in individual and group work; it is true for one school or multiple sites. Recently, school-based SLPs have begun to publish their insights and ideas on developing collaborative skills and its positive effect on students, schools, and professionals (Hoskins, 1990; Montgomery, 1990b; Reid, 1990; Simon, 1991). Sharing expertise with professional peers can be conducted on many levels. As discussed earlier in this chapter, SLPs use shared goals, and observation in classrooms, team teaching with educators, along with culturally sensitive assessment materials. Thoughtful explanations and frequent demonstrations of communication disorders to teachers to help them more accurately refer children is one form of collaboration. Of equal importance, however, is the need to become an active learner in the educational environment particularly by listening to teachers, children, and other professionals who know many aspects of curriculum and instruction that are comparatively unknown to SLPs. Many schools have begun to call themselves a "community of learners" to designate this attitude of lifelong learning and interaction with each other and with children. This attitude preserves dignity and enhances understanding.

The same collaborative style is effective for SLPs and audiologists outside of the school setting. It is not unusual for an SLP in private practice or a university clinic to make suggestions that are at odds with an original school-based assessment completed at school or with the school therapy program. In such a case, first steps often require that the school-based SLP ask for a meeting with the other professional either at school or at the SLP's office. Sometimes suggesting that the parent meet with both of you at the parent's home may facilitate a child-centered decision. As communication specialists we know the impact that context has on a conversation. The SLP should compare the information received from both reports to ensure that the communication disorder being discussed is relevant in both settings (see earlier section on determining eligibility for service in schools). In some school districts services can be combined in the school and private sector, although in others, students are restricted from receiving no-cost services from the school if another agency is providing the same type of related educational service. The SLP and audiologist need to know such local regulations before opening discussion with the entire team. Sometimes the two SLPs can work on different goals and accomplish twice as much; although a child may experience overload and confusion from stacked goals. Each professional encounter of this nature is a learning experience and will probably have a different outcome, based on the child's age and needs, the link to the curriculum of the school, and the relative expertise and collaborative skills of the clinicians.

In the same general way, parents and care providers are members of the educational team and work closely with the teachers and SLP. Good listening skills are important for these interactions with parents and evoke confidence in the flexibility of school-based programs to meet the needs of students with communication disorders within the scope of academic goals. Parents may misunderstand speech, language, and hearing programs that operate in a school program. The SLP needs to clearly state the type of assessment used, the design of the therapy program, and the expectations for the child. The SLP has an ethical responsibility to seek outside assistance for a student who has communication needs that cannot be appropriately addressed in a school setting. Parents and care providers may anticipate greater gains than can be expected for a certain child or they may not see the significance of language disabilities in academic performance. Supporting the interaction between language, cognition, and psychosocial development is a large part of the school-based SLP's program. Effectively conveying this to parents and other adults in the school environment can make a difference for the students who need these services.

SUMMARY

The changes in speech-language pathology and audiology service delivery in schools described in this chapter are strong indications that the discipline of human communication sciences and disorders will meet the future with fresh ideas and opportunities. School-based SLPs and audiologists will likely combine the most appropriate tools and procedures from the traditional models with the insight needed to assist students in a collaborative educational environment. SLPs and audiologists will merge educational measurement of academic gains with more authentic assessment of speech, language, and hearing behaviors. Both careful reflection and resolute action are needed at this critical transitional time to ensure a match between society's need for our services and the important learning opportunities that communication professionals can provide to students (Simon, 1991). The school-based speech, language, and hearing program remains a genuinely child-centered work setting with many service delivery challenges still ahead.

DISCUSSION QUESTIONS

1. Why does the definition of a communication disorder vary in schools? Why is this important?
2. Explain screening and assessment alternatives that are used in some schools.
3. School-based SLPs and audiologists work with many special populations. Name two of them and the type and nature of services provided.
4. Why are new models of service delivery being developed? List clinical, educational, economic, and political reasons. Describe three new models.

REFERENCES

American Speech-Language-Hearing Association. (1993). *ASHA omnibus survey.* Rockville, MD: Author.

Bardzik, P. (1990). Consult model for special education at the middle school. *The Middle Level News*, pp. 8–12. (Available from California League of Middle Schools, Sacramento, CA.)

Boyer, E. (1983). *A nation at risk.* Princeton, NJ: Carnegie Foundation for Education.

Christensen, S., & Luckett, C. (1990). Getting into the classroom and making it work! *Language, Speech and Hearing Services in the Schools, 21*(2), 110–112.

Eger, D. (1990). *Service delivery options for speech-language pathologists in the schools.* Presentation at the Special Education Innovation Institute, Lake Tahoe, CA.

Fischer, M., & Boncher, J. (1989). *Skills and strategies for integrating discourse, reading, and writing.* San Diego City Schools Inservice Course, San Diego, CA.

Hoffman, L. (1990). The development of literacy in a school based program. *Topics in Language Disorders, 10,* 81–92.

Hoskins, B. (1990). *Language literacy and self esteem.* Presentation for Developmental Learning Materials (DLM) Learning Consortium, Colorado Springs, CO.

IDEA. (1990). P.L. 101-476. Washington DC: U.S. Department of Education.

Lenich, J. (1993). The educational audiologist. In R.J. Lowe (Ed.), *Speech-language pathology and related professions in the school* (pp. 87–100). Boston, MA: Allyn & Bacon.

Montgomery, J. (1986). *End of the year report on special education.* (Available from Fountain Valley School District, 17210 Oak St., Fountain Valley, CA 92708)

Montgomery, J. (1987). *End of the year report on special education.* (Available from Fountain Valley School District, 17210 Oak St., Fountain Valley, CA 92708)

Montgomery, J. (1988). *End of the year report on special education.* (Available from Fountain Valley School District, 17210 Oak St., Fountain Valley, CA 92708)

Montgomery, J. (1989). *End of the year report on special education.* (Available from Fountain Valley School District, 17210 Oak St., Fountain Valley, CA 92708)

Montgomery, J. (1990a). Consultation/collaboration: Making the new model work! *Clinical Connection, 4*(3), 8–9.

Montgomery, J. (1990b). *Effective collaboration/consultation services for speech-language-hearing handicapped children.* Short course presented at the the the Annual Conference of the California Speech Language Hearing Association, Monterey, CA.

Moore-Brown, B. (1989). *The speech/language specialist—Critical support for teaching literacy.* Presentation at the Annual Conference of the California State Federation/Council for Exceptional Children, Costa Mesa.

Reid, B. (1990). *Communication in the classroom, or I'm dancing as fast as I can.* Presentation at the Annual Convention of the Alaska Speech Language Hearing Association, Fairbanks.

Rouse, M. (1993). *Special education: International perspectives.* Lecture at Cambridge University Summer Session, Cambridge, England.

Simon, C. (1991). A profession in transition: Thoughts on the speech language pathologist as a "school language specialist." *National Student Speech Language Hearing Association Journal, 18,* 26–33.

Stubbs, S. (1993). Executive Director, Save the Children Foundation, London England: personal communication.

Welsh, R. (1990). Unpublished report of activities of speech-language specialist using the in-class model of intervention. Bowley Elementary School, Fort Bragg Schools, Fort Bragg, NC.

Will, M. (1987). *Shared responsibility.* Washington, DC: U.S. Department of Education.

CHAPTER 18

Developing Policies and Procedures

■ PAUL RAO, Ph.D. ■
■ THERESE GOLDSMITH, M.S. ■

SCOPE OF CHAPTER

In preparing to educate students and colleagues about the particulars of policies and procedures (P&Ps) in audiology and speech-language pathology, the first author interviewed 28 graduate students on the topic (Rao, 1992). Each student was unfamiliar with the existence or location of the university clinic's P&P manual. There was also a general lack of familiarity with the need for a P&P manual, what might be covered in a P&P, and what difference a P&P makes in the operations of a clinic.

This chapter will familiarize you with what commonly constitutes a P&P manual and will answer the following questions: What is a policy and procedure? What should be included in a P&P manual? When, why, how, and by whom are P&Ps written? After reading this chapter, you will have a clearer idea of what is entailed in "managing by the book" in a variety of speech-language pathology and audiology employment settings. As the authors' expertise is in the area of hospi-

tal-based speech-language pathology, many illustrations will be derived from that area of clinical practice. However, much of the rationale, principles, and operational procedures which will be discussed may be applied to audiology as well as speech-language pathology, and to universities, schools, private practices, and other settings.

DEFINING TERMINOLOGY

WHAT IS A POLICY?

According to the Bureau of Business Practice (BBP) (Bureau of Business Practice, 1988), a policy is "a consistent guide to be followed under a given set of circumstances." The key word here is *guide*. A good policy will not force a manager into narrow or rigid decision making. Rather, it will provide guidance for handling a wide range of organizational issues and will establish a framework for both management and staff decision making. For example, a P&P on documentation in a hospital setting may state, "It is the policy of the Speech-Language Pathology Department to document a comprehensive evaluation in the medical record within 72 hours of the first patient contact." This statement is an explicit and measurable guide to policy and all clinical staff members should be cognizant of what the policy is. An example of a policy from a university setting might be a statement of the quality point average that must be maintained to continue graduate study.

The BBP (1988) describes good policies as: "broad, current, comprehensive, inviolate, written to specify responsibility for action, and used frequently" (p. 11). These attributes are essential ingredients of P&Ps if they are to be user-friendly and convey the mission, philosophy, and goals of a given program, department, or organization.

WHAT IS A PROCEDURE?

A procedure is a sequence of steps for completing a given activity. It may outline the manner in which a particular policy is to be implemented, but cannot take the place of that policy. Recall that a good policy is inviolate. Policies change slowly and infrequently. Procedures, on the other hand, change often, as dictated by any number of factors, such as staffing, equipment, space, and technology. The steps necessary for a graduate student to be advanced to candidacy, for example, constitute an academic procedure.

WHAT ARE INSTITUTIONAL, DEPARTMENTAL, AND PROGRAMMATIC P&PS?

All organizations should have an *institutional* P&P manual that applies to all employees. Such a manual includes a host of P&Ps that need not necessarily be restated in a departmental manual (e.g., the institution's policy on equal-employment opportunity).

Many institutions are organized by *departments* (e.g., Dietary or Medicine in a health care setting; Early Childhood Education or Speech-Language Pathology and Audiology

in a university setting). Each department is required to have its own P&P manual, including those P&Ps specific to the department. For example, in a hospital setting, only Audiology and Otorhinolaryngology may have a P&P on cerumen removal, while *all* patient care services have a P&P on documentation.

Other agencies and institutions may be organized along programmatic or product lines. In a rehabilitation facility, for instance, product lines such as a stroke program or a brain-injury program commonly exist. Patients with a given diagnosis (e.g., stroke) are admitted to a special geographic area in the institution (e.g., stroke unit). A number of professional disciplines, including Nursing, Physical Therapy, Occupational Therapy, Speech-Language Pathology, and others, form an interdisciplinary team to treat stroke patients. The services that the stroke team provides constitute the stroke *program*. The Commission on Accreditation of Rehabilitation Facilities (CARF) requires the various programs within an institution to have P&Ps, such as Entrance Criteria (how a patient gets into the program), Continued Stay Criteria (how long a patient remains in the program), Discharge Criteria (when and how a patient is discharged from the program), and Exit Criteria (when a patient is no longer followed by the program). Thus, each program must also have a P&P manual to guide the interdisciplinary team in delivering the desired programmatic care.

WHAT IS A P&P MANUAL?

For ease of access and use, all of the P&Ps for a given institution, department, or program should be kept together in a central manual. Frequently, this manual takes the form of a large three-ring binder, from which outdated P&Ps can be readily removed and into which new or revised ones can be easily inserted.

In addition to the P&Ps themselves, there are several manual components that facilitate consistent, efficient, and effective use. The first of these, according to the BBP *Personnel Policy Manual* (1988), is a complete and detailed *table of contents*, which lists major areas of policy and, under each major heading, the specific P&Ps in that area. In conjunction with a table of contents, the BBP suggests the use of a simple numbering system, whereby each major heading is assigned a corresponding section number (e.g., Clinical Policies = Section #200), and each subordinate P&P within that section has an individual subsection number (e.g., Client Referral and Assignment = #200.01). This system enhances an employee's or manager's ability to identify and locate the necessary P&P at a glance.

Other P&P manual components recommended by the BBP (1988) include a written explanation of the relationship between the P&P manual and other manuals, handbooks, and printed material in existence within the organization; a statement of the purpose of the P&P manual; and a statement of the organization's practice with regard to ensuring compliance with its policies and procedures.

NECESSITY AND VALUE OF POLICIES AND PROCEDURES

ACCREDITING AND REGULATORY REQUIREMENTS

A P&P manual is required by accrediting, certifying, licensing, and regulatory bodies such as the Joint Commission on Accreditation of Healthcare Organizations (JCAHO), the Commission on Accreditation of Rehabilitation Facilities (CARF), state licensing boards, state education agencies, and the American Speech-Language-Hearing Association's Professional Standards Board (ASHA PSB) and Educational Standards Board (ASHA ESB). These organizations establish and promote minimal standards that must be met by an institution seeking accreditation. Many of these standards must be translated into P&Ps for dissemination and implementation throughout the institution or practice setting.

Without a P&P manual, it is likely that the responsible program would be cited by PSB, ESB, JCAHO, CARF, or other accrediting or licensing agencies for not complying with a standard. Although the presence of a P&P manual is certainly no guarantee of quality—without it, an organization cannot become accredited (Rao, 1991).

LEGAL CONSIDERATIONS

We live in a litigious society in which nearly every decision can be called into legal question. Certainly in Audiology and Speech-Language Pathology, there is no shortage of potential litigants: clients, payers, and professionals. The P&P manual is a prerequisite for documenting compliance with existing laws. According to Applegate (1991),

> You want your policy manual to be as clear as possible because it often plays a key role in court if an employee sues you for wrongful termination or any other labor dispute. Many courts around the country have ruled that a policy handbook often serves as a contract between employees and employer. (p. C8)

The legal and regulatory climate, alone, has changed so rapidly during the past decade that a host of new policy areas has emerged. The Americans with Disabilities Act (ADA) [Public Law 101–336, 1990], which is intended to provide equal access to persons with disabilities, has resulted in a number of new legal requirements for employers and service providers. As will be discussed later in this chapter, the law mandates a number of changes in the P&P manuals of many organizations.

IDENTIFICATION AND DEFINITION OF ALL RELEVANT RULES AND REGULATIONS

The P&P manual is a comprehensive compendium of all relevant rules and regulations with which an organization must comply. Accreditation standards aside, a manager cannot operate effectively without written P&Ps. Although control of all management decisions may not be possible, a framework for managerial and clinical decision making is necessary. The P&P manual should not be designed to establish a set of rigid rules, but should enable managers to: (a) appreciate how far the impact of their decisions might reach, (b) encourage logical and consistent thinking, and (c) provide an opportunity for all employees to operate in a cohesive and consistent manner (Rao, 1991).

Many P&Ps are management protocols designed for the smooth and efficient operation of a department. The P&P manual should be the last word on what is required of an employee. It is designed to equip both employer and employee with a means to ensure compliance with all relevant rules and regulations.

WHAT TO INCLUDE IN A POLICY AND PROCEDURE MANUAL

There are a number of areas of administrative, clinical, and professional policy and operational procedures for audiology and speech-language pathology to be considered when generating, expanding, or revising a policy and procedure manual. Standards set forth by accrediting bodies, as well as legal requirements at the federal, state, and local levels, also serve as guidelines for many of the items to be incorporated as standard components of a P&P manual. Beyond these standards, requirements, and general areas of consideration, the content of a P&P manual is determined by the individual needs of a given program or department and by those of the institution in which it operates.

ACCREDITING BODY REQUIREMENTS

ASHA Professional Services Board (PSB)

Among the parameters considered essential by ASHA PSB (ASHA, 1992) for the provision of quality clinical services is the presence and utilization of current P&Ps in several areas. These areas include:

- The department's mission, goals and objectives
- The nature and quality of services provided
- The means of assessing the quality, effectiveness, and efficiency of services provided

- Administrative issues
- Financial resources and management
- Human resources issues

Specifically, ASHA PSB standards include the need for a written mission statement that describes the department's purpose and scope of practice and that remains up-to-date in relation to changing needs by means of periodic and systematic review. This mission statement, as well as corresponding measurable and attainable goals and objectives, is often located prominently in the first section of a department's P&P manual. The National Rehabilitation Hospital's (NRH) Speech-Language Pathology Service mission statement (National Rehabilitation Hospital, 1992) is

The mission of the Speech Language Pathology Service of the National Rehabilitation Hospital is to apply state of the art theory and knowledge in the realm of communication sciences to the quality care of persons with communication/swallowing disorders in order for them to achieve maximum independence and optimum functioning within the community. The Speech-Language Pathology Service is committed to the assessment and treatment of individuals exhibiting communicative/swallowing disorders; to educating and counseling patients and their families regarding the nature, cause, treatment, and prevention of conditions which may result in a communication disturbance; to educating the hospital and community at large regarding current concepts in the application of communication sciences to the communicatively impaired population; to expanding the knowledge base of the communication sciences through clinical research; and to serving as an advocate for persons with communication impairments. A continuous quality improvement program is the foundation of the Service's efforts to render the highest quality of care in an effective and efficient manner. All activities of the Speech-Language Pathology Service will be in accordance with the Code of Ethics of the American Speech-Language-Hearing Association and with legal and professional standards established for certification, licensure, accreditation, and protection of patient and staff rights. (p. 1)

ASHA PSB requires that the administration of an audiology and speech-language pathology department be based on established P&Ps

that are consistent with the department's stated mission and goals. ASHA maintains that any policies related to clinical decision making in the field must be established in consultation with persons holding a current ASHA Certificate of Clinical Competence (CCC) in the respective profession. PSB standards include the establishment of written P&Ps for client admission, evaluation, treatment, discharge, and follow-up, as well as for referrals to other professionals when a client's needs exceed the department's scope of practice. In addition, a P&P for evaluating the effectiveness and efficiency of service delivery and other aspects of program operations must be in place. Written personnel policies, as well as P&Ps related to the department's financial management (i.e., fee determination, accounting procedures, budgetary processes, and fiscal accountability), are also required by ASHA PSB (ASHA, 1992).

Joint Commission on Accreditation of Healthcare Organizations (JCAHO)

JCAHO requires that certain P&Ps be established for general and "non-bed therapy" services, such as Audiology and Speech-Language Pathology, within a health care organization seeking JCAHO accreditation. These include P&Ps regarding medical record documentation, fire and safety, infection control, equipment inspection and preventive maintenance, and special procedures (e.g., the P&P for calling a "code" in the event of a medical emergency) (Joint Commission on Accreditation of Healthcare Organizations, 1991). Other JCAHO requirements include a policy on orientation of new employees, evidence of a quality improvement plan with appropriate indicators addressing important aspects of care, the presence of an organizational chart and explanation of the relationship of the department to other hospital departments, and a statement of the scope of services provided. Specific to Audiology and Speech-Language Pathology Services, JCAHO also requires some mechanism whereby effectiveness of actions to improve a client's commu-

nication abilities is determined (Joint Commission on Accreditation of Healthcare Organizations, 1993).

Commission on Accreditation of Rehabilitation Facilities (CARF)

CARF has developed its own set of standards for rehabilitation organizations that wish to obtain CARF accreditation. Evidence that these standards are met must be present at the organizational level and also at the individual program level (e.g., Brain Injury Program), if the organization seeks specialty program accreditation. To the extent that audiology and speech-language pathology departmental policies and procedures may complement or reinforce organizational or specialty program P&Ps in meeting the standards of this and other accrediting bodies, you should consider them for inclusion in a departmental P&P manual.

CARF standards (Commission on Accreditation of Rehabilitation Facilities, 1992) that may have relevance for the audiology and speech-language pathology departmental P&P manual include, but are not limited to:

1. Evidence of active involvement in a process to remove architectural, attitudinal, employment, and other barriers to people with disabilities;

2. Evidence of opportunities for consumers to have an impact on the organization's systems and services;

3. Presence of a written plan to protect the health and safety of consumers and staff;

4. Use of a continuous program evaluation system to identify and evaluate the outcomes of the services provided;

5. Establishment and at least annual review of personnel policies that contribute to the effective function of the organization's personnel and into which staff members have input;

6. Development of and adherence to standards of qualifications of all staff, consultants, trainees/ interns, and volunteers;

7. Establishment of appropriate job descriptions for all staff members that are reviewed on a regular basis;

8. Presence of a policy for timely orientation of new staff members, volunteers, and trainees/interns;

9. Development and maintenance of a written policy and program regarding infection control;

10. Establishment of policies and procedures for orientation, informed consent, discharge, and follow-up of persons served;

11. Development of a policy that specifies time frames for entries into clients' medical records; and

12. Delineation of procedures for referral and/or recommendations to other services. (pp. 5–39)

FEDERAL, STATE, AND LOCAL REQUIREMENTS

In addition to the components of a P&P manual required by accrediting bodies, laws and regulations at the federal, state, and local levels may also dictate organizational and departmental P&Ps. The presence of and compliance with these P&Ps are not always regularly monitored through formal site visits or surveys. However, when compliance with the law is called into question in the form of litigation or other civil action, your ability to demonstrate the presence of and adherence to federal, state, and local regulations is of paramount importance.

Federal Requirements

As was discussed earlier, one of the most recent and relevant examples of a federal law that has had significant impact on P&P requirements is the Americans with Disabilities Act (ADA) (PL 101–336). This law prohibits discrimination on the basis of disability in employment; public services and transportation; privately operated public accommodations and services; and telecommunication services. P&Ps regarding recruitment, employment, promotion, and termination of employees; job descriptions, performance standards, and performance appraisals for staff; access to job training and continuing education opportunities; access to services provided; physical accommodations; and telecommunications, to name a few, must reflect compliance with the law by removing barriers to persons with disabilities through the provision of reasonable accommodations.

State and Local Requirements

Local requirements obviously vary between jurisdictions, but frequently have significant impact on P&Ps involving such areas as fire and safety, infection control, and/or the parameters of employees' entitlement to family/medical leave. State licensure requirements for audiology and speech-language pathology have been adopted in 43 states, although specific exemptions to these requirements sometimes exist. For example, school speech-language pathologists in Maryland are exempt from state licensure requirements, but are bound by the state's Department of Education standards. All such state and local requirements must be incorporated into the P&P manual (see Chapter 4 by Battle on certification and licensure).

OTHER NECESSARY POLICIES AND PROCEDURES

Administrative Issues

In addition to those previously mentioned as accrediting or regulatory body requirements, administrative issues for which you may wish to develop and maintain P&Ps include staff vacation, sick, and administrative leave; dress code for the workplace; access to secretarial support; staff productivity levels; staff meetings; and management reports.

A policy and procedure for the establishment and annual review of *job descriptions* that delineates the duties and responsibilities, lines of authority, working conditions, and required education and experience for each job title within the department is essential to a comprehensive P&P manual. Likewise, you should consider inclusion of an item that establishes the department's P&P regarding development and utilization of *performance standards* to be used to objectively measure performance within the critical components established for each job title. Sample performance standards for a staff speech-language pathologist are illustrated in Table 18–1 below.

Clinical Issues

As stipulated by JCAHO, CARF, and ASHA PSB, it is imperative that you establish a P&P that provides for a program of continuous evaluation and improvement of the quality of clinical care rendered to consumers. (See Chapter 19 by Frattali on quality improvement.) This particular P&P defines the parameters

within which a continuous quality improvement (CQI) program can be developed.

Other clinical issues for which you may consider developing a P&P include patient referral and assignment; general and/or specific evaluation and treatment protocols; treatment planning, implementation, and discontinuation; department-specific medical record documentation standards (for a concise review of this topic, refer to ASHA Professional Services Board, 1984); education and counseling of those who are served and their families; and

---

TABLE 18–1. SAMPLE PERFORMANCE STANDARDS FOR STAFF SPEECH-LANGUAGE PATHOLOGISTS.

A. Quality of Work

1. Accurately evaluates and assesses voice, speech, language, cognitive, and swallowing abilities of assigned patients.

   Outstanding: Consistently and independently demonstrates the ability to accurately administer, interpret, and integrate the results of both standard and nonstandard assessment measures for all patients assigned.

   Commendable: Consistently demonstrates the ability to accurately administer, interpret, and integrate the results of both standard and nonstandard assessment measures for most patients assigned with minimal supervisory guidance.

   Competent: Consistently demonstrates the ability to accurately administer and appropriately interpret standard test batteries for most patients assigned with minimal supervisory guidance.

2. Appropriately plans and organizes rehabilitative procedures for communicatively and swallowing impaired patients.

   Outstanding: Consistently demonstrates the ability to independently develop and implement a superior SLP treatment plan for all assigned patients and to effectively incorporate SLP rehabilitation procedures within the framework of an interdisciplinary treatment team.

   Commendable: Consistently demonstrates the ability to develop and implement an appropriate SLP treatment plan for most assigned patients with minimal supervisory guidance, and to effectively incorporate SLP rehabilitation procedures within the framework of an interdisciplinary treatment team.

   Competent: Consistently demonstrates the ability to develop and implement an appropriate SLP treatment plan for most assigned patients with minimal supervisory guidance.

3. Documents diagnostic and treatment services in a thorough, accurate, timely, and professional manner, in accordance with SLP policies, procedures, and guidelines.

   Outstanding: At least 95% of the time.

   Commendable: At least 90% of the time.

   Competent: At least 80% of the time.

Source: From "National Rehabilitation Hospital Performance Standards for Staff Speech-Language Pathologists" by P. Rao and T. Goldsmith, 1992. *National Rehabilitation Hospital Speech-Language Pathology Service Policies and Procedures Manual*, p. 220.04-D. Copyright 1992 by the National Rehabilitation Hospital. Reprinted by permission.

maintenance of standards of ethical practice. Perhaps more than in any other area of practice, additional P&Ps related to clinical issues may be largely determined by the individual needs of a particular clinical setting. For example, policies and procedures specifying evaluation protocols for particular communication disorders will be dictated by the clients served in a given setting.

Professional Issues

Beyond strictly administrative or clinical issues, examples of other areas for which you may develop written P&Ps include continuing professional education; student training; research activity; and professional presentations and publications. When issues arise requiring an administrative decision about these activities, or when questions of appropriateness, equity, or protocol are raised, it is extremely helpful to have ready and consistent access to clearly articulated P&Ps with regard to these areas of professional practice.

HOW TO WRITE POLICIES AND PROCEDURES

COMPONENTS AND FORMAT

Specific P&P components and format will vary from organization to organization, but within an organization or department, each P&P should reflect consistent documentation and presentation of policies, practices, and procedures. A sample format, as well as component definitions, utilized at the National Rehabilitation Hospital (NRH) in Washington, DC is provided below.

Section 1.0	Purpose:	a positive statement of the intention or aim of the policy conveyed to the reader in as few words as possible.

Section 2.0	Policy:	a brief descriptive statement articulating the policy.
Section 3.0	Responsibilities:	an explanation of the policy and expectations of personnel who implement it.
Section 4.0	Applicability:	a statement of those personnel to whom the policy and procedures apply.
Section 5.0	Procedures:	a sequence of prescribed steps for implementing the policy.
Section 6.0	References:	other existing documents or policies and procedures which are cited in, or related to, the policy and procedure. (NRH, 1991, #700.01)

Appendix 18A provides a sample P&P. The original effective date and latest revision date should be documented and clearly visible on each P&P within a department or organization. At NRH, revised P&Ps are disseminated to staff with an attached memo. This memo draws the reader's attention to the specific revisions made to the P&P.

STYLE

P&Ps should be written in clear, concise language that can be easily and quickly understood by all employees to whom the P&P applies. Technical or professional jargon and ambiguous statements should be avoided to minimize the possibility of misinterpretation. The Bureau of Business Practice (1988) recommends use of active voice when possible and suggests that exclusive passive voice use makes P&Ps sound "dull and pompous." The BBP also suggests that short, but not choppy, sentences enhance a P&P's "readability."

WHO SHOULD WRITE POLICIES AND PROCEDURES?

PRIMARY RESPONSIBILITY

In most cases, the department director has primary responsibility for drafting and revising departmental P&Ps. This task may be delegated to subordinate staff in some instances, but the responsibility for final review remains with the director. Other director-level responsibilities include assuring appropriate dissemination of and ready access to all applicable P&Ps, as well as assuring compliance with and enforcement of both department-specific and organizational P&Ps.

SOLICITATION OF INPUT

In many organizations, employees are encouraged to recommend new P&Ps, as well as to suggest revisions to existing P&Ps. A recent example in the authors' experience involved staff suggestions regarding access to departmental typing support. These suggestions prompted development of a related P&P. A regular practice of soliciting staff input on a P&P manual's usefulness and on suggestions for additions or changes to the manual is one mechanism of assuring that your manual is serving as the current, accurate, relevant, and authoritative resource for which it is intended.

ADMINISTRATIVE REVIEW AND APPROVAL

Although generally developed and/or approved at the department director level, department-specific P&Ps also frequently require review and approval by a member of an organization's senior management staff before dissemination and implementation. For P&Ps that involve or have impact on departments other than the one initiating the policy, review and approval by other affected department directors are also needed. Interdisciplinary clinical procedures, such as modified barium swallows, provide such opportunities

for interdepartmental collaboration. The originating department director is responsible for obtaining all necessary authorizations and signatures in accordance with the organization's policy.

WHEN SHOULD POLICIES AND PROCEDURES BE WRITTEN?

NEW POLICIES AND PROCEDURES

The need for new P&Ps may be prompted by a number of factors. Updates in the standards manuals of JCAHO, CARF, and ASHA PSB or ESB may include new or additional requirements that prompt new P&Ps. New P&Ps may also be dictated by federal, state, or local regulations. Recently, the Department of Labor required health care organizations to offer the hepatitis B vaccine to all employees. This federal regulation must ultimately be translated into policy for each health care institution. Installation of new technology and equipment also requires a P&P to clearly specify indications for application, responsibilities, and procedures. Development of an entirely new program or service within the department may be further grounds for development of a new P&P. If your department begins a home-care program, for instance, the department would clearly require a detailed P&P. Finally, evolving societal standards may prompt a P&P. One example in this area is a preemployment drug screening, which is becoming an increasingly common employment prerequisite because of the prevalence of drug use in society. If a drug screening practice is adopted, a corresponding P&P must be in place.

POLICY AND PROCEDURE REVIEW AND REVISION

Most organizations establish a schedule of P&P review which is at least as frequent as the minimum P&P review schedules mandated by accrediting bodies. JCAHO, for example, requires P&P review every 3 years and ASHA PSB's standard is every 5 years. Such review schedules are designed to assure that necessary and appropriate revisions to P&Ps are reflected in an organization's P&P manual.

Factors that might prompt the revision of a given policy are the same factors one would consider when drafting a new policy. For example, the NRH Speech-Language Pathology (SLP) Service recently revised its policy on documentation of progress notes. Originally, SLPs were responsible for writing inpatient progress notes every 2 weeks. However, because of a national trend toward shortened lengths of stay (LOS) for rehabilitation patients, along with a change in local standards (commercial insurance carriers were requesting more frequent notes), the department revised the policy from documenting progress every 2 weeks to documenting progress every 2 weeks to documenting weekly. The SLP Service has modified a number of other policies for a variety of reasons. Table 18–2 details that process, stating the nature of the policy, the nature of the change, and the primary reasons for revision of sample P&Ps.

P&P revision may also result from the quality improvement (QI) data of the institution, program, or department. These QI data may have identified a problem in the structure or process of a given P&P. For example, after a comprehensive analysis of the NRH system for scheduling patients, it was determined that cancelled therapy time was excessive. Once barriers to patient flow were identified and removed, improved patient care was obtained. When the revised scheduling process was fine-tuned and staff were trained, the revised P&P was documented and disseminated hospital-wide.

TABLE 18–2. ORIGINAL POLICY, REVISED POLICY, AND REASON FOR REVISIONS IN NRH SLP'S 1992 P&P MANUAL.

Original Policy	Policy Revision	Reason for Revision
Biweekly inpatient progress summaries	Weekly inpatient progress summaries	Shortened length of stay (LOS)
Discharge Summary within 48 hours of discharge	Discharge Summary within 24 hours of discharge	Referring institutions request more timely data
		Physicians request data for medical discharge summaries
		Social Workers request more timely reports to enhance continuity of care
Written Evaluation Report within 5 working days of initial contact	Written Evaluation Report within 3 working days of initial contact	Shortened LOS External Case Managers' request
Uniform staff working hours from 8:00 am to 4:30 pm	Establishment of flexible schedule options	Staff retention Expand tour of duty to reach patients' families
Modified Barium Swallow studies conducted off-site	Modified Barium Swallow studies conducted on-site	New equipment at NRH precluded the need to go off-site

Source: From *The National Rehabilitation Hospital Speech-Language Pathology Service Policies and Procedures Manual* by P. Rao and T. Goldsmith, 1992, pp. 220.01–220.40. Copyright 1992 by the National Rehabilitation Hospital. Reprinted by permission.

ACCESS TO POLICIES AND PROCEDURES

It should be clear from this chapter that the P&P manual is designed to be a dynamic management tool—consulted often, revised periodically, and available to all staff. Familiarity with the P&P manuals of an institution, program, and department can be accomplished by following several steps:

■ **Orientation:** All new employees should be provided with an opportunity to read the P&P manual and to ask questions about its contents during the first weeks of employment. Written verification by the employee that he or she has read the P&Ps and agrees to abide by them is standard practice in many organizations. In addition to this initial orientation to existing P&Ps, new or revised P&Ps must be circulated through all current staff, and written verification of an awareness and understanding of the new and/or revised P&P should be obtained.

■ **Location:** The P&P manual must be located where all staff within a given program or department have easy access. It is suggested that a sign-out sheet for the P&P manual be maintained in a central location (e.g., the secretary's bulletin board) so that the manual can be readily located if it is in use.

■ **Promulgation:** In addition to orienting new employees to the entire P&P manual, and current employees to new and revised P&Ps, the department director is strongly encouraged to regularly highlight or note important policy issues in staff meetings. If the director has observed confusion about a given P&P, an informational review and discussion is a necessary first step in promulgating the policy. Another method of updating employees on P&Ps is to write a "Did You Know?" column as a regular feature in your institution's newsletter. Such a column can highlight certain P&Ps and clarify any common problems or misinterpretations. Managing *by* the book is easier if staff know what's *in* the book.

SUMMARY

A policy and procedure manual is perhaps the single most important tool a manager can have, to the extent that it:

1. Clearly articulates the department's and the organization's mission, philosophy, and goals;
2. Documents compliance with all applicable laws, rules, regulations, and standards; and
3. Provides a sound framework for logical and consistent decision making.

This chapter defined the terms policy, procedure, and P&P manual; argued for the necessity and value of P&Ps; provided guidelines for writing P&Ps; and offered suggestions regarding what to include in a P&P manual. Because a policy and procedure manual is *useful* only to the degree that it is *used*, recommendations were also made for the regular review and revision of P&P manuals, as well as for the promulgation of P&Ps to all applicable staff.

DISCUSSION QUESTIONS

1. Why establish a P&P manual rather than simply maintain a notebook of memoranda?
2. You have been hired to establish a new audiology and speech-language pathology clinic. What P&Ps would you develop first and why?
3. In your current academic and/or clinical setting, identify a new P&P that needs to be established and a current one that needs to be revised and discuss why.
4. Recall one instance in your practice when a disagreement or debate ensued over a particular institutional practice. Was the P&P instrumental in resolving this conflict? How could the conflict have been avoided?

REFERENCES

American Speech-Language-Hearing Association Professional Services Board. (1984). Organization and maintenance of records for clinical service delivery. *Asha, 26,* 49.

American Speech-Language-Hearing Association, Council on Professional Standards. (1992). Standards for professional service programs in audiology and speech-language pathology. *Asha, 34,* 63–70.

Applegate, J. (1991, September 23). Succeeding in small business. *Baltimore Evening Sun,* p. C-8.

Bureau of Business Practice. (1988). *Personnel policy manual.* Englewood Cliffs, NJ: Prentice-Hall.

Commission on Accreditation of Rehabilitation Facilities. (1992). *Standards manual for organizations serving people with disabilities.* Tucson, AZ: Author.

Department of Labor, Occupational Safety and Health Administration. (1991). Occupational exposure to bloodborne pathogens: Final rule. *Federal Register, 56,* 235.

Joint Commission on Accreditation of Healthcare Organizations. (1991). *Survey preparation for physical rehabilitation services* (2nd ed.). Oakbrook Terrace, IL: Author.

Joint Commission on Accreditation of Healthcare Organizations. (1993). *Accreditation manual for hospitals* (Vol. I). Oakbrook Terrace, IL: Author.

National Rehabilitation Hospital. (1991, June). Policy and procedure on policies and procedures, #700.00. Washington, DC: Author.

National Rehabilitation Hospital. (1992, August). Speech-language pathology service mission statement. Washington, DC: Author.

National Rehabilitation Hospital. (1992, December). Performance standards for staff speech-language pathologists. Washington, DC: Author.

Rao, P. (1991). The policy and procedure manual: Managing by the book. In C. Frattali (Ed.), *Quality improvement digest.* Rockville, MD: ASHA.

Rao, P. (November, 1992). Interview with graduate students on policies and procedures. Baltimore, MD: Loyola College.

APPENDIX 18A

National Rehabilitation Hospital
Speech-Language Pathology Service

Policy & Procedures on Infection Control	**Effective Date:** 7-1-85
#220.34	**Latest Revised Date:** 9-30-92

Section 1.0   <u>Purpose</u>:   To establish a policy for infection control precautions to be observed by Speech-Language Pathology Service staff.

Section 2.0   <u>Policy</u>:   All Speech-Language Pathology (SLP) Service staff and practicum students shall adhere to universal precautions during patient care activities involving actual or potential contact with blood or body fluids, and shall adhere to all other NRH policies, procedures, and guidelines with regard to infection control.

Section 3.0   <u>Responsibility</u>:   The Director of the Speech-Language Pathology Service shall be responsible for ensuring adherence to this policy. The SLP Clinical Supervisor charged with the responsibility of CE Coordinator shall be responsible for tracking and documenting SLP staff attendance at required annual infection control inservice training.

Section 4.0   <u>Applicability</u>:   All Speech-Language Pathology Service staff and practicum students.

Section 5.0   <u>Procedures</u>:   5.1   All newly hired SLP employees and all SLP graduate practicum students shall attend the training program on universal precautions which is included in the new employee orientation program coordinated by Human Resources. Thereafter, all SLP clinical staff shall attend an annual infection control inservice. "SLP clinical staff" is defined as including employees in the following positions:

- Director
- Assistant Director
- Clinical Supervisor
- Senior Speech-Language Pathologist
- Staff Speech-Language Pathologist
- Speech-Language Pathology Assistant

5.2   SLP clinical staff shall adhere to universal precautions during patient care activities involving actual or potential exposure to blood or body fluids. These activities include, but are not limited to:

- oral peripheral speech mechanism examination
- dysphagia/therapeutic feeding team evaluations and treatment
- modified barium swallow studies
- thermal stimulation to the mouth or pharynx
- oral facilitation or manipulation procedures
- oral appliance or prosthesis contact
- physical contact with patients who expectorate tracheal secretions or who exhibit drooling
- physical contact with patients who have open wounds or drainage of body fluids, or physical contact with any patient when the clinician has an open wound or drainage of body fluids

5.3   All episodes of SLP staff occupational exposure to blood or body fluids shall be immediately reported to the Director of SLP and to Employee Health.

Section 6.0   References: 6.1   NRH Policy and Procedure #800.09, "Guidelines for Protection of NRH Health Care Workers from the Hepatitis-B Virus (HBV), Human Immunodeficiency Virus (HIV) and other Blood Borne Pathogens.

6.2   NRH Isolation Manual.

6.3   AIDS/HIV: Implications for Speech-Language Pathologists and Audiologists, Asha, December, 1990.

CHAPTER 19

Quality Improvement

■ CAROL FRATTALI, Ph.D. ■

SCOPE OF CHAPTER

Quality improvement, to many practitioners in the health care and education systems, is an elusive concept. Historically, the problem lies in the lack of agreement on an operational definition of quality care and the transient nature of various quality improvement approaches (e.g., implicit review, patient care audit, problem-oriented studies, and ongoing monitoring of clinical indicators). In recent years, however, a promising and more scientific approach to improving quality has gained widespread recognition in the human services. It often is labeled total quality management (TQM). Although the approach is regarded as new in the human services, it has been in place in the manufacturing industry for the last 50 years (Deming, 1986, 1993). Some call it continuous quality improvement; others call it quality process control. The nomenclature is unimportant. What is important are its basic tenets. Modern principles and methods for improving quality are

● consumer driven;
● process oriented; and
● continuously applied

To be consumer driven, you must direct your attention to the needs and expectations of your clients, as well as others who receive the results of your work. These "others" include referral sources, families, payers, regulators, and other professionals and support staff with whom you interact. To be process oriented, you must recognize that all work is a process. Thus, when you study and improve work processes, you increase the likelihood of a positive outcome. In a clinical context, the work process involves inputs (what it takes to provide quality care; for example, qualified staff, adequate physical space, well-functioning equipment, appropriate test and treatment materials) and methods (when to do what and how to provide care; for example, defined clinical indications for performing clinical procedures, assessment and treatment methods based on accepted standards of practice) to reach desired outcomes (the end result of care; for example, accurate diagnoses, functional communication, swallowing ability that results in adequate nutrition, hearing status that allows the ability to respond in an emergency, client satisfaction with treatment). Finally, you must do this continuously, never being satisfied that your professional services are good enough.

This chapter includes definitions of "quality" from varying perspectives, explores modern principles of improving quality in contrast to earlier ones and introduces quality improvement models and specific tools for data collection/analysis and problem solving. A case example will illustrate how you can apply a quality improvement model to a commonly encountered problem in a multidisciplinary setting.

QUALITY DEFINED

In a clinical context, quality care relates to the degree to which desired client outcomes are achieved. For a broader definition, however, the work of the late W. Edwards Deming (1986) is noteworthy. Deming was an American statistician credited with leading, through his teachings on management methods and statistical process control, the post-World War II industrial revolution in Japan. He believed quality had meaning only in terms of the customer. In other words, it is the customer who defines quality and the customer who judges the value of a product or service.

Cast in the field of health care or education, quality implies differing perceptions and depends on the particular constituency defining it (Donabedian, 1980; O'Leary, 1986). Among these constituencies are practitioners and clients. Practitioners often define quality of care in terms of their *technical* skill, or their proficiency in conducting clinical procedures. Clients, in contrast, tend to define quality by practitioners' *interpersonal* skills, or their more human characteristics. These divergent views were highlighted recently in an article and subsequent letter-to-the-editor in *Asha* (Wender, 1990). Dorothea Wender, a person with aphasia who underwent a course of treatment, offered her perspective on quality care. She described a "good therapist" and a "bad therapist." The good therapist spoke to her as an intelligent adult, smiled often, was warm and gentle, and talked to her daughters. The bad therapist reportedly was rigid in clinical

style, insensitive to her failed communication attempts, used child-like test materials, and appeared more interested in finishing a test than responding to Wender's feelings. The article prompted letters to the editor from the "bad therapist's" peers. Said one colleague, "The person described as a 'bad therapist' was actually an outstanding aphasiologist . . . . If the reader only knew that the speech-language pathologist is so highly regarded, the article would have been so much more useful" (p. 3).

The point is that both technical and interpersonal aspects of care should be weighted equally in your definition of quality care. When focused on consumer needs and expectations, the interpersonal aspects of care take on added importance and could make a notable difference in your treatment outcomes. A client who perceives that he or she is being treated with respect and caring will more likely adhere to a treatment regimen and, thus, will have a better treatment outcome.

Another consumer group, third-party payers, should be considered in defining quality. Not surprisingly, payers define quality, not in technical or interpersonal terms, but in terms of cost efficiency. Explained a third-party payer (Adamczyk, 1991) to an audience of rehabilitation professionals:

We want to know what we are getting for our money. We [therefore] want a quantitative measure [functional outcome measure] of a qualitative product [rehabilitative services]. . . . If I give you [X number of dollars], I get one point on the functional measure. If others can give me two points [greater functional gains for the same number of sessions], I'll buy from them. I'm a buyer. I want to get more for my money.

Lest the payer's perspective seem ignoble, Donabedian (1980) and Schumacher (1991), both respected experts in quality measurement and management, also address cost in their perspectives on quality. Donabedian says quality of care consists of the ability to achieve desirable objectives using legitimate means. Schumacher says quality is efficiency. He also believes inefficient care is unethical.

Using a profile of health care expenditures as a percent of the gross domestic product (GDP) (now more than 14% and rising at a rate more than twice that of inflation), along with the 37 million Americans who are uninsured and receiving inadequate health care, Schumacher maintains our responsibility is one of efficiency. Donabedian, too, uses an ethically defensible definition of quality care. He believes that practitioners are responsible not just for their individual clients, but also for the welfare of an entire population in need of services. According to Donabedian, the inefficient care provided to one may deprive another of the most basic care. Given limited resources, then, the highest quality of care would be that which yields the highest net utility for the entire population in need.

A final definition of quality merits mention. Philip Crosby (1979, 1984), an American theorist credited with advancing quality management approaches in the manufacturing industry, defines quality as conformance to requirements. Quality of care, then, can be measured against a set of clinical standards or guidelines. These yardsticks of quality allow comparison of actual care against a predetermined "gold standard" by which to judge quality. Within the professions of speech-language pathology and audiology, practice guidelines developed by the American Speech-Language-Hearing Association (ASHA) (ASHA, 1991), and ASHA's Preferred Practice Patterns (ASHA, 1993a), which specify basic clinical processes and expected outcomes (among other parameters), can be used as so-called gold standards against which to measure the quality of care.

In summary, positive client outcomes, technical and interpersonal aspects of care, clinical effectiveness and efficiency, and conformance to requirements all define quality. Additional dimensions of quality care, identified by the Joint Commission on Accreditation of Healthcare Organizations (JCAHO) (Joint Commission on Accreditation of Healthcare Organizations, 1994), include efficacy, appropriateness, availability, timeliness, continuity, safety, efficiency, and respect and caring in its standards relating to improving organizational performance. These dimensions of performance, as detailed in Table 19–1, encompass doing the right thing and doing the right thing well. They can serve as a guide in targeting areas for improvement and selecting the most appropriate models and quality measurement tools.

FROM "QUALITY ASSURANCE" TO "QUALITY IMPROVEMENT"

To appreciate the distinction between earlier and more current approaches to improving quality, the work of Roberts and Schyve (1990) is pertinent. They contrast the concepts of quality assurance (QA) (an earlier concept) and quality improvement (QI) (a current concept) in the framework of a multidisciplinary setting. These distinctions, as described in an earlier article by this author (Frattali, 1991), are summarized below and listed in Table 19–2.

- Compared with QI, QA has a more negative orientation by focusing on problems and people. Often QA is driven by alleged incompetence, threats of malpractice, and accusations that people are to blame for poor outcomes. QI is focused on the work process, not people, and on improvement, not problems.
- QA's narrow focus on clinical care implies that the outcomes of care are dictated exclusively by diagnostic and therapeutic decisions. QI expands the focus to consider how, for example, the activities of the governing board, management, and support services influence the outcome of care. In this broader sense, quality is the end product of *all* activities of the organization.
- QA often is activated by an impending site review, and deactivated after the review team gives its approval. In contrast, QI is internally driven by the continual search for better ways to deliver care. There are no end points.
- QA closely follows the organizational structure, rather than the flow of client care that crosses departmental boundaries. QI erases departmental lines and fosters interdepart-

TABLE 19–1. DIMENSIONS OF PERFORMANCE.

I. Doing the Right Thing

The **efficacy** of the procedure or treatment in relation to the patient's condition

The degree to which the care/intervention for the patient has been shown to accomplish the desired/projected outcome(s)

The **appropriateness** of a specific test, procedure, or service to meet the patient's needs

The degree to which the care/intervention provided is relevant to the patient's clinical needs, given the current state of knowledge

II. Doing the Right Thing Well

The **availability** of a needed test, procedure, treatment, or service to the patient who needs it

The degree to which appropriate care/intervention is available to meet the patient's needs

The **timeliness** with which a needed test, procedure, treatment, or service is provided to the patient

The degree to which the care/intervention is provided to the patient at the most beneficial or necessary time

The **effectiveness** with which tests, procedures, treatments, and services are provided

The degree to which the care/intervention is provided in the correct manner, given the current state of knowledge, in order to achieve the desired/projected outcome for the patient

The **continuity** of the services provided to the patient with respect to other services, practitioners, and providers and over time

The degree to which the care/intervention for the patient is coordinated among practitioners, among organizations, and over time

The **safety** of the patient (and others) to whom the services are provided

The degree to which the risk of an intervention and the risk in the care environment are reduced for the patient and others, including the health care provider

The **efficiency** with which services are provided

The relationship between the outcomes (results of care) and the resources used to deliver patient care

The **respect and caring** with which services are provided

The degree to which the patient or a designee is involved in his/her own care decisions and to which those providing services do so with sensitivity and respect for the patient's needs, expectations, and individual differences

Source: From *Accreditation Manual for Hospitals* (p. 52) by Joint Commission on Accreditation of Healthcare Organizations, 1994, Oakbrook Terrace, IL: Joint Commission on Accreditation of Healthcare Organizations. Copyright 1994 by JCAHO. Reprinted by permission.

TABLE 19–2. DISTINCTION BETWEEN "QUALITY ASSURANCE" AND "QUALITY IMPROVEMENT."

Quality Assurance	Quality Improvement
Focused on problem solving	Focused on continuous improvement
Focused on clinical care	Focused on all activities of an organization
Externally driven	Internally driven
Follows organizational structure	Follows client care
Delegated to a few	Embraced by all
Focused on individuals	Focused on work processes
Actions decided by committee	Actions decided by team
Creates defensiveness	Promotes team spirit
Works toward end points	Has no end points
Dividend analysis of effectiveness/efficiency	Integrated analysis of effectiveness/efficiency

Source: Adapted from "Chairman's Address: Improving Healthcare Quality in the New Global Community" by W. Jessee, 1991, at Eighth International Symposium on Quality Assurance in Health Care.

mental concern for client care. Thus, all are working toward a common aim, rather than specific aims within a specific department.

■ Whereas QA historically has been delegated to a coordinator or a committee comprising managers or department heads, QI enlists the support of all employees. Decisions are made by cross-departmental teams.

■ QA, with its narrow and punitive focus on clinical activities and individuals, discourages an integrated analysis of effectiveness and efficiency. Integration, allowing for effective care in an efficient fashion, is the focus of QI.

As part of the JCAHO's Agenda for Change, these principles were incorporated into a recast set of accreditation standards (Joint Commission on Accreditation of Healthcare Organizations, 1994) for health care settings. The new standards, which can apply to any work setting, shift the primary focus from the performance of individuals to the performance of the organization's systems and processes. The new standards do not require adoption of any particular management style, subscription to any specific model of improving quality, or use of specific quality improvement tools. Thus, they provide exceptional latitude in how quality is measured and improved. Nevertheless, the new JCAHO standards reflect the need for:

■ Commitment from the organization's leaders to provide the stimulus, vision, and resources to permit successful implementation of quality improvement activities

■ Measurement on a continuing basis to understand and maintain the stability of systems and work processes

■ Measurement of outcomes (including the judgments of clients and their families or significant others)

■ Assessment of individual competence and performance (including by peer review), when appropriate

In principle, the shift from quality assurance to quality improvement makes good common sense. But how do you proceed from principle to practice? The discussion that follows introduces you to some current quality improvement models and tools, and provides a simple case example to illustrate the application of a model and some related tools.

QUALITY IMPROVEMENT MODELS

Many models for improving quality are found in the literature, for example, the JCAHO Ten-step Model (JCAHO, 1992b), Hospital Corporation of America's (HCA's) FOCUS-PDCA (Hospital Corporation of America, 1991), and a Model for Improvement designed by Associates in Process Improvement (Langley, Nolan, & Nolan, 1992). The Ten-step Model, which relies on comparisons of actual care to predetermined quality indicators and thresholds for evaluation, is summarized in Table 19–3. The FOCUS aspect of the HCA model, which is an acronmym for Find-Organize-Clarify-Understand-Select, helps individuals narrow their attention to a discrete opportunity for improvement; the PDCA aspect of the model, which stands for Plan-Do-Check-Act, allows individuals to act on that opportunity. Finally, the Model for Improvement, suggested by Associates in Process Improvement (API), assists individuals in focusing and acting to improve systems by asking three questions: What are we trying to accomplish? How will we know that a change is an improvement? What changes can we make that will result in improvement? Figure 19–1 provides a schematic of API's model (Langley et al., 1992).

Both the HCA and API models incorporate what is known as the Shewhart Cycle (also called the PDCA Cycle for Plan-Do-Check-Act, PDSA Cycle for Plan-Do-Study-Act, or the Deming Cycle, because it was Deming who introduced it in Japan). This circular (and thus continuous) process is named for Walter Shewhart, a statistician who worked for Bell Telephone Laboratories in the 1920s. The four steps are briefly described:

Plan: The first step is to study a work process to decide what change might improve it. Organize the appropriate team. What data are necessary? Do the data already exist or is it necessary to collect and organize data to understand the current situation? Once current knowledge is acquired, determine what changes can be made or tested. Are tests necessary? Do not proceed without a well-defined plan.

Do: Carry out the test, or make the change—preferably on a small scale.

Study: Observe the effects, using the same measures used to document the current situation. Did the change result in improvement?

Act: What did you learn? If the change resulted in improvement, standardize the change on a full-scale basis. If the change did not result in improvement, decide what other changes can be tested. Thus, the cycle starts again.

The PDSA Cycle is not unfamiliar to clinicians. It, in fact, mirrors the clinical process. We collect baseline data to understand a client's current communication abilities and develop a plan of treatment to improve com-

TABLE 19–3. JCAHO TEN-STEP MODEL.

1. Assign responsibility for quality improvement activities.
2. Delineate the scope of care.
3. Identify the important aspects of care.
4. Identify quality indicators for monitoring the important aspects of care.
5. Establish thresholds for the indicators that trigger evaluation of that care.
6. Collect and organize data for each indicator.
7. Evaluate care when thresholds are reached to identify opportunities to improve care or correct problems.
8. Take actions to improve care or correct identified problems.
9. Assess effectiveness of the action and document improvement in care.
10. Communicate the results to relevant individuals, departments, or services and to the organization-wide quality improvement program.

Source: From *Using Quality Improvement Tools in a Health Care Setting* (p. 14) by Joint Commission on Accreditation on Heatlhcare Organizations, 1992, Oakbrook Terrace, IL: Joint Commission on Accreditation of Heatlhcare Organizations. Copyright 1992 Joint Commission on Accreditation of Healthcare Organizations. Reprinted by permission.

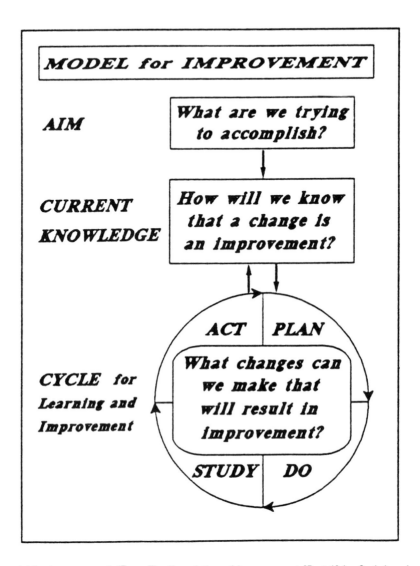

Figure 19–1. A model for improvement. (From The Foundation of Improvement [Part 1] by G. J. Langley, K. M. Nolan, and T. W. Nolan, 1992 Silver Spring, MD: Associates in Process Improvement, Inc., p. 4. Copyright 1992 Associates in Process Improvement. Reprinted by permission.)

munication (Plan), carry out the plan (Do), observe the effects to determine if treatment results in improved communication (Study), and apply what is learned to either continue with or modify the plan of treatment (Act), thus, starting the cycle again. On a broader scale the PDSA cycle can be applied not only to clinical processes, but to administrative, teaching, research, and supervisory processes as well.

QUALITY IMPROVEMENT TOOLS

Once you select a model for improving quality, you will need to use specific data collection/analysis and problem-solving tools to proceed through the steps of the quality improvement process. Germane to the Deming method is the need to base decisions on accurate and timely data, not on hunches, assumption, or "experience" (Walton, 1986).

Quality improvement involves the use of basic tools to study and improve work processes. They often are referred to collectively as statistical process control tools. Some of these tools, however, are not statistical tools but merely ways to organize information or ideas. You may find it helpful to think of these tools as pictorial means to display and analyze information.

Brassard (1988) calls these tools graphical problem-solving techniques. They identify variations in work processes, the root causes of problems, the relative importance of problems to be solved, and the impact of subsequent changes.

THE SEVEN QUALITY CONTROL TOOLS

The graphical techniques associated with quality improvement include:

- **Flow charts:** Pictorial representations showing sequentially all steps of a work process;
- **Fishbone diagrams:** Also called cause-and-effect diagrams that show the relationship between an effect (or outcome) and all the possible causes influencing it;
- **Pareto charts:** A special form of vertical bar graphs, showing the frequency of events in descending order to help determine which problems to solve and in what order;
- **Run charts:** Visual representations of data that display points on a graph to show levels of performance over time;
- **Histograms:** Bar graphs that display the distribution of data or the number of units in each category;
- **Scatter diagrams:** Pictorial representations of the possible relationship between two variables; and
- **Control charts:** Run charts with statistically determined upper and lower control

limits, drawn as lines on either side of the process average.

Excellent resources to learn more about these tools include *Total Quality Management: A Continuous Process for Improvement* (American Speech-Language-Hearing Association, 1993b), *The Memory Jogger* (Brassard, 1988) (a pocket guide of tools for continuous improvement), and *A Pocket Guide to Quality Improvement Tools*, (Joint Commission on Accreditation of Healthcare Organizations, 1992b). ASHA's publication addresses applications of these seven quality control tools using specific examples in speech-language pathology and audiology.

CONSUMER SATISFACTION MEASURES

In addition to the tools mentioned above, another tool deserves your attention—consumer satisfaction surveys. As quality improvement methods shift the focus to the needs of and judgments of quality by consumers, use of these outcome measures is becoming standard protocol in health care and education settings. These surveys solicit judgments about the quality of care from clients, families, or other consumers such as referral sources. Many such tools have been developed for commercial publication and quietly by individual programs or institutions. One that is available for speech-language pathology and audiology services was developed by ASHA's former Committee on Quality Assurance (American Speech-Language-Hearing Association, 1989). ASHA's Consumer Satisfaction Survey is a one-page mailable questionnaire that addresses the degree of patient satisfaction with timeliness of service, physical setting, interactions with staff, and service outcomes. A sample of the tool is shown in Appendix 19A.

TEAMWORK

Now knowing a little about principles, models, and tools, you should recognize that quality improvement activities are irrelevant without teamwork. In most instances your work is interdependent. That is, your work intersects with that of other service providers, and thus, the quality of your work will depend on how well others do their jobs. If you work in a health care setting, others can include, for example, physicians, nurses, physical therapists, occupational therapists, technicians, aides, social workers, transporters, and dietitians. If you work in a school, others can include, for example, teachers, nurses, secretaries, guidance counselors, special educators, psychologists, and principals. When all are working toward a common aim, it becomes necessary to engage in quality improvement activities that involve a team of individuals, each playing a vital role in the work process targeted for improvement.

Teamwork does not happen naturally. Rather, it requires specialized knowledge and skills in group dynamics and use of problem-solving and decision-making tools. Every quality improvement team should have a leader, advisor, recorder, and members who play key roles in the work process(es) under study. The leader sets the agenda, facilitates discussion and decision making, and moves the team through the agenda. The advisor, an expert in quality improvement techniques, trains team members in the use of the tools and provides technical assistance as necessary. The recorder, usually a rotating position, keeps minutes and records delegation of duties. The team members participate in discussions and complete assigned projects (Frattali, 1993; Joint Comission on Accreditation of Healthcare Organizations, 1992b).

Some effective techniques to facilitate group decision making and problem solving are **brainstorming, multivoting,** and **nominal group technique** (Scholtes, 1988).

Brainstorming is a free form approach to generating ideas. Every team member contributes ideas without the restriction of discussion or judgment. No one is allowed to criticize another's ideas. All ideas are recorded for team review.

Multivoting is a way to select the most important or popular items from the list of ideas generated. Thus, it often follows a brainstorming session. Multivoting is accomplished through a series of votes, each cutting the list in half. It results in identification of items worthy of immediate attention.

Nominal group technique is a more structured approach than either brainstorming or multivoting. It is used to generate and narrow a list of options. Each team member is asked to generate ideas in silence and write them down. Each participant reads one idea from his or her list. The process continues until everyone's list has been shared. All ideas are recorded on a flipchart. Afterwards, individual ideas are clarified and discussed. The list is then narrowed by having members record a limited number of choices and assign a point value to each, based on their preferences. The votes are tallied and the values are added. The item with the highest point total is the group's selection.

Finally, you must address the issue of group dynamics. When any process involves a team of individuals, you can anticipate varying levels of participation, "hidden agendas," and some personality conflicts. Addressing these variables up front and allowing time for the team to coalesce will be crucial.

A CASE EXAMPLE

By way of a simple example, application of a model for improvement and selected tools are described. A multidisciplinary team convenes to address the problem of low productivity resulting from missed treatment sessions for both inpatient and outpatient rehabilitative services. Members of the improvement team include all key people who are involved in the process of treatment. These individuals include an audiologist, speech-language pathologist, physical therapist, occupational therapist, rehabilitation aide, transporter, and administrative director of rehabilitation services. The team decided to apply the Model for Improvement by Associates in Process Improvement (Langley et al.,

1992). Thus, the team attempted to answer three fundamental questions.

1. What are we trying to accomplish? The team agreed that the aim of this project was to reduce the frequency of missed treatment sessions. Thus, it decided to address in the first cycle for improvement the performance dimensions of treatment availability and timeliness.

2. How will we know that the change is an improvement? To answer this question, the team decided to organize historical data from client satisfaction surveys and client schedule logs. The team plotted a **run chart** for a 6-month period and found that the frequency of missed treatment sessions ranged from 10% to 28% per month, with a 20% average monthly frequency of missed sessions. Descriptive data taken from client satisfaction measures completed during the same 6 months documented that 3 of 30 clients complained that "therapists did not always show up for my therapy," or "two different therapies were sometimes scheduled at the same time and I had to miss one," or "I couldn't find a parking space." The team then constructed a **flow chart** of rehabilitation treatment scheduling to identify potential breakdowns in the scheduling process. It also constructed a **cause-and-effect diagram** to determine the causes of missed sessions. These causes included scheduling conflicts, parking problems, medical complications, lost or late referrals, lack of coverage during practitioner absences, hospital transport service problems, and cancellations because of bad weather.

To determine which causes were accounting for most of the problems, the team constructed a **Pareto chart.** They found that 80% of the missed sessions was caused either by scheduling conflicts with other rehabilitation providers or by inpatient transportation problems. In addition, the parking problems reported by some outpatients occurred as a result of construction, which had been completed by the time the team process had begun.

3. What changes can we make that will result in improvement? Using the above information, the team brainstormed solutions to the two primary problems. Solutions included the use of a master schedule board prominently mounted in the rehabilitation department and communication with the transportation service director. The transportation director agreed to assign two transporters to the rehabilitation service for a trial period to determine if this change would result in fewer missed sessions.

Once these changes were implemented, the team again plotted the patterns of missed sessions on a run chart for 6 months. The frequency of missed sessions dropped to a range of 3% to 15%, with an average monthly frequency of 7%. Client satisfaction surveys during the same time documented only one related complaint among 35 surveys completed. The team constructed a new flow chart to document the changes to the scheduling process.

The graphic displays of improvement were shared with staff, as well as with upper management. The team continued to work together to develop yet better ways to reduce the frequency of missed treatment session and to determine if the increased treatment attendance rate resulted in better functional outcomes at the time of patient discharge. Thus, the cycle began once again (this time to address the performance dimensions of availability, timeliness, and treatment effectiveness).

SUMMARY

A more systematic and data-based approach to improving quality is perhaps the most promising way to amass objective evidence of quality care. We no longer can ethically defend the provision of services without knowledge of appropriateness, timeliness, effectiveness, safety, efficiency, and so forth. Use of quality improvement methods affords you the opportunity to acquire new knowledge along the dimensions of performance as identified by JCAHO (1992b). Along with clinical research, quality improvement methods can help you answer clinical questions that can shape new and more cost-effective patterns of service delivery. Does clinical intervention make a difference in the client's functional communication? According to whom? The client? The family? Can fewer treatment sessions result in the same functional outcomes? Can use of alternative treatment methods (e.g., use of support personnel, inclusion models in the classroom, cotreatment) result in the same outcomes? These are reasonable questions, given today's consumer-oriented and cost-conscious climate, and they merit your continual attention and investigation.

DISCUSSION QUESTIONS

1. Discuss the differences between the principles associated with "quality assurance" and "quality improvement."
2. Who are your consumers?
3. What dimensions of performance can be measured?
4. Describe the PDSA cycle and apply it to the clinical process.
5. What might be the benefits of incorporating quality improvement activities into your routine professional activities? What might be the consequences if you do not apply methods to improve quality?

REFERENCES

Adamczyk, J. (1991, June). Relevance of CIQI measures of quality and outcome to the payor/insurer—How to "buy smart." Presentation at Rehabilitation Medicine: Continuous Interdisciplinary Quality Improvement Conference sponsored by the Buffalo General Hospital and State University of New York at Buffalo, NY.

American Speech-Language-Hearing Association. (1989). *Consumer satisfaction measure.* Rockville, MD: Author.

American Speech-Language-Hearing Association. (1991). *ASHA desk reference—revised.* Rockville, MD: Author.

American Speech-Language-Hearing Association. (1992). *How to establish a quality improvement process: A ten-step model.* Rockville, MD: Author.

American Speech-Language-Hearing Association. (1993a). Preferred practice patterns for the professions of speech-language pathology and audiology. *Asha Supplement.*

American Speech-Language-Hearing Association. (1993b). *Total quality management: A continuous process for improvement.* Rockville, MD: Author.

Brassard, M. (1988). *The memory jogger.* Methuen, MA: GOAL/QPC.

Crosby, P. (1979). *Quality is free: The art of making quality certain.* New York: McGraw-Hill.

Crosby, P. (1984). *Quality without tears: The art of hassle-free management.* New York: NAL Penguin.

Deming, W. E. (1986). *Out of the crisis.* Cambridge, MA: Massachusetts Institute of Technology, Center for Advanced Engineering Study.

Deming, W. E. (1993). *The new economics.* Cambridge, MA: Massachusetts Institute of Technology, Center for Advanced Engineering Study.

Donabedian, A. (1980). *The definition of quality and approaches to assessment.* Ann Arbor, MI: Health Administration Press.

Frattali, C. M. (1991, November). From quality assurance to total quality management. *American Journal of Audiology, 1,* 41–47.

Frattali, C. M. (1993). Professional collaboration: A team approach to health care. *Clinical Series #11.* Rockville, MD: National Student Speech Language Hearing Association.

Hospital Corporation of America. (1991). *Hospitalwide quality technology network.* Nashville, TN: Author.

Jessee, W. (1991, April). *Chairman's Address: Improving healthcare quality in the new global community.* Eighth International Symposium on Quality Assurance in Health Care, Washington, DC.

Joint Commission on Accreditation of Healthcare Organizations. (1991). *Transitions: From QA to CQI.* Oakbrook Terrace, IL: Author.

Joint Commission on Accreditation of Healthcare Organizations. (1992a). *A pocket guide to quality improvement tools.* Oakbrook Terrace, IL: Author.

Joint Commission on Accreditation of Healthcare Organizations. (1992b). *Using quality improvement tools in a health care setting.* Oakbrook Terrace, IL: Author.

Joint Comission on Accreditation of Healthcare Organizations. (1994). *Accreditation manual for hospitals.* Oakbrook Terrace, IL: Author.

Langley, G. J., Nolan, K. M., & Nolan, T. W. (1992). *The foundation of improvement (Part 1).* Silver Spring, MD: Associates in Process Improvement, Inc.

O'Leary, D. (1986, April). *JCAHO quality assurance standards.* Keynote address presented at the 1986

National Association of Quality Assurance Professionals, Fort Worth, TX.

Roberts J. S., & Schyve, P. M. (1990, May). From QA to QI: The views and role of the Joint Commission. *The quality letter for healthcare leaders*. Rockville, MD: Bader & Associates.

Scholtes, P. R. (1988). *The team handbook*. Madison, WI: Joiner Associates, Inc.

Schumacher, D. (1991). *Linking clinical and financial data to improve quality and efficiency*. Session presented at the Eighth International Symposium on Quality Assurance in Health Care, Washington, DC.

Walton, M. (1986). *The Deming management method*. New York, NY: Putnam.

Wender, D. (1990). Quality: A personal perspective [Letter to the editor]. *Asha, 32*, 41–44.

RESOURCES FOR ADDITIONAL INFORMATION

PERIODICALS

The Joint Commission Journal on Quality Improvement in Healthcare
[monthly publication]
Joint Commission on Accreditation of Healthcare Organizations
One Renaissance Boulevard
Oakbrook Terrace, IL 60181

ASHA's *Quality Improvement Digest*
[quarterly publication]
American Speech-Language-Hearing Association
Health Services Division
10801 Rockville Pike
Rockville, MD 20852

Journal of Health Care Quality
[bimonthly publication]
National Association for Healthcare Quality
5700 Old Orchard Road
First Floor
Skokie, IL 60077-1057

Hearsay
Journal of the Ohio Speech and Hearing Association
Theme Issue: Quality Improvement in Speech-Language Pathology and Audiology (Vol. 7, No. 1, 1992)
OSHA Business Secretary
9331 Union Road, South
Miamisburg, OH 45342

Quality Assurance in Health Care
International Society for Quality Assurance in Health Care
Pergamon Press, Inc.
Maxwell House, Fairview Park
Elmsford, NY 10523

ACCREDITATION AGENCIES

Joint Commission on Accreditation of Healthcare Organizations
One Renaissance Boulevard
Oakbrook Terrace, IL 60181
(708) 916-5600

Commission on Accreditation of Rehabilitation Facilities
101 North Wilmot Road, Suite 500
Tucson, AZ 85711
(602) 748-1212

American Speech-Language-Hearing Association
Professional Services Board
10801 Rockville Pike
Rockville, MD 20852
(301) 897-5700

PROFESSIONAL ASSOCIATIONS AND GROUPS

National Association for Healthcare Quality
5700 Old Orchard Road
First Floor
Skokie,IL 60077-1057
(708) 966-9392

International Society of Quality Assurance in Health Care
ISQA Secretary
CBO, National Organisation of Quality Assurance in Hospitals
PO Box 20064
3502 LB Utrecht
The Netherlands

American Society for Quality Control
P.O. Box 3005
Milwaukee, WI 53201-3005
(800) 952-6587

Quality Improvement Study Section
Special Interest Division #11: Administration and Supervision
American Speech-Language-Hearing Association
10801 Rockville Pike
Rockville, MD 20852
(301) 897-5700

APPENDIX 19A: American Speech-Language-Hearing Association Consumer Satisfaction Survey

American
Speech-Language-Hearing
Association

Quality
Assurance

Consumer Satisfaction Measure

After answering all items, detach here and return

READ each item carefully and CIRCLE the one answer that is best for you.

SA - Strongly Agree   **N** - Neutral   **SD** - Strongly Disagree

A - Agree   **D** - Disagree   **NA** - Not Applicable

1. It is important that we see you in a timely manner.

A. My appointments were scheduled in a reasonable period of time.   SA   A   N   D   SD   NA

B. I was seen on time for my scheduled appointments.   SA   A   N   D   SD   NA

2. It is important that you benefit from Speech-Language Pathology and/or Audiology Services.

A. I am better because I received these services.   SA   A   N   D   SD   NA

B. I feel that I have benefited from speech-language pathology and/or audiology services.   SA   A   N   D   SD   NA

3. You are important to us; we are here to work with you.

A. The support staff (e.g., secretary, transporter, receptionist, assistant) who served me was courteous and pleasant.   SA   A   N   D   SD   NA

B. The clinician who served me was courteous and pleasant.   SA   A   N   D   SD   NA

C. Staff considered my special needs (age, culture, education, handicapping condition, eyesight and hearing).   SA   A   N   D   SD   NA

D. Staff included my family or other persons important to me in the services provided.   SA   A   N   D   SD   NA

4. Our Speech-Language Pathology and Audiology staff is highly trained and qualified to serve you.

A. The clinician was prepared and organized.   SA   A   N   D   SD   NA

B. The services were explained to me in a way that I could understand.   SA   A   N   D   SD   NA

C. My clinician was experienced and knowledgeable.   SA   A   N   D   SD   NA

5. It is important that our environment is secure, comfortable, attractive, distraction free, and easy to reach.

A. Health and safety precautions were taken when serving me.   SA   A   N   D   SD   NA

B. The environment was clean and pleasant.   SA   A   N   D   SD   NA

C. The environment was quiet and distraction free.   SA   A   N   D   SD   NA

D. The building and treatment areas were easy to get to.   SA   A   N   D   SD   NA

6. It is important that we provide you with efficient and comprehensive services.

A. I feel that the length and frequency of my service program was appropriate.   SA   A   N   D   SD   NA

B. My clinician planned ahead and provided sufficient instruction and education to help me retain my skills after my program ended.   SA   A   N   D   SD   NA

C. I feel that my program was well-managed, involving other services when needed (e.g., teachers, dentist, doctor).   SA   A   N   D   SD   NA

7. We respect and value your comments.

A. Overall, the program services were satisfactory.   SA   A   N   D   SD   NA

B. I would seek your services again if needed.   SA   A   N   D   SD   NA

C. I would recommend your services to others.   SA   A   N   D   SD   NA

D. Check the services you received.

Speech-Language Pathology ☐   Audiology ☐

Comments: _____

_____

Thank you for your time.

CODE [   ] Please staple/seal the questionnaire so that the Center's address is on the outside and return it to us.   © 1989

Reprinted with permission from American Speech-Language-Hearing Association (1989). Consumer Satisfaction Survey. Rockville, MD.

■ CHAPTER 20 ■

Marketing

■ ANGELA LOAVENBRUCK, Ed.D. ■

SCOPE OF CHAPTER

Marketing is a term that has many meanings. For speech-language pathologists and audiologists, marketing in its broadest sense is a philosophy—an approach to practicing our professions that involves the analysis, planning, implementation, and control of programs designed to bring our services and products to consumers. It encompasses a broad range of coordinated activities where the focal point is the consumer. Specifically, marketing involves identifying the needs and wants of consumers of our services and products, determining *how* to provide these services and products, persuading consumers to buy those services (and to buy from you or your agency), and finally to do all of this in a financially viable way. For professionals in audiology and speech-language pathology, the marketing process must also be considered within the framework of codes of ethics to which we ascribe—both as members of state and national professional organizations and as governed by state licensure guidelines. Therefore, the purposes of this chapter are to help you and your practice site to determine your marketing needs and develop an overall marketing plan.

BALANCED MARKETING—A COMPREHENSIVE APPROACH

A comprehensive marketing program involves at least four steps: (a) research; (b) identifying marketing problems; (c) setting goals and objectives with some means to measure progress; and finally (d) identifying and planning an appropriate mix of promotional activities designed to attain the goals and objectives that have been set.

MARKETING RESEARCH TASKS

There are four major marketing research tasks that must be accomplished: (a) market identification and segmentation; (b) analysis of the needs of consumers and referral sources within these markets; (c) analysis of competitors and (d) analysis of the larger environmental issues that might impinge on the ability to provide services or products to the identified markets.

Market identification and segmentation involves identifying and defining the consumer that the marketing program will be designed to reach. Analysis must include both consumers and potential referral sources. For example, audiologists might design a program to reach hearing impaired adults aged 50 to 70. This potential market could be segmented further by income, residence, or interest group. The term "market" need not refer to individuals. Programs could be designed to reach certain industries or certain referral sources. A speech-language pathologist might wish to target adults who stutter or preschool children with speech-language delays. School-based practitioners may want to target groups that have decision-making power over program or funding—the school board, school superintendents, or other administrators.

Once the market groups have been identified and segmented, questions that might be asked include:

1. What is our profession's image to the target market?
2. Do they know about our training?
3. Do they perceive us as capable of meeting their needs?
4. What educational tools would best raise their familiarity level with our professional roles?
5. What factors determine consumers' satisfaction with our professional services/products?
6. Who is the real consumer of our services?
7. What is really for sale?
8. Are there differences between our professionally perceived notions of consumer "needs" and self-perceived needs?
9. What tools can be used to answer these questions?

In addition, the availability of payment sources for the services and products that will be provided to various markets must be analyzed. Finally, practitioners need to identify the particular strengths and weaknesses of their practice settings for meeting the needs of the identified markets.

The marketing research task must also include an analysis of competitors and of larger environmental issues. With respect to competitors, analysis must be done of the competencies of major competitors for the identified market segments. An important question to be answered is how the practitioner or practice setting can maintain distinctiveness in the eyes of consumers and referral sources. Larger environmental issues include social/psychological barriers for potential clients to obtain our services, funding barriers, attitudes toward aging and disabilities, and laws and other regulations that serve to limit or define our services. For example, Public Law 99-457 has been expanded to include services to preschool children and in some states services have been extended to infants. If a practice setting has focused on providing services to children now covered by publicly funded programs, the defining characteristics of this "market" change, and practitioners in various settings must redefine the strategies needed to remain focused on this preschool market.

For both speech-language pathologists and audiologists, regardless of practice setting, our ability to successfully market our services is substantially limited and defined by historical factors. For example, third-party reimbursement of speech-language pathology services is often limited. Many managed health care policies limit coverage to 60 days—seldom enough to treat a problem. Other insurance companies restrict coverage to disorders clearly related to an illness or accident and expect rapid progress. Still others deny coverage for children by insisting that most speech-language pathology services are "educational" in nature and, therefore, the responsibility of the schools. Similarly, Medicare coverage for speech-language pathology services is limited to agency-provided services. As speech-language pathologists are not considered autonomous or independent practitioners under Medicare law, direct marketing efforts to consumers have limited usefulness. Instead, the marketing efforts must be directed toward referral sources who can provide access to Medicare caseloads. For audiologists, Medicare coverage is restricted solely to diagnostic procedures administered as part of a medical evaluation, and this fact limits the kind of marketing that can be directed at this particular consumer population. All of these "macro-environmental" factors impinge on the provision of audiology and speech-language pathology services and must be included in marketing decisions.

Similarly, recent focus group research conducted by the American Speech-Language-Hearing Association (ASHA), as part of its audiology marketing program (Powell, Adams, & Rinehart, 1991), delineated significant information gaps about hearing loss, audiology, and audiologists among the consumers surveyed. Lack of information or misinformation among consumers represents a barrier to marketing efforts individual practitioners or agencies may engage in. Marketing research activities, then, lead to a clearly defined target market that may be further segmented into smaller target groups, each requiring specific strategies, goals, objectives, and activities.

MARKETING PROBLEMS

Once target markets are clearly defined, it is possible to delineate the problems that exist in reaching each particular market. The practitioner can analyze the "demand" state that exists in that particular market for the products or services available. Demand states include high demand (services are desired by many consumers), low demand (services are desired by few consumers), latent demand (there is demand, but it needs to be stimulated or identified for consumers), negative demand (consumers actively resist the service or product), or no demand (the service is not needed). For example, the practitioner might determine that, in the age group 50 to 70, the demand for audiological services is quite low. In that case, both consumer resistance and referral source resistance would need to be studied. Negative demand for hearing aids is an ongoing marketing problem for audiologists.

The analysis of demand states leads to the development of more precise and definable marketing tasks. For example, if a speech-language pathologist determined that the demand for poststroke services was low and further analysis indicated that potential referral sources were not aware of the efficacy of speech-language pathology services for that group of clients, it then becomes possible to develop specific goals and strategies to solve this particular problem. Although the research task sometimes seems tedious and time-consuming, it is far better to facilitate focused activities than to engage in shotgun strategies that miss the mark.

SETTING GOALS AND OBJECTIVES

Goals and objectives should be set for each identifiable market segment. For example, an objective might be to increase the number of initial audiological evaluations to hearing impaired adults aged 50 to 70, with a goal of 10 new clients per week. Further analysis of this objective would identify the barriers to attaining the goal. Specific barriers might be that Medicare law limits coverage for audiological evaluations or that many individuals in the target group belong to a managed care plan that the practitioner does not participate in. It is important to identify and concentrate on the barriers that can be realistically removed. In the above example, although the practitioner might choose to support efforts to change Medicare law, becoming a participating provider in the managed health care network, and reaching out to referral sources, is a far more realistic strategy.

MARKETING ACTIVITIES—THE FOUR Ps: PRODUCT, PRICE, PLACE, PROMOTION

The final step in a marketing program is the most enjoyable—delineating the four Ps:

1. product,
2. price,
3. place,
4. promotion.

With research completed, the practitioner can identify and refine the "product" to be sold, such as speech-language evaluations and therapy for stroke patients or comprehensive amplification services. The "price" of the service is determined, as well as the mechanisms to insure payment. If the market segment is a private paying market, the "price" must be perceived as reasonable by that market. If the market segment is mainly composed of participants in a managed care network, the "price" will be defined by the insurance company. The practitioner must then be certain that the predetermined payment amounts are fair and justify the time, effort, and expense of providing the service. Next, the practitioner decides the "place" where services will be provided. This is a critical decision—for example, offering home-based as opposed to office-based services can represent a substantial benefit to some target market groups. Finally, the practitioner must design a "promotion" strategy to attain the goals and objectives set.

PROMOTIONAL ACTIVITIES: THE MARKETING MIX

Promotional activities must be designed to reach the measurable goals that have been set. The major promotional methods are public relations, personal contact, and advertising. Each practice setting must choose the array of activities that fit best into its budget and overall philosophy. A well-rounded marketing program will include activities in each category. Advertising is paid promotional activities and includes office brochures; newspaper, television and radio advertisements; yellow pages advertisements; and newsletters. Public relations activities are unpaid promotional activities that center on community services. They reflect the philosophy that, when a practice setting acts in the best interest of the public, it also acts in its own best interest. Public relations activities are particularly well suited to a marketing philosophy that emphasizes the professional nature of the services provided by speech-language pathologists and audiologists.

Advertising

BROCHURES. The design and content of your office brochure carries a critical message to the consumers you wish to reach. Practice brochures can be used to answer commonly asked practical questions about the office or agency such as office hours, directions to the location, insurance and payment information, and types of services offered. In addition, the brochure can provide information about the professional background of staff. There are a number of excellent publications that offer good advice about creating effective office brochures. Matthews (1993) discusses the importance of copy style, brochure design, cover photography and art work, color and type style, and size and shape of the brochure. An important objective of an office brochure is to provide information about the unique benefits of obtaining services from a particular office. It is important to consider the target market of the brochure. It is often necessary to create one brochure for consumers of your services and another for referral sources.

NEWSPAPER AND OTHER MEDIA ADVERTISING. Effective newspaper, radio, and television advertising is the most expensive form of promotion. To create the kind of familiarity that typical name-brand advertising ensures, large amounts of money need to be budgeted. In addition, the most critical "product" offered by speech-language pathologists and audiologists is information, service, and professional expertise, not a tangible product per se. Therefore, media advertising becomes more expensive. It is difficult to create one-liners or brief copy that conveys the more intangible nature of our work. Informational type advertising (e.g., an "Ask the Expert" type newspaper or radio format) is more appropriate. To be effective, however, this type of advertising must appear regularly and prominently and, therefore, must be part of an ongoing budget. As our national organizations begin to engage in nationwide advertising campaigns that stress the professional expertise of speech-language pathologists and audiologists, the advertising task of local practitioners will become easier. For example, ASHA is carrying out a nationwide audiology advertising campaign in nine national magazines during 1993 and 1994 and has also prepared a marketing kit so that audiologists can coordinate local advertising efforts with the national campaign. Similar materials exist for speech-language pathologists. Because newspaper and other media advertising generally is the most expensive promotional activity, it is wise to coordinate it with national advertising efforts and with other types of promotional activities on a local level.

NEWSLETTERS. The use of a newsletter can be effective in accomplishing a number of marketing goals. It allows practitioners to maintain regular contact with an existing client list. In that way, new products and services and, most importantly, information about relevant topics can be presented to a target market group already familiar with the services of the speech-language pathologist or audiologist. Newsletters can increase name recognition and can serve as additional reminders about the importance of follow-up care or yearly evaluations. They are a way to remind clients of the expertise of the practitioner. For referral sources, newsletters mailed on a regular basis serve much the same purpose—they keep the practitioner's name up front and remind the referrer of the practitioner's expertise and of the importance of continuing referrals. Separate newsletters need not be written for consumers and referral sources. It is helpful to send a cover letter to referral sources with the first several newsletters asking them to share the newsletter with clients by placing it in their reception area. In that way, the referral sources see the newsletter and their reception areas become additional "marketing" sites for the audiologist or speech-language pathologist.

Production of newsletters is time-consuming, however, and to be effective they must be prepared on a regular basis. Practitioners often err by thinking that an effective newsletter has to be expensively produced. In fact, a single page newsletter on the practice's usual stationary is probably as effective as a fancy printed newsletter. The important goal is to send it regularly, to include interesting and timely information, and to keep the letter concise. Including regular features gives the newsletter writer an outline to work from and makes the writing task easier. Newsletters can also be purchased from companies that prepare them and customize them for individual practices. ASHA prepares a newsletter that appears regularly in *Asha* magazine ("Let's Talk") that can be copied, in whole or part, or purchased in bulk with a blank section for personalized messages from individual practices. A particular benefit of newsletters is that they allow far more information to be presented economically, compared to the cost of more expensive newspaper or other media advertisements.

Public Relations

Public relations (PR) activities are defined as unpaid promotional activities. These activities center on community services. A public relations program developed as part of an overall promotional plan allows staff to inform the public about all aspects of speech-language pathology and audiology services. The use of public relations activities is an organized way to counter the lack of information or misinformation about our services that may exist for both consumers and our referral sources. Public relations activities are sometimes thought of as "free" advertising. However, although these activities generally require the expenditure of little or no "out-of-pocket" money, they require a sizable investment of practitioners' time. For many practice settings in speech-language pathology and audiology, PR activities can serve as core activities around which other promotional activities can be scheduled.

Effective public relations tools include public speaking, consumer advocacy activities, special events such as open houses and health fairs, letters to the editor of local newspapers, participation in charitable events, and media releases and interviews.

PUBLIC SPEAKING. In most practice settings, it is important for staff members to make active efforts to contact public libraries, service organizations, local professional groups such as medical societies, medical specialists' study groups, nursery school organizations, charities, private schools, Parent-Teacher Associations, business services groups, and senior citizen organizations. It is helpful to join several community service organizations, such as Rotary Clubs, Lions Clubs, or Sertoma Clubs. Some of these organizations have targeted hearing and speech disorders as part of their charitable mission. Whether this is or is not the case, participation in service organizations links practitioners to their communities, serves as a valuable networking mechanism, and often leads to additional opportunities to broaden the community's information about an audiology or speech-language pathology practice.

Service groups all have regularly scheduled meetings, yearly luncheons or dinner meetings, or consumer programs and generally are delighted to have speakers and programs offered. Although the general topic should be some aspect of hearing, speech, or language disorder, dinner and meeting speeches are most successful when tailored to consumers and to the particular group's needs and interests. Written materials should always be included in the presentation—public speaking engagements present excellent opportunities to distribute office brochures and newsletters.

Use every opportunity to garner speaking invitations. For example, if an interesting client has been seen, call the referring physician to discuss the results and suggest that the case might make an interesting short presentation for the next hospital medical meeting or as part of a continuing education program presented at the hospital. It is also helpful to ask clients if they are members of organizations that might be interested in a speech, language, or hearing health care program. Successful clients are often the best promoters of these activities. Public relations activities should be part of every staff member's responsibility. Time must be alloted in staff schedules to encourage public relations programs and outreach.

In school-based settings, public relations activities can include informative programs given to the psychology, special education, or regular teaching staff about some aspect of audiology or speech-language pathology. Most school systems have conferences or continuing education activities for staff at various times of the year. These represent excellent opportunities to provide colleagues with useful information about referral criteria, effects of various communication disorders on learning, interesting products or service innovations, or new diagnostic methods.

In many practice settings, it is also useful to include other audiology or speech-language pathology facilities in public relations programs. Joint presentations add to the credibility of a program and reduce the possibility that the public relations activities will be viewed as merely self-serving. When presentations are made, it is also useful to provide information to the audience about all audiology or speech-language pathology services available in the community. Because the office organizing the presentation is spotlighted, however, it is likely to be chosen by new clients.

CONSUMER ADVOCACY. A worthwhile marketing goal is to be identified in the community as an "expert" about speech, language, hearing, or related problems. With that goal in mind, it is useful to establish good relationships with local, state, and federal political representatives. Political representatives and their staffs are always eager for good information about communication disorders and other aspects of speech-language pathology and audiology practices. For example, presentations made before local legislators about legal requirements for assistive listening devices can establish the practitioner or facility as a source of information about the needs of hearing impaired individuals. These presentations can lead to newspaper stories and other good publicity about the advocacy efforts. The return on this kind of investment of time is immeasurable and satisfying. Not only do these kinds of efforts often result in improved accessibility for individuals with communication impairments or increased public information about audiology and speech-language pathology services, but the members of the audience (or their families) often become clients. Another benefit of consistent contact with legislators is that it becomes easier to stay current on potential legislation that may have an impact on our professional practices.

SPECIAL EVENTS. Audiology and speech-language pathology facilities can sponsor, organize, or participate in many special events such as health screening days, nursery school screenings, round-table public television and radio programs about various health problems, senior citizen information programs, and health awareness programs at local hospitals or libraries. Again, it is best to participate in these programs as generic representatives of the audiology or speech-language pathology professions rather than as specific representatives of a particular office or agency. At many of these kinds of events, it is not necessary to "sell" an individual practitioner or agency; it is the benefits of our professional services that are being sold. The events offer an opportunity for practitioners to showcase their expert knowledge and benefit from the public relations activity in an indirect, but often quickly measurable way.

Local cable television stations present an excellent opportunity to present information to the public. Two recent productions in the New York City area spotlighted stuttering and hearing loss. There are problems, however, with these programs. They may be aired at strange hours with little advance publicity. But, a videotape of the program can be used in other presentations. The office newsletter can be used to alert your clients about an upcoming program. The idea is to use materials and events to build a constant presence in the perception of potential consumers or referral sources.

Local radio stations often have daily talk programs with listeners calling in with questions. These present excellent opportunities for joint guest "appearances" with other practitioners from the community. Everyone benefits. In programs such as these, participants need to be

gregarious, informative, articulate, and able to respond quickly to questions. The best advice is to over-prepare. Take notes to the studio for reference, especially for radio appearances. Use anecdotes to illustrate points about speech-language pathology or audiology services. If questions cannot be answered immediately, offer to send more information by mail. Be assertive. Have definite opinions backed by facts. Radio and television programs are fun and offer excellent vehicles to disseminate information to various target markets.

LETTERS TO THE EDITOR AND OTHER NEWSPAPER WRITING. Scour the newspaper for opportunities to comment about matters that affect consumers of our services or our professions. For example, your local newspaper publishes an Associated Press story about brainstem evoked response (BSER) testing of infants. This is an excellent opportunity to write a letter commending the newspaper for publishing the story. Include more information about innovative test procedures for infants or add information about the effects of hearing loss on language development. Include information about the unique capabilities of audiologists in these endeavors. Then sign your name and that of your office or agency. This is excellent "free" advertising. This type of newspaper coverage is priceless, and the benefits to the practice are far-reaching and cumulative.

In working with newspaper writers and editors, persistence pays off. Identify the writers responsible for health or education information. Begin sending information about hearing loss or communication disorders to those writers. Human interest stories are always more interesting than generic articles. Material developed jointly with other agencies or practitioners from several settings is often more desirable than material developed by a single office or practitioner. Newspapers want to appear to be fair and not to be promoting one office over another.

OFFICE STAFF AND OFFICE ENVIRONMENT. Often the first "public relations" activity performed in the name of a practice setting is the appearance of the waiting room and the behavior of the office staff members who greet clients on the telephone or as they enter the door. It is extremely important to be constantly mindful of what these PR activities say about you to your public. Clearly, if clients are greeted poorly (or not at all), if telephones are answered curtly or rudely, if clients' complaints or problems are not promptly addressed, if inquiries are handled in an untimely or incomplete way, if the waiting room is not a welcoming place, then all of the best formal public relations efforts are diluted. It is helpful to remind both professional and office staff that personal contact with clients is our most important promotional activity. Periodic reviews and client questionnaires on their perception of office staff and policies are helpful methods of identifying problem areas. (See Chapter 19 by Frattali on Quality Improvement for more discussion of client feedback.)

PERSONAL CONTACT. Finally, the most critical public relations activities for any practice setting occur in the personal contact between consumers or referral sources and practitioners. The questions that must be asked involve how consumers perceive the personal image of the professionals with whom they interact. For speech-language pathologists and audiologists, personal attributes such as professional, knowledgeable, concerned, decisive, confident, and personable are all important. In interacting with clients, it is important to be straightforward about the procedures to be administered and the fees to be charged. Treatment options and recommendations should be presented clearly. Both consumers and referral sources appreciate practitioners who have an opinion and can make reasoned recommendations. Reports should be clear, short, and helpful. When warranted, referrals to colleagues for second opinions or for special skills will be appreciated by consumers and convey concern for their well-being. Prompt thank-you letters and reports are always appreciated by referral sources. Direct interactions with both consumers and referral sources allow clinicians to display self-confidence, joy in their work, and the overall philosophy that the needs of the consumer are paramount. Personal contact is a powerful marketing tool. Best of all, this aspect of marketing is virtually cost free.

SOURCES OF MARKETING HELP

ASHA has a number of publications and marketing kits that are helpful in organizing a marketing plan in any practice setting. In addition, ASHA offers frequent marketing workshops throughout the country. The August 1993 issue of *Asha* contains several articles about marketing in different practice settings. The Small Business Administration also offers free booklets about various aspects of marketing for service organizations and professionals. Marketing is a popular topic for presentations at state and national conferences. Because marketing is all about information and communication, the more sophisticated and knowledgeable we become about marketing our expertise and our services, the more informed our various "publics" will become about speech-language pathologists and audiologists and the services we provide.

SUMMARY

A successful marketing program is the sum of many parts. Marketing research tasks lead to careful identification of potential consumers and their needs, as well as analysis of competitors and other factors that affect practitioners' ability to deliver services for these consumers. Research enables practitioners to identify the problems that must be solved to allow the services they wish to provide to be delivered to the consumers who need and want them. Measurable goals can then be set, and promotional activities—a blend of advertising, public relations activities, and personal contact—can be planned to attain these goals.

DISCUSSION QUESTIONS

1. What are some of the factors that would differentiate a marketing program for a speech-language pathology or audiology practice from that of a commercial enterprise?
2. What factors might be considered in the analysis of competitors? How might the characteristics that differentiate one practice from a competitor's practice be conveyed to consumers?
3. How would the Code of Ethics of ASHA and/or your state professional licensure rules and regulations affect the development of a comprehensive marketing program?

REFERENCES

Academy of Dispensing Audiologists. (1990). *Directions in marketing audiology: Turning up the volume.* Columbia, SC: Author.

American Speech-Language-Hearing Association. (1993). *Asha, 35*(8).

Matthews, C. B. (1993). *Marketing speech-language pathology and audiology services–A how-to guide.* San Diego, CA: Singular Publishing Group.

Powell, Adams, & Rinehart [Public Relations Firm]. (1991). *Audiology marketing program focus group research: Final report.* Rockville, MD: American Speech-Language-Hearing Association.

CHAPTER 21

Infection Prevention

■ ROSEMARY LUBINSKI, Ed.D. ■

SCOPE OF CHAPTER

Little did you know on entering the professions of audiology or speech-language pathology that, in addition to your professional knowledge base and clinical skills, you would need to know about such topics as communicable diseases and universal precautions. Whether you practice in a health care institution; educational setting; community speech, language or hearing clinic; or private practice, it is essential to know procedures to protect yourself, your family, and your clients from the spread of infectious diseases. Although infectious diseases are not new or unique to the populations with whom we work, the changing demographics of our society, mainstreaming into educational settings, increase in service to high-risk populations, and increase in certain conmmunicable diseases are a few of the factors that prompt serious attention to risk management. Therefore, this chapter will provide a rationale for protecting yourself and others, present a basic discussion of infection pathways and types, outline ways of incorporating a hygiene plan into your clinical practice with all clients, and, finally, discuss some special situations related to the topic of infection prevention.

This chapter encourages you to use a common sense approach to creating a hygienic environment that minimizes the potential of infection transmission.

IMPORTANCE OF INFECTION PREVENTION TO SPEECH-LANGUAGE PATHOLOGISTS AND AUDIOLOGISTS

Although those of you who practice in health care facilities are likely to be aware of clean practices or risk management, this subject is often "ignored" by professionals working in other settings such as schools or private practice (McMillan & Willette, 1988). This is most unfortunate because clients with infectious diseases can range from toddlers in preschool programs to elderly persons seeking a hearing aid from a dispensing audiologist. Changing demographics of our client population suggest that you are likely to work with individuals who may be at high risk for contracting or transmitting an infection, including inpatients who are acutely ill and those with communicable diseases such as hepatitis B, human immunodeficiency virus (HIV, the virus that causes acquired immune deficiency syndrome or AIDS), tuberculosis, and cytomegalovirus. All of these individuals are in high-risk populations, usually because of repressed immune systems or complicated medical conditions. In addition, speech-language pathologists have created new roles in shock trauma centers, high-risk neonatal programs, and AIDS programs, and have become responsible for swallowing management programs where the focus may be on working with critically ill patients. In addition, audiologists have created special hearing health programs for such populations.

Relatively recent federal legislation (i.e., Public Law [P.L.] 99-142, Section 504 of the Rehabilitation Act, and P.L. 99-457) and various state laws focus on the right of disabled individuals to a free, appropriate public education in the least restrictive environment (ASHA, 1991).This means that children with compromised health resistance may be attending public schools and may be in need of communication services. Thus, speech-language pathologists and audiologists in educational settings need to be as aware as colleagues in health care institutions of risk-management procedures. (See Chapter 16 by Montgomery for more in-depth discussion of federal education legislation.)

The increase in the prevalence of diseases also necessitates such awareness. Although AIDS may be the best known infectious disease, other diseases are more prevalent, such as herpes simplex and hepatitis B. Contact with individuals with certain infectious diseases such as cytomegalovirus may have health implications for professional women who work during pregnancy.

The nature of our "hands on" contact with clients during speech mechanism examinations, respiratory and laryngeal assessments, inspection of the outer ear, hearing aid fittings, swallowing assessments and treatments, and care of clients with laryngectomies and tracheostomies also increases the risk for infection transmission. Any procedure that brings you in direct contact with body fluids necessitates precautions.

Lest we forget, speech-language pathologists and audiologists, themselves, may be sources of infections that can be transmitted to clients. The state of low resistance to illness of many of our clients already mentioned makes them more susceptible to the infections that we might transmit to them. For example, what may appear to be a "common cold" to you, may result in bronchitis or pneumonia for frail elderly residents of a nursing facility. These illnesses, in turn, may result in increased nursing care, additional medications, relocation to an acute care hospital, prolonged illness, or death. You may also have a more serious communicable disease that requires the use of precautions to protect your clients.

Further, McMillan and Willette (1988) remind us of the ethical responsibility we have to protect our patients from all health and safety dangers. The most basic ethical responsibility you have regarding spread of infection is to reduce the probability of its occurrence to its lowest possible level in your interactions with clients. When a patient suffers an infection, "progress is slowed, revenue may be decreased due to absence, and the risk of malpractice accusation may increase" (p. 37). Dixon (1987) estimates that in 1984 hospital-acquired infections resulted in more than $2.5 billion in direct hospital costs. He added that indirect costs such as loss of income are incalculable but likely to be high. Various hospital and rehabilitation program accrediting bodies, such as the Joint Commission on Accreditation of Healthcare Organizations (JCAHO), require that facilities have ongoing, comprehensive infection control procedures in place to maintain their accreditation.

According to the American Speech-Language-Hearing Association (ASHA) Code of Ethics any certified professional must provide services to high-risk individuals, including those with HIV. ASHA's Legislative Council passed the following resolution in 1988 (ASHA, 1989).

RESOLVED, That it is the position of the American-Speech-Language- Hearing Association that persons with HIV disease (including individuals with AIDS, ARC, and individuals who are seropositive) and those who are regarded by others as having the disease,should be entitled to civil rights protections under Section 504 of the Rehabilitation Act of 1973, as amended (LC-29-88).

INFECTION AND ITS PATHWAYS

An infection is an "invasion of host tissue by one or more microbial species usually detrimental to the host, with the resulting production of clinical disease" (Fuchs, 1979, p. 4). Although infections may be acquired in any setting, those acquired *after admission* to a health care institution such as a hospital, nursing facility, psychiatric setting, or outpatient program, are called nosocomial infections.

The transmission of an infection follows a predictable pathway. There must be a source of infection, a means of transmission, and a susceptible host. This is referred to as the chain of infection (Castle & Ajemian, 1987). The source of infection may be a person, for example, the client or clinician; or it can be an inanimate object such as equipment that has been contaminated by an infected person. Thus, clinicians and clients may infect each other, or one client can infect a second client through indirect contamination of inanimate objects such as toys, a microphone, or speculum (McMillan & Willette, 1988). Clients can also infect themselves (autoinfection). There are many ways an infection can be transmitted, for example: (a) touching another person, particularly with your hands during assessment, intervention, or daily care; (b) touching one infected client and then using the same hand to touch the oral area of another client; (c) touching an inanimate object that has been contaminated; (d) coughing or sneezing; (e) ingestion of contaminated food or water; and (f) through animals or insects.

The final link in the chain of infection is the availability of a susceptible host. It is known that individuals become more vulnerable to contracting an infection when they have reduced immunological defense systems because of their illness(es) and malnourishment. Procedures such as radiation therapy and insertion of medical equipment (e.g., catheters or intravenous tubes) may also increase susceptibility. Infants, the elderly, and those with chronic debilitating diseases are more susceptible to infection by the very nature of their frailty.

EXAMPLES OF COMMUNICABLE DISEASES

Examples of infections are so numerous that a complete discussion of all agents is beyond the scope of this chapter. In this chapter seven common chronic communicable diseases are introduced: Hepatitis B, HIV/AIDS, cytomegalovirus, herpes, tuberculosis, scabies, and influenza.

HEPATITIS B VIRUS (HBV)

Hepatitis B Virus (HBV) is a common potentially life-threatening blood-borne infection affecting about 300,000 newly diagnosed persons per year in the United States (Occupational Safety and Health Administration [OSHA], 1992). The incubation is 120 days on average, and the onset of acute disease is insidious. Symptoms include anorexia, malaise, nausea, vomiting, abdominal pain, and jaundice (Heeg & Coleman, 1992; OSHA, 1992). Individuals at high risk for harboring or contracting hepatitis B include sexually active individuals, intravenous drug users, patients of hemodialysis units, hemophiliacs, residents of some institutions for the mentally or developmentally disabled and prisons, and immigrants from areas of high endemicity, including east Asia, Africa, most Pacific Islands, parts of the Middle East, and the Amazon basin (OSHA, 1992). Health care workers who come in contact with blood or secretions containing blood are potentially among the high-risk groups for contracting HBV. Twelve thousand health care workers in the United States are infected with HBV each year, and about 250 die (Centers for Disease Control, 1989). It should be remembered, however, that the risk of contracting hepatitis B is much greater than that for HIV.

HIV/AIDS

HIV, the virus that causes AIDS, is generally well known by the public. Since the first clinical cases were identified in Los Angeles and New York in 1981, about 270,000 cases of HIV/AIDS in the United States have been reported to the Centers for Disease Control and Prevention (CDCP). A far greater number of individuals are HIV-positive but are asymptomatic. Those at highest risk for contracting HIV include sexually active individuals, intravenous drug users, and unborn children of an infected mother. Transmission is through direct sexual contact and the bloodstream. HIV turns on a mechanism whereby the immune system self-destructs. Once turned on, the destruction continues even if the virus itself is killed. This gives hope that new pharmaceutical approaches to the treatment of the disease may be designed in the future, such as drugs that may not be as harmful as the current ones.

Symptoms of active HIV infection tend to cluster and may include prolonged fever, lymph node enlargement, night sweats, prolonged diarrhea, unexplained weight loss, fungal infections, and persistent cough (Fauci, 1983). Children infected with HIV may also show chronic lung infections, failure to thrive, otitis media, and rashes. Numerous physiological, neurological, and psychological disorders are likely to result including sensory perceptual changes, dysphagia, dementia, cognitive deficits, and depression (ASHA, 1989, 1990). Conductive and sensorineural hearing impairments are also common and may necessitate the use of a hearing aid or other assistive listening device (Flower, 1991). Communication difficulties include voice disorders related to Karposi's sarcomas in the larynx, motor speech disorders, language disorders, and general withdrawal from socialization. In addition, should the patient be intubated, an assistive communication device

may be necessary (Flower & Sooy, 1987). For a more in-depth discussion of HIV/AIDS and communication disorders, see Flower (1991).

CYTOMEGALOVIRUS (CMV)

Cytomegalovirus (CMV) is a common infection in less developed areas of the world and is more prevalent among young children, organ transplant patients, and AIDS patients (Sherertz & Hampton, 1987). Populations at risk include unborn children of CMV-infected mothers and adults with immunodeficiency (ASHA, 1991). CMV is a member of the herpes virus group (cold sores, chickenpox, shingles, and mononucleosis) (Crawford & Studebaker, 1990). Transmission is primarily through contact with body fluids such as urine, genital secretions, and eye and nose secretions. Cytomegalovirus is of concern for women of child-bearing age if they contract the disease during pregnancy (ASHA, 1991). The affected individual may appear asymptomatic or have a protracted mononucleosis-like illness. Any employed woman who is pregnant and who works with young children may wish to be tested to determine susceptibility to CMV infection. In general, frequent hand-washing and appropriate disposal of diapers helps to minimize the spread of infection. For an in-depth discussion of CMV and hearing loss, see Crawford and Studebaker (1990).

HERPES SIMPLEX VIRUS (HSV)

Herpes Simplex Virus (HSV) may take two forms: Type 1 (herpes labialis) usually manifests itself by cold sores or fever blisters in the oral facial region. Type 2 is often a genital infection. Both forms of the infection may be recurrent. The virus is contagious during the blister and wet ulcer stages and can be transmitted through saliva, urine, genital secretions, or contact with broken skin or mucous membranes. Individuals with herpes labialis should refrain from working with infants, burn patients, or immunocompromised patients (Valenti, 1992). Type 2 genital herpes can be spread during vaginal delivery or sexual activity.

TUBERCULOSIS

In the mid-1980s a resurgence of tuberculosis (TB) became evident in the United States after 30 years of decline. Its resurgence is attributed primarily to the increase in antibiotic-resistant strains of the disease, the HIV epidemic, and also to an increase in immigration from Asian countries, physician non-adherence in prescribing recommended drug regimen, and few resources for prevention and care. Although TB can affect anyone of any age, it more often is seen in older people who have been exposed to tuberculosis and immunocompromised individuals. Populations at highest risk for incurring tuberculosis are those living with the consequences of poverty, such as poor nutrition, poor ventilation, cramped quarters, poor hygiene, and so on. Of particular concern is that the tuberculosis rate of nursing home patients is four times higher than that of age-matched community residents (Boscia, 1986).

The primary symptoms of pulmonary tuberculosis are coughing which spreads the Mycobacterium tuberculosis through the air (LaForce, 1992), night sweats, low-grade fever, and weight loss. Should you work in a hospital or nursing home, an annual tuberculosis screening may be mandatory. Treatment for the infection includes a program of medications. Compliance with the medication program is essential because noncompliance leads to treatment failure and may result in drug resistance, continuing transmission, increasing disability, and death (Hellman & Gram, 1993).

SCABIES

Scabies is an infectious skin rash caused by infestation with the mite Sarcoptes scabiei. Transmission is through skin-to-skin contact with an infected individual. Control measures include mass cleaning of patient bedding, clothing, and food tray, and skin application of a pesticide, usually lindane, for all employees or others who have come in contact with the infected individual (Sherertz & Hampton, 1987). Universal precautions including adequate hand-washing, gloving, and gowning are essential when working with an infected client (Polder, Tablan, & Williams, 1992).

INFLUENZA VIRUSES

It is especially important to prevent transmission of type A and type B influenza viruses to high-risk groups such as the elderly and patients of all ages with chronic cardiac, pulmonary, renal, or metabolic diseases. Outbreaks of influenza in acute care and chronic care hospitals as well as nursing homes can have serious health care and morbidity implications. Symptoms include fever, headache, and cough (LaForce, 1992). Prevention includes yearly vaccine immunization and measures to limit the spread of the disease, including universal precautions, restrictive admission to a facility, separation of infected patients, and prohibition of individuals with respiratory symptoms from visiting high-risk patients (Fedson, 1987). Should you contract influenza, it is critical that you check with your employer's infection control personnel for guidelines regarding client contact.

PROGRAM FOR INFECTION PREVENTION

Most settings in which you practice as a speech-language pathologist or audiologist will have an infection prevention program in place. The general purpose of such programs is to minimize the potential of infection transmission to clients and staff members. Although plans differ according to settings, certain commonalities exist across infection prevention programs. Staff need to (a) be aware of potential risks associated with their settings and professional procedures; (b) know their institutional and departmental infection prevention management plans for minimizing infection spread; (c) know how to implement the infection prevention management plan; (d) know how to modify the plan to meet individual situations; and (e) know when and to whom to report incidents.

Should you work in a health care institution such as a hospital or nursing home, there will be a multidisciplinary Infection Control Committee (ICC) that is responsible for reduc-ing the occurrence of infections through the establishment and monitoring of general policies and procedures for infection control. These rules usually emanate from standards established by federal and state governments and agencies, professional organizations, and accreditation agencies such as the Joint Commission on Accreditation of Healthcare Organizations. The ICC is charged with approving programs of prevention, and investigating, reporting, and monitoring of infections (Castle & Ajemian, 1987). In addition to complying with general infection prevention procedures established for the entire institution, individual departments such as speech-language pathology or audiology will be required to state in writing specific policies and procedures for ensuring infection prevention during their contact with clients. (See Chapter 18 by Rao and Goldsmith on policies and procedures.)

Settings other than hospitals should also have infection prevention programs. For example, home health care programs, educational settings, private practices, and community speech, language, or hearing clinics should each have and implement a systematic written program for ensuring, to the highest extent possible, the prevention of infection transmission between staff and clients or among clients. Committees similar to the ICC implement and monitor the infection prevention program and provide orientation and continuing education on this topic for all staff.

PRE-EMPLOYMENT SCREENING AND FOLLOW-UP

A pre-employment medical evaluation is one of the requirements of employment in most organizations and certainly in all health care institutions . The purpose of this examination is to identify any individual who may serve as a source of an infectious agent and, therefore, compromise clients, staff, or families with whom they would come in contact. The most important aspects of the screening focus on identification of rubella, hepatitis B, and tuberculosis (Castle & Ajemian, 1987). The pre-employment evaluation usually includes a communicable disease history, a history of immunization, and a physical examination. Most organizations also have established policies for immunizations, yearly medical reevaluations, protocols for documentation of employees exposed to communicable diseases, and guidelines for return-to-work for these individuals. Information regarding such protocols can be found in your employee handbook or obtained from your institution's infection prevention committee.

ORIENTATION AND TRAINING IN INFECTION PREVENTION

One of the first tasks you will be required to do on employment in most institutions is to participate in a general orientation. Part of this orientation will be devoted to understanding infection prevention needs and protocols. During this orientation you will become familiar with the management or hygiene plan designed for your department, its rationale, and specific ways to implement the plan into daily practice. Inservice education programs to update an existing hygiene plan will also occur as needs arise.

HYGIENE PLAN

The hygiene plan designed for your department will focus on creating an environment with every reasonable effort made to limit exposure to infectious agents. Potential infectious agents include all body fluids, including blood, semen, drainage from scrapes and cuts, feces, urine, vomitus, respiratory secretions, and saliva as well as anything that has come in contact with body fluids (e.g., bandages, prostheses, and instruments). In general, hygiene plans will have as their cornerstone the adoption of universal precautions. The underlying premise of universal precautions is that one adopts practices that minimize and, if possible, eliminate the risk of transmitting any infection, whether potential or actually present. Thus, every clinician, including trainees, working with every client in every setting must assume a preventive approach to reducing infection transmission. A universal approach to clients ensures that all are treated equally, without discrimination, and with confidentiality regarding their medical status.

HYGIENE PLAN TECHNIQUES

The hygiene plan techniques presented here focus on what you can do to help prevent the transmission of an infectious disease. The first technique discussed, hand-washing, is considered the most basic approach to infection prevention. Other techniques include barrier techniques such as the use of gloves, masks, gowns, and lab coats. Finally, sterilization and disinfection are discussed as additional priority methods.

Hand-washing

There is no substitute for hand-washing in the prevention of infection transmission. This is a simple and cost-effective means of preventing the spread of infectious agents to noncontaminated areas and personnel. The goal of hand-washing is to reduce as much as possible the presence of contaminating organisms on hands that touch clients or objects in the environment that might be contaminated. Simply, you should wash your hands thoroughly before and after contact with each client even when gloves are worn. Wearing gloves does not negate the need for hand-washing. The American Speech-Language-Hearing Association (ASHA, 1989, p. 35) also lists other times when you should wash your hands:

■ Upon arrival at work;
■ Immediately, if they are potentially contaminated with blood or body fluids;
■ Between patients;
■ After removing gloves;
■ Before and after handling in-patient care devices;

■ Before preparing or serving food;
■ Before and after performing any personal body function;
■ When hands are obviously soiled—such as after a sneeze, nose blowing, using the bathroom;
■ Before leaving your worksetting;
■ For isolation patients; before removing gown and mask; after removing gown and mask.

The following procedures for hand-washing are adapted from those recommended by several sources (e.g., ASHA, 1989; Palmer, 1984). Should water conservation be an issue in your geographical area, adaptations in the continuous flow of water will be needed.

■ Remove all jewelry, except for plain wedding bands;
■ Obtain paper towel from dispenser;
■ Slightly lean forward over the sink and avoid touching the sink with clothing;
■ Turn on water to a comfortably warm, but not overly hot or cold temperature;
■ Wet your hands and forearms;
■ Apply liquid antiseptic soap (usually preferable to bar soap);
■ Use a vigorous mechanical action to wash the palms, backs of hands, and fingers—taking between 30 and 60 seconds for this step;
■ Wash your wrists and forearms with soap;
■ Thoroughly rinse your forearms, wrists, and hands;
■ Dry hands, then wrists and forearms using a paper towel;
■ Do not rub hands so hard that chapping occurs to avoid creating small cracks in skin;
■ Use a clean paper towel to turn off the faucet if foot or electronic controls are not available;
■ Dispose of all paper towels in an appropriate container;
■ Use your favorite emollient to decrease the risk of skin cracking.

If you do not have access to a water source, you can use disposable antiseptic wipes or towelettes.

Barrier Techniques:
Gloves, Masks, Goggles, and Gowns

Gloves, masks, goggles, and gowns, otherwise known as personal protective equipment (PPE), are used to prevent the possibility of transmitting airborne or spattered infectious agents, such as droplets of blood or other body fluids, onto your skin or clothes. Gloves provide a barrier, although not an impermeable one, to microorganisms that may be transmitted between client and clinician. Wearing gloves becomes particularly important during an oral–facial examination, during middle ear testing, when handling or fabricating earmolds and other prostheses, during swallowing assessments and therapies, and during assessments of respiratory and laryngeal functioning. Gloves should be worn during each of these tasks. Speech-language pathologists and audiologists are most likely to use disposable, nonsterile gloves. Palmer (1984) suggests that the method for putting on disposable, nonsterile gloves should be as consistent as the methods for sterile gloves. If nonsterile gloves are used, hands should be washed before and after gloving. All gloves should be changed before each new client contact. Finally, gloves should be discarded in a properly marked container after each use or when torn during contact with a client.

An acceptable method for putting on nonsterile gloves when no gown is used is recommended by Palmer (1984). Remember not to touch any surface with a contaminated glove that you will later touch without gloves, for example, doorknobs, telephones, and pens. Failure to take this precaution may result in harmful exposure to disease for yourself, co-workers, and clients.

- Wash and dry hands first;
- Grasp the inside of the right glove with left hand;
- Insert the right hand into glove and pull glove on;
- Place the left hand into the left glove and pull glove on;

- Remove gloves by pulling the contaminated outer side in onto itself;
- Discard gloves in appropriate place;
- Wash and dry hands after gloves are removed.

Remember that masks should only be worn once, donned prior to gown or gloves, and discarded when they become moist . Palmer (1984) suggests that the strings must be tied securely for a snug fit. "If you wear glasses, the mask should fit snugly over your nose and under the edge of your glasses to prevent fogging" (p. 57). Your hands should be washed before and after removing the mask. Isolation gowns must be worn when working with an infected patient or when a patient is in protective isolation. In donning a gown, touch only the inside of the gown. All of these protective clothing items should be disposed of in proper containers. Finally, if washable lab coats are used, they should be changed daily or as needed throughout a day, if contaminated. Otherwise, you should use disposable gowns and, after use, dispose of them properly. The Occupational Safety and Health Administration (OSHA, 1992) mandates that any clothing worn as personal protective equipment should be laundered, maintained, or disposed of by the employer and not sent home with the employee for cleaning.

Cleaning, Sterilization, Disinfection

Cleaning is the removal of any obvious foreign material from objects through washing. This step may precede both disinfection and sterilization (Rutala, 1987). During sterilization there is a complete destruction of infectious agents through physical or chemical processes (Rutala, 1987). This can be done by use of a steam autoclave, dry heat oven, chemical vapor sterilization, or immersion in a chemical sterilant for 10 hours. Items such as impedance probe tips, otoscopic specula, and other heat-sensitive instruments must be cleansed of debris prior to being sterilized in a chemical sterilant although mirrors can be sterilized by the first methods (McMillan & Willette, 1988, p. 36).

Disinfection involves cleansing the surfaces of materials and furniture touched by a client. Materials include all therapy materials, toys, games, and other items used in assessment or therapy. All surfaces of table tops, chairs, and chair arms should be disinfected after each use. All equipment or materials used during an oral–facial evaluation that are not inserted in the oral cavity should be disinfected after each use. Metal surfaces should be cleaned by using a registered germicide, and nonmetal surfaces can be disinfected with a solution of household bleach at a 1:10 dilution with water. The items should be sprayed, vigorously washed, lightly misted again, and left moist (McMillan & Willette, 1988). Any paper towels used, should be disposed of in proper containers. It is important to point out that the use of any cleaning, disinfection, or sterilization of materials or equipment should adhere to the manufacturers' instructions.

Toys

Toys are such a common part of our interaction with pediatric clients that special mention should be made about their place in infection prevention. Whenever possible, toys that have washable surfaces should be used, especially when working with children in diapers. If possible, each group of children should have its own toys. Avoid furry or fabric dolls and stuffed animals. All toys, game boards and pieces, materials, and furniture should be washed and disinfected after each assessment or therapy session. Toys that have been mouthed by a child should be isolated immediately from other children and then properly washed and disinfected before use with other children.

REGULATED WASTE CONTAINERS

Your setting will have specific guidelines for what is considered "regulated waste" in that agency. The Occupational Safety and Health Administration (1992) defines regulated waste as liquid or semiliquid blood or other potentially infectious material (OPIM), items contaminated with blood or OPIM, contaminated sharp objects (sharps), and pathological and microbiological wastes containing blood or OPIM. Individual containers for such regulated waste must be closable, suitable to contain the type of materials enclosed, prevent leakage, and labeled with the biohazard symbol or color coded (usually red) to warn employees of the potential hazards within. Local and state laws govern where and how regulated wastes will be disposed. You should check your department's policy and procedure manual section on infection prevention as to appropriate disposal methods for items you use.

ISSUES OF SPECIAL CONCERN

There are several special issues that you should be aware of regarding infection control. These include high-risk settings and populations. This discussion should help you become more sensitive to infection control in the settings in which you work. Also considering the high proportion of women who practice as audiologists or speech-language pathologists during child-bearing years, this group should have a solid knowledge base about infection control and its relationship to pregnancy. Finally, you should know your setting's procedures for reporting an exposure incident.

EDUCATIONAL SETTINGS

A practical issue that arises in an educational setting, such as a public school, is how to apply universal precautions. Hand-washing between students may not be easily available or possible because of the location of a therapy room or inability to leave a child or children unsupervised in a room while you go to another room for washing. When possible, the speech-language pathologist or audiologist in this setting should seek a room with or very near hand-washing facilities. A possible alternative to hand-washing is to cleanse hands with disposable antiseptic wipes. Hand-washing with soap and water should be done as soon as possible thereafter. Professionals in education should be acutely aware of the need to disinfect tables, chairs, and clinical materials between use and appropriate disposal of gloves, tongue blades, or any other potentially infected clinical materials. It is also important that any cleaning materials be kept out of the reach of children at all times.

NURSING HOMES

Although less attention has been paid to nosocomial infections in nursing homes as compared with acute care hospitals, the resident population in this setting is considered a high-risk group. The increased risk for nosocomial infections among this population is due to living in closed quarters, participation in numerous group activities, malnutrition and dehydration, underlying systemic diseases, use of indwelling devices such as catheters, immobility, fecal incontinence, impaired cognitive skills, decreased ability to maintain personal hygiene, and frequent use of sedatives and tranquilizers (Garibaldi & Nurse, 1992; Gross & Levine,1987) . Risk also increases because of decreased staffing and staff who may be unaware of infection prevention procedures. In a study of over 500 residents in a nursing home, Garibaldi, Brodine, and Matsumiya (1981) found that 16.2% of the residents had some type of infection. The most common types included infected decubitus ulcers, conjunctivitis, urinary tract infections, and pneumonia. They related this prevalence, in part, to the nursing home staff, particularly the high ratio of patients to staff, lack of compensation to staff for sick leave, inadequate immunization requirements, and frequent turnover of nonprofessional employees. Infections that occur at epidemic rates in nursing homes include respiratory tract infections, gastroenteritis, and urinary tract infections (Garibaldi & Nurse, 1992). Thus, if you work in this setting, consider the higher possibility of transmitting an infection to or contracting one from the population of the institution.

DAY CARE CENTERS

Children attending day care centers or nursery programs are at increased risk for contracting and transmitting a variety of diseases (Sherertz & Hampton, 1987). The reasons why infections may spread so easily in this setting are similar to those discussed for nursing home settings. Professionals who work in these settings or whose own children attend them should be aware of the increased potential for contracting and transmitting infections.

Of particular concern in day care centers is the issue of proper diapering techniques. The Fountain Valley School District, Fountain Valley, California, provides the following guidelines for diapering and suggests that similar guidelines be used with children who use potty chairs. Be sure to wear gloves during this procedure and dispose of them and the diaper in accordance with your setting's guidelines.

■ The child lays on a disposable towel;
■ The soiled diaper touches only your hands;
■ The diaper is disposed in a plastic bag to be taken home or to an appropriate receptacle;
■ There is proper cleansing of the child's bottom;
■ There is proper disposal of the washcloth or towelette;
■ The child's hands are washed;
■ The diapering area and equipment are cleaned and disinfected;
■ The caregiver's gloves are disposed of properly;
■ The caregiver's hands are washed thoroughly.

A second concern in day care centers is how to identify a child who is ill and subsequent procedures. An in-depth discussion of this topic is beyond the scope of this chapter. The reader is referred to an excellent resource *What You Can Do to Stop Disease in the Child Day Care Center* (Centers for Disease Control,Department of Health and Human Services, 1984).

STAFF WHO ARE PREGNANT

Staff who are pregnant may be concerned about contracting an infection that may affect their unborn child. Infections that have the greatest potential for affecting a fetus include those due to rubella, enterovirus, hepatitis B, syphilis, toxoplasma, cytomegalovirus, and varicella. Recommendations range from use of appropriate isolation precautions for direct patient care to conducting only indirect patient care to conducting no patient care.

REPORTING EXPOSURE INCIDENTS

According to the Occupational Safety and Health Administration (OSHA, 1992) you should immediately report any situation in which you have been exposed to a potentially infectious agent. Early reporting will help you receive the medical care you may need, help prevent the spread of the infection to others, and assist your employer in assessing the situation surrounding the exposure incident in an effort to prevent further occurrences. Your employer must provide you with a free medical evaluation and treatment if the exposure occurred during your employment. Again, should you be exposed to a potentially infectious agent, check your departmental policy and procedure manual for specific guidelines for how and to whom to report the incident.

SUMMARY

An important aspect of risk management in any setting in which you work is to prevent, to the highest degree possible, the transmission of infectious diseases between those with whom we work, ourselves, and others. The source of an infection can be a person or an inanimate object. Infections are spread through direct contact with the body fluids of another person, through cross-contamination involving the clinician as the means of transmission from one client to another, through airborne transmission of agents, or through direct contact with inanimate objects that have been contaminated by another person. The best precaution to prevent infection transmission is to adhere to universal precautions with all clients, regardless of known or unknown pathology. Universal precautions include rou-

tine vigorous hand-washing before and after client contact; use of gloves, masks, and gowns as necessary; and appropriate disposal of and disinfection/sterilization of clinical tools and materials. The ASHA Code of Ethics requires that all individuals with infectious diseases who require speech-language pathology or audiology services receive those services, although you should be notified as to the presence of any known infectious disease so that you can take appropriate precautions. Confidentiality regarding any client's health status must always be maintained. Remember that infection prevention is a necessary component of quality service delivery.

DISCUSSION QUESTIONS

1. Consider your present employment or training setting. What routine precautions do you take to prevent the transmission of infections? How did you learn about these precautions?
2. Why is hand-washing one of the best ways to prevent transmission of infections?
3. Suppose you worked with a colleague who had a severe cold and cold sores around the lip area. You notice that the co-worker does not observe any special precautions to prevent the transmission of her infections to pediatric clients. What would you do?
4. You work in a hospital at which you frequently get referrals to assess patients with AIDS. What ethical and legal issues should you consider in working with these patients?
5. What are some populations and settings that are at high risk for infection transmission? Why is the risk higher with these populations?

REFERENCES

American Speech-Language-Hearing Association. (1989). AIDS/HIV: Report: Implications for speech-language pathologists and audiologists. *Asha, 29,* 33–37.

American Speech-Language-Hearing Association. (1990). AIDS/HIV: Implications for speech-language pathologists and audiologists. [Report update]. *Asha, 30,* 46–48.

American Speech-Language-Hearing Association. (1991). Chronic communicable diseases and risk management in the schools. *Language, Speech, and Hearing Services in Schools, 22,* 345–352.

Boscia, J. (1986). Epidemiology of bacteriuria in an elderly ambulatory population. *American Journal of Medicine, 80,* 208–212.

Castle, M., & Ajemian, E. (1987). *Hospital infection control: Principles and practice.* New York: John Wiley and Sons.

Centers for Disease Control. (1984). *What you can do to stop disease in child day care centers.* Washington, DC: Author

Centers for Disease Control. (1989). Guidelines for prevention of human immunodeficiency virus and hepatitis B to health care and public safety workers. *Morbidity and Mortality Weekly Report, 38,* S-6.

Crawford, M., & Studebaker, G. (1990). Cytomegalovirus: A disease of hearing. *The Hearing Journal. 43,* 25–30.

Dixon, R. (1987). Costs of nosocomial infections and benefits of infection control programs. In R. Wenzel (Ed.), *Prevention and control of nosocomial infections* (pp. 19–25). Baltimore, MD: Williams & Wilkins.

Fauci, A. (1983). The acquired immune deficiency syndrome: The ever broadening clinical spectrum. *Journal of the American Medical Association, 249,* 2375–2376.

Fedson, D. (1987). Immunizations for health care workers and patients in hospitals. In R. Wenzel (Ed.), *Prevention and control of nosocomial infections* (pp. 116–174). Baltimore, MD: Williams & Wilkins.

Flower, W. (1991). Communication problems in patients with AIDS. In J. Mukand (Ed.)., *Rehabilitation for patients with HIV disease.* New York: McGraw-Hill.

Flower, W., & Sooy, C. (1987). AIDS: An introduction for speech-language pathologists and audiologists. *Asha, 27,* 25–30.

Fuchs, P. (1979). *Epidemiology of hospital associated infections.* Chicago: American Society of Clinical Pathologists.

Garibaldi, R., Brodine, S., & Matsumiya, S. (1981). Infections among patients in nursing homes: Policies, prevalence, and problems. *New England Journal of Medicine, 305,* 731–735.

Garibaldi, R. L., & Nurse, B. (1992) Infections in nursing homes. In J. Bennett & P. Brachmann (Eds.), *Hospital infectons* (pp. 491–532). Boston: Little, Brown.

Gross, P., & Levine, J. (1987). Infections in the elderly. In R. Wenzel (Ed.), *Prevention and control of nosocomial infections.* Baltimore, MD: Williams & Wilkins.

Heeg, J., & Coleman, D. (1992). Hepatitis kills. *Registered Nurse, 55,* 60–66.

Hellman, S., & Gram, M. (1993). The resurgence of tuberculosis. *American Association of Occupational Health Nurses Journal, 41,* 66–71.

LaForce, F. M. (1992). Lower respiratory tract infections. In J. Bennett & P. Brachman (Eds.), *Hospital infections* (pp. 611–640). Boston: Little, Brown.

McMillan, M., & Willette, S. (1988). Aseptic technique: A procedure for preventing disease transmission in the practice environment. *Asha, 31,* 35–37.

Occupational Safety and Health Administration Fact Sheet. (1992). Washington, DC: Author.

Palmer, M. (1984). *Infection control: A policy and procedure manual.* Philadelphia: W.B. Saunders.

Polder, J., Tablan, O., & Williams, W. (1992). Personnel health services. In J. Bennett & P. Brachman (Eds.), *Hospital infections.* Boston: Little, Brown.

Rutala, W. (1987). Disinfection, sterilization, and waste disposal. In R. Wenzel (Ed.), *Prevention and control of nosocomial infections* (pp. 257–282). Baltimore, MD: Williams &Wilkins.

Sherertz, R., & Hampton, A. (1987). Infection control aspects of hospital employee health. In R. Wenzel, (Ed.), *Prevention and control of nosocomial infections* (pp. 116–174). Baltimore, MD: Williams & Wilkins.

U. S. Government Manual. (1992/1993). Washington, DC: Office of the Federal Register National Archives and Records Administrations.

Valenti, P. (1992). Selected viruses of nosocomial importance. In J. Bennett & P. Brachman (Eds.), *Hospital infections* (pp. 789–822). Boston: Little, Brown.

RESOURCES

Centers for Disease Control and Prevention (CDCP)
1600 Clifton Road
Atlanta, GA 30333
404-629-3291

Established in 1973, the Centers for Disease Control and Prevention is a federal agency within the U.S. Public Health Service. The CDCP is responsible for national programs aimed at prevention and control of communicable and airborne diseases and other preventable conditions. The agency is composed of nine major divisions that consult with related state and local health programs; develop programs for chronic disease prevention, environmental health, and occupational safety and health; and focus on research, education, information, and epidemiological data collection and analysis. The agency also provides international consultation on these topics. The CDCP can issue recommendations but is not a standard-setting body (U.S. Government Manual, 1992/1993).

Occupational Safety and Health Administration
Labor Department
200 Constitution Avenue, N.W.
Washington, DC 20210

Part of the U.S. Labor Department, the Occupational Safety and Health Administration (OSHA) develops policies, disseminates information, and enforces occupational safety and health standards. This agency also determines compliance with occupational safety and health standards through inspections and determines and enforces penalties for noncompliance (U.S. Government Manual, 1992/1993).

■ CHAPTER 22 ■

Service Delivery Issues for Multicultural Populations

■ HORTENCIA KAYSER, Ph.D. ■

SCOPE OF CHAPTER

During the past 25 years, speech-language pathologists and audiologists have become increasingly aware of the needs of multicultural populations. Clinicians are faced daily with the challenge of providing appropriate assessment and treatment to populations that, historically, have received little attention. This chapter provides an overview of issues you will confront as a speech-language pathologist or audiologist working with multicultural populations.

The chapter begins with a discussion of the demographic profile of minority individuals in the United States, the prevalence of communication disorders in multicultural populations, and factors that affect assessment and influence treatment efficacy. The chapter then focuses on an historical review of minority concerns. Finally, you will be introduced to factors that define and affect practice such as monolingual clinicians' use of paraprofessionals and interpreters and cultural sensitivity of professionals.

ISSUES AFFECTING MULTICULTURAL POPULATIONS

COMMUNICATION DISORDERS: DEMOGRAPHICS AND DEFINITIONS

Multicultural populations, which include American-Indian, Asian-Americans, African-Americans, and Hispanic-Americans, are expanding rapidly and becoming an increasingly important factor in sociocultural, economic, and educational planning in the United States. The 1990 census reported that the nation's culturally diverse population exceeds 60 million persons. Both immigration and the high birth rate will contribute to the rapid increase of this segment of the population (U.S. Census, 1991). Battle (1993) reported that, if current trends in immigration continue, the Hispanic population will increase by 21%, the Asian population by 22%, and the African-American population by 12%. In contrast, the Anglo population will increase only by 2%. This will eventually turn the combined minority population into the majority population of this country. By the year 2000, one fourth to one third of the United States population will be African-, Hispanic-, and Asian-American (Allen & Turner, 1990).

The American Speech-Language-Hearing Association (ASHA) estimates that approximately 10% of the U.S. population have communication disorders (Battle, 1993). The same figure may be used to estimate the prevalence of communication disorders among culturally diverse populations, translating into a possible figure of 6 million Americans. This estimate may be conservative from nondominate groups with communication disorders, considering that many diverse groups have health and social problems particular to their race or ethnicity, such as hypertension and sickle cell anemia among African-Americans, diabetes among Hispanics, and the high incidence of otitis media among American Indians. The U.S. Department of Health and Human Services (DHHS) (1985) reported that economically disadvantaged populations are more likely to be predisposed to causes of disorders related to environmental, teratogenic (causing developmental malformations), nutritional, and traumatic factors than other groups. Children born into poverty are often urban and multiracial, including as many as 13 million children (Kozol, 1990). According to Hodgkinson (1985) these children are more likely to be judged by teachers to need remedial or special education than children from middle class families. These and other variables, such as child abuse in low-income families, single-parent families, homelessness, teen pregnancies, and low educational achievement, may increase the number of multicultural individuals with communication disorders.

Our knowledge about communication disorders in multicultural populations is limited. A hindrance to our knowledge is evidenced in how we define a communication disorder. Traditional definitions, originating from our study of mainstream English-speaking individuals, may skew our efforts in identifying communicatively disordered persons from culturally diverse backgrounds. The definition must include the person's and that individual's community's expectation of communicative competency and deviancy (Battle, 1993; Taylor, 1986). A culturally sensitive definition of communication disorder is developed only after experience with the particular culture and after gaining an understanding of the community's expectations for the development and use of speech and language.

Language and Phonological Disorders

The characteristics of a language disorder are specific to individuals (Hubbell, 1981). When these language features are compared with the community norm, individuals can readily be identified as either language-impaired or within normal range. Consistent with this, Taylor (1986) revised Van Riper's (1978) standard definition of communication disorder to comply with the "community norm." Taylor states that the indigenous culture or language group must consider the communication of an individual as defective and as operating outside the norms of acceptability for that population. Thus, understanding the cultural norms for communicative competency for any culturally and linguistically diverse population is the first step to appropriately defining communication disorders.

Identifying a communication disorder becomes problematic with individuals who are acquiring a second language. Bilingual individuals may be identified inappropriately as speech- or language-impaired when they are experiencing societal effects.

Linares (1983) states that a language disorder in bilingual children exists when comprehension and/or expression is unlike the language used by peers and interferes with communication. If a person is learning two languages and developing communicative competency for two cultures, bilingualism may complicate the identification of a language disorder (Kayser, 1989). The development of two languages includes natural phenomena that affect the receptive and expressive abilities of the individual. Therefore, these abilities must be considered in assessment and treatment. These phenomena include language loss, transference of features from one language to the other, language mixing, and code switching.

Language loss is defined as the loss of a first or second language because of lack of use (Baetens Beardsmore, 1986). Language loss occurs frequently in children. While they are learning to speak English, they lose the ability to speak their native language within 1 to 2 years. Unfortunately, these children may not develop the ability to communicate proficiently in English, a skill that facilitates effective participation in school (Kayser, 1993).

Transference of features or interference at the phonological, morphological, syntactic, semantic, and pragmatic levels occurs in both weaker and stronger language use (Valdes-Fallis, 1978). The bilingual individual is aware of these momentary "errors" and may either self-correct or continue speaking. It is important to note that these are not confusion difficulties.

Language mixing is the intermingling of one language into another because the individual may not know the word needed to complete an utterance. This occurs frequently in children who are becoming bilingual (Valdes-Fallis, 1978). The frequency of language mixing decreases as the child becomes proficient in the second language (Grosjean, 1982). Code switching is the alternate use of two languages at the word, phrase, or sentence levels when there is a complete break between languages in phonology (Valdes-Fallis, 1978). Bilingual communities code switch for a variety of reasons. Children learn these rules as they become proficient in two languages (Hudelson, 1983). Each of these phenomena occurs in bilingual speakers and must be considered when assessing or treating these individuals.

Fluency Disorders

Conrad (1992) offers a summary of the current knowledge about fluency disorders in multi-cultural populations. First, the ratio of males to females among those who stutter is not the same for all cultural groups. For example, among African-American males the ratio is 2:1 as compared to 4:1 for white males. Second, the nature of stuttering behaviors is influenced by cultural factors. The response to stuttering behaviors varies among cultures; some cultures accept the disfluencies, others do not. Third, the frequency and loci of stuttering behaviors are influenced by the nature of the language spoken. Bilingual persons who stutter will have differing frequency and loci of stuttering because of the form or structure of their language. Finally, the parameters of the language spoken influence stuttering behaviors. For example, in Spanish, the person who stutters may insert a subject pronoun that is nonobligatory. Thus, we cannot assume that what is known about fluency disorders in the white population is true and valid for other races and ethnic groups. There are many unanswered questions regarding assessment and treatment in the area of fluency among multicultural populations. What may be acceptable fluency assessment and treatment procedures for one population may not be acceptable for another.

Voice disorders

Agin (1992) suggests that vocal dynamics exhibit dialectic variation. Studies of vocal dynamics and disorders currently are limited and based largely on clinical observations and anecdotal evidence. Few studies, in fact, identify subjects by race or ethnicity. Available data suggest, however, a higher incidence of vocal disorders in African-American and Hispanic adolescents and higher incidence of laryngeal cancer in African-American males when compared to age-matched white populations. Agin (1992) warns that traditional clinical methods employed in the treatment of dysphonic persons of most white cultures do not equally serve persons from other cultures.

Hearing Disorders

Two diseases have been reported to be of higher incidence among multicultural populations: sickle cell anemia among African-Americans and otitis media among American Indians. Observations and limited reports have suggested that these populations have a higher incidence of hearing loss.

Sickle cell anemia is a genetic abnormality of the hemoglobin molecule found in red blood cells. Once oxygen is removed from abnormal hemoglobin, red blood cells become sickle-shaped (Scott, 1986). These sickled cells do not circulate and may clog the capillaries throughout the body. Sickle cell anemia has an estimated prevalence rate of between 0.3% and 1.3% in African-Americans (Lin Fu, 1972). Crawford et al. (1991) reported that 41% of adults with sickle cell disease had a sensorineural hearing loss. Buchanan, Moore, and Counter (1993) state that there may also be central auditory nervous system involvement in persons with this disease.

Otitis media is one of the most common health problems of children. Buchanan et al. (1993) report that approximately 70% of children in the general population have one or more episodes of otitis media by the age of 5. Stewart (1992) reports that, among American-Indians, the disease is from 4 to 13 times more prevalent than in the general population. The prevalence of hearing loss is, therefore, higher for American Indians than for the general population, with 3.3% reported for conductive hearing loss and 13.3% reported for sensorineural hearing loss. Buchanan et al. (1993) state that American Indians and Asian/Pacific-Americans have the highest prevalence of otitis media, followed by Hispanics, whites, and African-Americans with the lowest prevalence rate.

STANDARDIZED TESTS

Test instruments are important for accurate and objective assessment of individuals with communication disorders. They help determine the client's communication strengths and weaknesses by comparing the subject's performance to a "normal" population. Norms are usually developed from a population that is primarily middle class, English speaking, and of European background. When clinicians assess individuals who do not fit this "norm," accurate assessment is not possible for a variety of reasons: (a) inappropriate use of English tests with their English norms; (b) faulty translation of test instruments, thus, compromising test validity and reliability; and (c) the use of nonprofessionals as interpreters. An extreme measure by a clinician may be to withhold services to minority individuals. Not providing services to any individual on the basis of an inability to meet their needs is unethical, and for school-age children is illegal (P.L. 94-142). The clinician without appropriate measures or clinical resources should always refer these clients to another agency or individual who is better equipped to meet the individual's needs.

The use of tests that are insensitive to the diversity of the population results in invalid data. Culture must play a dominant role in the development of any diagnostic or behavioral test. Taylor (1986) states that clients may perform differently when tested because of their cultural background. Because of a client's linguistic differences, results in levels of communicative competence may vary from those of the mainstream population.

Test instruments are likely to reflect the culture of the test developer and present speech and language stimuli thought to be familiar to all individuals. A minority client may not, however, have had the same cultural and language experiences as the majority population. Therefore, a test may be translated into the native language, but this poses other problems. The test may be translated into words unfamiliar to the client. For example, a language test for school-aged children may be translated and then administered to two Spanish-speaking children. The first child may be urban-born in the United States and the other rural-born and a new immigrant from Mexico. Those two Spanish-speaking children have two very different world experiences. Administration of a translated test developed for English-speaking students from the United States may result in two different profiles for these two children. The urban child may recognize objects and concepts that are seen in stores, billboards, books, and television. Thus, this child may perform well. The child from rural Mexico may appear to be severely delayed in Spanish because of the child's unfamiliarity with American culture.

Using a nonprofessional as an interpreter may seem to be an adequate solution, but interpretation, too, may be problematic. Langdon (1988) reports that interpreters may omit or add information, use the wrong word, or transpose information. Interpreters must be carefully trained before they participate in client-family conferences, assessment, and treatment.

Vaughn-Cooke (1983) suggests seven alternatives to traditional tests: (a) standardize existing tests on nonmainstream English speakers; (b) include a small percentage of minorities in the standardization sample when developing a test; (c) modify or revise existing tests in ways that will make them appropriate for nonmainstream speakers; (d) utilize a language sample when assessing the language of nonmainstream speakers; (e) use criterion-referenced measures when assessing the language of nonmainstream speakers; (f) refrain from using all standardized tests that have not been corrected for test bias when assessing the language of nonmainstream speakers; and (g) develop a new test that can provide a more appropriate assessment of the language of nonmainstream English speakers. Although, these suggestions appear feasible, Vaughn-Cook cautions that each has potential problems for implementation.

A practice that has received considerable attention is the use of nonstandard or modified procedures in the assessment of minority clients (Erickson & Iglesias, 1986; Kayser, 1989). The clinician administers a test using standardized procedures, then readministers the test by altering the procedures to allow more response time or allow for more dialectal variation. Other modified procedures include rewording instructions, providing more examples, having the child explain the "error" response, administering items beyond the test ceiling, and allowing other similar test responses.

Another suggestion is to adapt a test instrument so that it becomes culturally appropriate for the target population (Kayser, 1989). The test instrument is adapted so that the content and/or tasks become culturally familiar to the client. For example, the vocabulary may be adapted to words used in the community. The task used to elicit a response may be unfamiliar or unnatural to the individual; therefore, a change can be made so that the area of speech and language tested can be assessed using a more culturally acceptable task. Once tests are adapted, the original test no longer exists, and therefore, the norms are invalid and inappropriate for comparison. The danger of adapting a standardized test is loss of standardization, thus minimizing validity and reliability. The clinician must then describe the performance of the individual and compare this performance to known developmental norms for a particular population. Kayser (1989, 1993) provides a detailed discussion concerning the assessment of bilingual clients using adapted tests and modified procedures.

INTERVENTION

Intervention for a client is based on comprehensive assessment involving identification of strengths and weaknesses in the areas of voice, phonology, fluency, language, and hearing. Through the development of goals and objectives, intervention is aimed at meeting a client's communication needs. Treatment planning for the client from a minority population should involve three considerations: (a) the clinician and client's cultural backgrounds and the influence of each on the clinical process; (b) the choice of language for instructing the non-English-speaking client; and (c) culturally sensitive treatment procedures.

The Clinician and Client Interaction

The basis for all clinical decisions and treatment results rests with the interaction between the clinician and the client. Taylor (1986) states that all clinical interactions are cultural events. Therefore, the clinician should view the clinical situation as a social communicative event with cultural rules for appropriate clinician and client interactions. The clinician should also be aware of potential sources of miscommunication resulting from the client's assumptions and norms. These possible miscommunications should be prevented during the course of intervention. Taylor (1986) states that the client's culture should be taken into consideration, which, in turn, increases the clinician's sensitivity to diversity. Taylor further suggests that clinicians should use culturally appropriate procedures, materials, activities and subject matter of interest to their culturally diverse clients. Recognition that minority clients are different in their communication style is the first step toward improvement of services to culturally diverse populations.

Clinical services for the bilingual client who requires treatment in his or her first language may be problematic for the monolingual clinician. Juarez (1985) suggests that monolingual clinicians may facilitate treatment through: (a) inservice training on cultural diversity for educators, aides, and resource personnel; (b) consulting with the bilingual instructional unit on a regular or on-call basis; (c) training minority aides to collect data, such as language samples, and adapt materials for intervention. Kayser (1993) also suggests that treatment with minority clients include family counseling about client rights, future bilingualism for the client, and parental, spouse, or caregiver contributions to developing the client's communication abilities.

The Language of Intervention

English has been the language of choice for intervention for most minority clients, whether or not the client speaks English.

Choice may not exist, however, when a bilingual clinician or paraprofessional is not available. Even if intervention in the home language is possible, a number of issues must be considered. Ortiz (1984) identifies these issues as follows: (a) the language preference of the parent and client; (b) age; (c) type and severity of the communication problem; (d) availability of bilingual personnel; (e) length of residency in the United States; (f) motivation for learning a new language; and (g) attitudes toward Americans and instruction in English. Innate abilities, such as language aptitude and general intellectual abilities, are also important. Finally, the time allocated for treatment and progress in therapy in the chosen language may determine whether the second language should be included in the treatment process.

Bilingual individuals constitute a heterogeneous group. Their use of two languages will vary depending on their exposure to each language and their interests in maintaining their bilingualism. Additionally, bilingual individuals may have differing attitudes toward each of the languages. Therefore, the combination of language proficiency and attitudes may influence the outcome of treatment. Determining which language to use for treatment must take the individual client into consideration and the person's particular needs and desires.

Therapy Content

Cultural sensitivity has been the theme among advocates for culturally and linguistically diverse individuals with communication disorders (Harris, 1986; Kayser, 1993; Saville-Troike, 1986). This cultural sensitivity may then affect the content of therapy. Kayser (1985) describes the participation of Hispanic children in therapy when a white clinician used a culturally sensitive art activity. The children were to make cascarones (dried egg shells filled with confetti used to crack over a person's head during a festival) in therapy. The clinician, who had recently learned about this art form, used this as part of the therapy plan. She was surprised and delighted to see the recognition, active response, and participation of the children in the session. Kayser (1993) states that background research about a culture may be necessary to appropriately plan therapy that is culturally sensitive. Preparation may include observations of the community and discussion with bilingual professionals and families to understand aspects of culture that may be unfamiliar, offensive, and inappropriate in the therapy session.

ISSUES AFFECTING PRACTICE IN SPEECH-LANGUAGE PATHOLOGY AND AUDIOLOGY

ASHA POSITION STATEMENTS

Three ASHA position statements have had a major impact on service delivery to multicultural populations. These statements embody several years of discussion among clinicians and researchers.

Social Dialects

The purpose of the Position Paper on Social Dialects (ASHA, 1983) was to clarify the association's view on social dialects. The policy document makes it clear that dialectal variation of English is not a communication disorder. According to the position, all social dialects are adequate, functional, and effective varieties of English. Thus, children and adults are not to be admitted to treatment programs or identified as disordered solely on the basis of their dialect. However, individuals who speak a nonstandard English dialect may elect to have speech and language services to use standard English. If a speech-language pathologist does provide this service, the practitioner must work to preserve the integrity of the client's dialect.

Clinical Management of Communicatively Handicapped Minority Language Populations

The purpose of the Clinical Management position statement (ASHA, 1985) was to "recommend competencies for assessment and remediation of communicative disorders of minority language speakers and to describe alternative strategies that can be utilized when those competencies are not met" (p.29). Five competencies were identified as necessary for the assessment and remediation in a minority language. These include: (a) language proficiency (native or near native fluency in both the minority language and the English language); (b) normative processes (the ability to describe the process of normal speech and language acquisition for both bilingual and monolingual individuals and how those processes are manifested in oral and written language); (c) assessment (the ability to administer and interpret formal and informal assessment procedures to distinguish between communication difference and communication disorders); (d) intervention (the ability to apply intervention strategies for treatment of communicative disorders in the minority language); and (e) cultural sensitivity (the ability to recognize cultural factors that affect the delivery of speech-language pathology and audiology services to the minority language speaking community).

The position paper acknowledged that there may be difficulty in acquiring bilingual personnel to serve minority language individuals; therefore, five alternative strategies for using bilingual personnel were included: (a) establish contact (find consultants who can provide the service); (b) establish cooperatives (a group of agencies or school districts could share one bilingual speech-language pathologist or audiologist); (c) establish networks (ties could be developed between agencies and university programs that might have bilingual students; these students can then be recruited by the agencies); (d) establish Clinical Fellowship Year and graduate practicum sites (bilingual graduates can be utilized to assist personnel in school and other facilities); and (e) establish interdisciplinary teams (a team approach could be developed among the monolingual speech-language pathologist or audiologist and bilingual professionals, such as teachers, psychologists, and nurses who are knowledgeable of nonbiased assessment procedures and development of the minority language).

The final recommendation in the position paper covered use of interpreters or translators. Interpreters are recommended only when competent bilingual professionals are not available. Interpreters can be recruited from language banks, bilingual professional staff, family members, or friends of the client. Note that use of family or friends is the last resort when using an interpreter. Interpreters should be trained and have knowledge of clinical procedures.

This position statement was of particular importance because it served as the basis for curriculum development for many minority-emphasis programs. Although the majority of the competencies of clinicians who serve minority language clients are clear, the language proficiency competency is not as well-defined.

Bilingual Speech-Language Pathologists and Audiologists

The primary purpose for this ASHA position paper was to define the term "bilingual" and thus to protect the public from clinicians who claim to have bilingual abilities (ASHA, 1989). The ASHA definition offers guidelines for bilingual professionals as well as professionals who aspire to become bilingual.

The definition states that speech-language pathologists or audiologists who call themselves bilingual must be able to speak their primary language and to speak (or sign) at least one other language with native or near-native proficiency in semantics, phonology, morphology/syntax, and pragmatics during clinical management.

Many bilingual professionals have attempted to meet the intent of this definition and, through continuing education, have met the academic competencies as outlined in the 1985 position statement (ASHA, 1985). Lan-guage competencies can be evaluated through testing services of university language programs or by state education agencies that certify bilingual education teachers. No matter how clinicians choose to document bilingual competencies, they are bound by the ASHA Code of Ethics, to provide quality services to all clients (ASHA, 1992).

PARAPROFESSIONALS AND INTERPRETERS

Paraprofessionals and interpreters provide two separate clinical roles that require different training. The *paraprofessional* (also referred to as support personnel), as defined by ASHA (1983), is any person who, after receiving on-the-job or academic training, provides clinical services that are prescribed and directed by a certified speech-language pathologist or audiologist. An *interpreter* is one who conveys information from one language to another in the oral modality; a *translator* conveys information in the written modality (Langdon, 1992). Both paraprofessionals and interpreters should have a minimum of a high school diploma with communication skills adequate for the tasks assigned by the clinician. Interpreters should have oral and written abilities in English and the minority language. These skills are not easily acquired by all bilingual persons. Rather, professional interpreting requires training and advance linguistic skills in at least two languages (Kayser, 1993). Langdon (1992) states that the role of the interpreter requires an ability to stay emotionally uninvolved with the discussions. The interpreter must maintain confidentiality and neutrality, accept the clinician's authority, and be able to work with other professional staff (Kayser, 1993). When a family member or friend serves in this role, information relayed to the family may be omitted or misunderstood (Kayser, 1993). Unfortunately, interpreting is not yet recognized as a profession in our field.

The paraprofessional/interpreter's role may include screening of speech, language, and/or hearing, treatment activities that do not require clinical decision making, chart recording, clinical record maintenance, preparation of clinical materials, and testing of hearing aids. The paraprofessional and/or interpreter should not be responsible for interpreting data, determining caseloads, transmitting clinical information to other professionals, preparing reports, referring clients to other professionals, or use a title other than that assigned by the professional.

SUMMARY

The purpose of this chapter was to introduce you to issues that confront speech-language pathologists and audiologists working with culturally and linguistically diverse populations with communication disorders. Issues discussed included communication disorders in multicultural populations, assessment, and treatment. The roles of minority and nonminority speech-language pathologists and audiologists were discussed, as well as ASHA position statements concerning culturally and linguistically diverse populations. Each of these issues has a direct impact on the quality of service provided to multicultural populations. ASHA has been a leader among professional associations in providing its membership with information concerning culturally and linguistically diverse populations. As the population demographics for the United States continue to change, the professions must continue to heighten sensitivity in clinical practice to meet the needs of the multicultural population.

ACKNOWLEDGMENT

This chapter was funded, in part, by Research and Training Center Grant 1P60 DC-01409 from the National Institute on Deafness and Other Communication Disorders. National Center for Neurogenic Communication Disorders, University of Arizona, Tucson, Arizona.

DISCUSSION QUESTIONS

1. List and explain the ASHA position statements concerning minority populations and discuss implications for your practice as a speech-language pathologist or audiologist.
2. Discuss the pros and cons of standardized testing for minority groups.
3. Describe your options in providing treatment services to an individual who does not speak English.
4. How do you think your own cultural background affects your provision of clinical services?
5. What are some ways you have (or could) increase your own sensitivity to other cultures?

REFERENCES

Agin, R. (1992). *Voice disorders in diverse cultural populations.* A paper presented to the Working Group, Research and Research Training Needs of Minority Persons and Minority Health Issues. Washington, DC: National Institute on Deafness and Other Communication Disorders.

Allen, J. P., & Turner, E. (1990). Where diversity is. *American Demographics, 12*(8), 34–38.

American Speech-Language-Hearing Association. (1983a). *Guidelines for the employment and utilization of supportive personnel.* Rockville, MD: Author.

American Speech-Language-Hearing Association. (1983b). Position of the American Speech-Language-Hearing Association on social dialects. *Asha, 27,* 23–25.

American Speech-Language-Hearing Association. (1985). Clinical management of communicatively handicapped minority language populations. *Asha, 27,* 29–32.

American Speech-Language-Hearing Association. (1989). Definition: Bilingual speech-language pathologists and audiologists. *Asha, 31,* 93.

American Speech-Language-Hearing Association. (1992). Code of ethics. *Asha, 34*(3, Suppl. 9), 1–2.

Baetens Beardsmore, H. (1986). *Bilingualism: Basic principles* (2nd. ed.). San Diego: College-Hill Press.

Battle, D. (Ed.). (1993). *Communication disorders in multicultural populations.* Boston: Andover Medical Publishers.

Buchanan, L. H., Moore, E. J., & Counter, S. A. (1993). Hearing disorders and auditory assessment. In D. Battle (Ed.), *Communication disorders in multicultural populations* (pp. 256–286). Boston: Andover Medical Publishers.

Conrad, C. (1992). *Fluency disorders in culturally diverse populations.* A paper presented to the Working Group, Research and Research Training Needs of Minority Persons and Minority Health Issues. Washington, DC: National Institute on Deafness and Other Communication Disorders.

Crawford, M. R., Gould, H. J., Smith, W. R., Beckford, N., Gibson, W. R., & Bobo, L. (1991). Prevalence of hearing loss in adults with sickle cell disease. *Ear and Hearing, 12,* 349–351.

Education for All Handicapped Children Act of 1975. PL No. 94-142, 20 U.S.C. Section 1401 et seq. (Supp. 1984).

Erickson, J., & Iglesias, A. (1986). Assessment of communication disorders in non-English proficient children. In O. Taylor (Ed.), *Nature of communication disorders in culturally and linguistically diverse populations* (pp. 181–218). San Diego: College-Hill Press.

Grosjean, F. (1982). *Life with two languages: An introduction to bilingualism.* Cambridge: Harvard University Press.

Harris, G. (1986). Barriers to the delivery of speech, language, and hearing services to Native Americans. In O. Taylor (Ed.), *Nature of communication disorders in culturally and linguistically diverse populations* (pp. 219–236). San Diego: College-Hill Press.

Hodgkinson, H. L. (1985). *All one system: Demographics of education—Kindergarten through graduate school.* Washington, DC: Institute for Educational Leadership, Inc.

Hubbell, R. (1981). *Children's language disorders: An integrated approach.* Englewood Cliffs, NJ: Prentice-Hall.

Hudelson, S. (1983). Beto at the sugar table: Code switching in a bilingual classroom. In T. Escobedo (Ed.), *Early childhood bilingual education: An Hispanic perspective* (pp. 32–49). New York: Teachers College Press.

Hymes, D. (1962). The ethnography of speaking. In T. Gladwin & W. C. Sturtevant (Eds.), *Anthropology and human behavior* (pp. 13–53). Washington, DC: Anthropological Society of Washington.

Juarez, M. (1983). Assessment and treatment of minority language handicapped children: The role of the monolingual speech-language pathologist. *Topics in Language Disorders, 3,* 57–65.

Kayser, H. (1985). *A study of speech-language pathologists and their Mexican American language disordered caseloads.* Unpublished doctoral dissertation, New Mexico State University, Las Cruces.

Kayser, H. (1989). Speech and language assessment of Spanish-English speaking children. *Language, Speech and Hearing Services in Schools, 30,* 226–244.

Kayser, H. (1993). Hispanic cultures. In D. Battle (Ed.), *Communication disorders in multicultural populations* (pp. 114–157). Boston: Andover Medical Publishers.

Kozol, J. (1990). The new untouchables. *Newsweek,* pp. 48–53.

Langdon, H. (1988, August). *Working with an interpreter/translator in the school setting. Dimensions of appropriate assessment for minority handicapped students: Recommended practices.* Presented at the State Conference for School Superintendents, Tucson, AZ.

Langdon, H. (1992). Speech and language assessment of LEP/bilingual Hispanic students. In H. Langdon & L. R. L. Cheng (Eds.), *Hispanic children and adults with communication disorders* (pp. 201–271). Gaithersburg, MD: Aspen Publishers.

Linares, N. (1983). Management of communicatively handicapped Hispanic American children. In D. R. Omark & J. G. Erickson (Eds.), *The bilingual exceptional child* (pp. 145–162). San Diego: College-Hill Press.

Lin-Fu, J. S. (1972). *Sickle cell anemia: A medical review.* Washington, DC: U.S. Department of Health, Education, and Welfare.

Ortiz, A. (1984). Choosing the language of instruction for exceptional bilingual children. *Teaching Exceptional Child,* pp. 208–212.

Saville-Troike, M. (1986). Anthropological considerations in the study of communication. In O. Taylor (Ed.), *Nature of communication disorders in culturally and linguistically diverse populations* (pp. 47–72). San Diego: College-Hill Press.

Scott, D. (1986). Sickle-cell anemia and hearing loss. In F. H. Bess, B. S. Clark, & H. R. Mitchell (Eds.), *Concerns for minority groups in communication disorders* (pp. 69–73). *ASHA Reports, 16.*

Stewart, J. L. (1992). *Hearing science and cultural diversity: Native Americans.* Paper presented to the Working Group, Research and Research Training Needs of Minority Persons and Minority Health Issues. Washington, DC: National Institute on Deafness and Other Communication Disorders.

Taylor, O. (1986). Historical perspectives and conceptual framework. In O. Taylor (Ed.), *Nature of communication disorders in culturally and linguistically diverse populations* (pp. 1–19). San Diego: College-Hill Press.

U.S. Bureau of the Census (1991). *Statistical Abstract of the United States.* 111th Ed. No. 1434. Washington, DC: Government Printing Office

U.S. Department of Health and Human Services. (1985). *Report of the secretary's task force on black and minority health* (Vol 1, Executive Summary, Publication 491-313/44706). Washington, DC: Government Printing Office

Valdes-Fallis, G. (1978). Code switching and the classroom teacher. *Language in education: Theory and practice* (Vol. 4). Arlington, VA: Center for Applied Linguistics.

Van Riper, C. (1978). *Speech correction.* Englewood Cliffs, NJ: Prentice-Hall.

Vaughn-Cook, F. (1983). Improving language assessment in minority children. *Asha, 25,* 29–34.

RESOURCES FOR FURTHER READING

Battle, D. (Ed.). (1993). *Communication disorders in multicultural populations.* Boston: Andover Medical Publishers.

Cheng, L. L. (1987). *Assessing Asian language performance.* Rockville, MD: Aspen.

Hamayan, E. V., & Damico, J. S. (1991). *Limiting bias in the assessment of bilingual students.* Austin, TX: Pro-Ed.

Langdon, H. W., & Cheng, L. L. (Eds.). (1992). *Hispanic children and adults with communication disorders.* Gaithersburg, MD: Aspen Publishers.

Taylor, O. (Ed.). (1986). *Nature of communication disorders in culturally and linguistically diverse populations.* San Diego: College-Hill Press.

MULTICULTURAL RESOURCES

American Speech-Language-Hearing Association. (1987). *Concerns for minority groups in communication disorders* (Report 16, #01 10911). Rockville, MD: Author.

American Speech-Language-Hearing Association. (1990). *Directory of bilingual speech-language pathologists and audiologists 1990–91* (#01 11404). Rockville, MD: Author.

American Speech-Language-Hearing Association. (1987). *Linguistic minority populations: Selected annotated bibliography* (#01 11358). Rockville, MD: Author.

American Speech-Language-Hearing Association. (1992). *Marketing to multicultural audiences kit (Speech-language pathology)* (#01 11652). Rockville, MD: Author.

American Speech-Language-Hearing Association. *Marketing to multicultural audiences kit (Audiology)* (#01 11649). Rockville, MD: Author.

American Speech-Language-Hearing Association. (1990). *Minority focus: Selected abstracts from ASHA conventions 1980–1990* (#01 11457). Rockville, MD: Author.

American Speech-Language-Hearing Association. (1987). *Multicultural professional education in communication disorders: curriculum approaches* (#01 11460). Rockville, MD: Author.

American Speech-Language-Hearing Association. (1987). *Resource guide to multicultural tests and materials* (#01 11359). Rockville, MD: Author.

■ CHAPTER 23 ■

Supervision and the Supervisory Process

■ JUDITH A. RASSI, M.A. ■

SCOPE OF CHAPTER

As with any discipline in which the understanding of core concepts is enhanced through observation and practice, the communicative disorders (CD) field uses such methods in the education of its university students. This involves supervision. Beyond the preparation stage, the professions of speech-language pathology and audiology, like comparable professions, call for skilled individuals who can carry out complex processes and procedures efficiently and effectively. This, too, involves supervision.

In that supervision is such an integral part of CD education and of audiology and speech-language pathology practices, the participants—the educators and students, the administrators and practitioners, as well as others—are wise to familiarize themselves with the supervisory process. Being informed about its various components can help to make your work and study experiences more enriching and productive. This, in turn, creates opportu-

nities for upgrading professional quality. Insight into the process can also provide direction for those of you who aspire to supervisory positions in your professional careers.

In the next section of this chapter, definitions of supervision are stated and discussed. Past events that have contributed to the current status of CD supervision are delineated in the succeeding chapter section. This is followed by sections on the roles of supervisors and supervisees; the elements of supervision; the continuum of the supervisory process; and supervision research. Finally, future directions in CD supervision are considered.

DEFINITIONS

Even for those who engage daily in the supervisory process, defining exactly what they do is not an easy task. This is understandable because there are many different kinds of supervision activities and these vary greatly from person to person, setting to setting, and situation to situation. Still, the variations have a common theme. To supervise, according to dictionary definition, is to superintend or oversee; whereas supervision is defined as the action, process, or occupation of supervising, especially critical watching and directing (*Webster's Ninth New Collegiate Dictionary*, 1990).

These generic definitions do capture the general notion of supervision but, in doing so, they promote a popular misconception that supervision focuses narrowly on the overseeing of a subordinate's activities. Supervision can be, should be, and often is much more. As will become apparent in later discussions, the entire supervisory process, as studied and practiced at either the student or practitioner level, incorporates assorted roles and tasks that change with time and circumstance.

For purposes of this overview chapter, the often-cited definition statements from a status report of the American Speech-Language-Hearing Association (ASHA) Committee on Supervision in Speech-Language Pathology and Audiology (ASHA, 1978) will constitute the base of reference. The committee, in recognizing the variety of titles, duties, and work settings that apply to CD supervisors, has defined supervision as it relates to these two primary task categories, clinical teaching and program management. According to the committee (1978):

> Clinical teaching is defined as the interaction between supervisor/supervisee [person being supervised] in any setting which furthers the development of clinical skills of students or practicing clinicians as related to changes in client behavior. Traditionally this interaction has consisted of observation and conferences. . . . Program management is defined as those activities that relate to the administration or coordination of programs, for example scheduling, budgeting, program planning, employing, or dismissing personnel. (p. 479)

It is important to add that there are many CD professionals who function as supervisors and supervisees in nonservice, nonacademic roles and circumstances where neither clinical skill development nor actual program management is part of supervising. For example, some form of supervision takes place in interactions between individuals at different levels within hierarchical organizations, regardless of setting or work unit; between team leaders and their groups; and between advisers, consultants, or mentors and those they guide. If these combinations are included in the scope of our supervision context, it can be seen that most CD professionals are likely to be involved in supervisory interactions from time to time throughout their careers.

THE CD SUPERVISION MOVEMENT

Supervision has been recognized as part of CD education and practice since the field's beginning. For developmental milestones during the early years, you are referred to comprehensive accounts of the evolution (Anderson, 1988; Farmer, 1989a; Ulrich, 1987). Highlighted here are some of the major events occurring since the 1960s, when concerted effort to examine the process began taking hold.

SIXTIES: BREAKTHROUGH

This decade saw the emergence of supervision offerings in various formats. Among those presented at the national level were: a seminar on supervision of clinical practicum (Villareal, 1964); a conference on guidelines for the internship year—later to become the Clinical Fellowship Year (CFY) (Kleffner, 1964); two conferences on supervision in school settings (Anderson & Kirtley, 1966; Kirtley, 1967); and a symposium on supervision (Miner, 1967). The reports and articles emanating from these proceedings constituted the first major phase of writings on the topic. Also contributing to the new literature base were a monograph (Darley, 1961) and an article on supervision issues (Halfond, 1964).

SEVENTIES: ACCELERATION

During these years, movement accelerated rapidly. Nationally, another conference (Anderson, 1970) and workshop (Turton, 1973) were held. Working groups (ASHA, 1972; Conture, 1973) and an ASHA committee on supervision were established (ASHA, 1975b). Out of this committee's work came the previously mentioned status report. Whereas most earlier efforts had concentrated on supervision in the schools, a broader perspective took shape during these years. The Council of College and University Supervisors of Practicum in the Schools (CCUSPS), a national organization founded in 1970 (Staff, 1975), soon expanded its membership base in 1974, becoming CUSPSPA, the Council of University Supervisors of Practicum in Speech-Language Pathology and Audiology (ASHA, 1975a). The Council started distributing its own quarterly newsletter, *SUPERvision*, to the membership.

For the first time, books on supervision in the field were published (Oratio, 1977; Rassi, 1978; Schubert, 1978). CD programs began to offer formal graduate-level course work specifically designed to prepare individuals for the supervisor role. Indeed, in 1972, doctoral education with an emphasis on analysis of and research in the supervisory process, as well as the training of supervisors, became available at Indiana University (Anderson, 1981). From this and other CD educational programs came dissertations and related published articles. Supervision papers made their appearance in ASHA convention sessions.

EIGHTIES: MOMENTUM

This momentum continued into the 1980s, beginning with a unifying conference on supervisor preparation (Anderson, 1980) that brought together for the first time many of the individuals who were to become instrumental in moving supervision forward in the years ahead. CUSPSPA established a networking system, SUPERNET, for the purpose of connecting supervisors through the development of supervisor professional groups at regional, state, and local levels; exchange of information across the country; and promotion of cooperative research (Staff, 1982). In conjunction with the Canadian Association of Speech-Language Pathologists and Audiologists (CASLPA), a supervisors' group in Canada also became active during this time period (Godden, 1990-1991).

Four significant events took place later in this decade. A conference held by directors of graduate programs was devoted primarily to student supervision (Bernthal, 1985). CUSPSPA held its first national conference on supervision (Farmer, 1987), and following another name change to reflect the inclusion of all CD supervisors in all settings at all levels—the Council of Supervisors in Speech-Language Pathology and Audiology (CSSPA)—held a second national conference (Shapiro, 1989). In 1989, ASHA also sponsored a workshop on supervision across work settings (ASHA, 1990b). Proceedings of all the conferences have been published.

ASHA certification and accreditation boards began recognizing the need for quality supervision through stipulations in their requirements for educational and service programs (ASHA, 1980, 1981, 1983). The association also developed a position statement in which supervision tasks and competencies for effective clinical supervision were delineated (ASHA, 1985). ASHA convention programs expanded coverage of supervision, devoting substantial program segments to the topic. Two group presentations—one on supervisor preparation models (Anderson et al., 1989) and the other on supervision of the clinical fellow (McCready et al., 1989)—were later summarized in articles, calling special attention to these important issues.

An unprecedented number of supervision research articles, many based on dissertations, made their debut in refereed professional journals, outside as well as inside the field. The end of this decade produced five major books, each analyzing CD supervision from a unique perspective (Anderson, 1988; Casey, Smith, & Ulrich, 1988; Crago & Pickering, 1987; Farmer & Farmer, 1989; Leith, McNiece, & Fusilier, 1989).

NINETIES: DIRECTION

The course of the CD supervision movement is taking new direction in the 1990s, as is necessary and appropriate amidst the rapidly changing climate of our field and professions. Although proceeding at a sometimes uneven pace, the evolution continues unabated nonetheless. For example, as a consequence of changes in the ASHA's governance, the Committee on Supervision has been disbanded. Even so, supervision is now represented, along with administration, in the ASHA special interest division structure as Special Interest Division 11, Administration and Supervision (ASHA, 1990b). Furthermore, CSSPA, as an official ASHA related professional organization (RPO), takes part in an annual meeting held for such groups and is a recognized member of the consortium (ASHA, 1991).

Effective since January 1, 1993, the Standards and Implementations for the Certificates of Clinical Competence as well as the Clinical Certification Board's accompanying interpretations address the need for supervision quality. This is particularly evident in the newly required Clinical Fellowship Registration Agreement and formal evaluation procedure for clinical fellows (ASHA, 1992). Clinical fellowship requirements and procedures are detailed in a special section of the ASHA Membership and Certification Handbook (ASHA, 1992), and an information packet is now sent to every clinical fellowship supervisor, thereby providing more guidance for both the supervisor and the clinical fellow than has been the case in the past.

Information on CD supervision continues to be disseminated through convention presentations and articles, although the numbers of comprehensive research investigations and dissertation-producing doctoral students appear to have decreased. The CSSPA is at-tempting to involve more supervisors in research through a special support network, Research SUPERNET (Peaper, 1991), and a new publication, *The Supervisor's Forum* (Staff, 1991–1992). In the CSSPA's third national conference, contemporary themes such as total quality management (TQM) and women's approaches to supervision were explored. Again, the proceedings were published (Dowling, 1992c). Thus far in this decade, two books have been produced—one combining theory and practice in implementation (Dowling, 1992b), and the other addressing supervision within the larger context of education in the field (Rassi & McElroy, 1992b).

SUPERVISOR AND SUPERVISEE ROLES

As suggested in definition statements, a supervisor's work is likely to be multifaceted, resulting in a gamut of roles that are setting- and situation-dependent. Personal preferences and philosophical views also appear to influence individual role choices and how they are carried out. When based on past supervisory experiences and information from other sources or simply on an individual's notion of how supervision ought to be approached, roles can reflect what Brasseur (1987) calls "preconceived stereotypes of supervision" (p. 145). Supervisees also may bring their own set of preconceptions to the supervisory relationship (Larson, 1982).

ROLE DIVERSITY

Regardless of the underlying rationale behind particular role choices, it is useful to know what some of the many options are. Identifying supervisor and supervisee roles helps to describe the process, providing clues about its scope and complexity (Rassi & McElroy, 1992a). Farmer (1989b), for example, sees supervisors operating within the broad array of distinct roles as professional, researcher, academic and clinical educator, administrator, and clinician. Rassi and McElroy (1992a), in examining the roles of a student practicum supervisor, view those of clinical instructor, expert, master clinician, facilitator, counselor, and mentor to be contributory. Examples reported elsewhere have found the supervisor serving variously in evaluator, feedback provider, collaborator, and consultant roles (Anderson, 1988); as one who assists, shares information, models, and demonstrates, according to the ASHA position statement (ASHA, 1985); as coach (Hagler, 1991); and as colleague (Cogan, 1973). This brief listing illustrates the range and diversity of possible roles.

ROLE INTERDEPENDENCE

It would appear to be axiomatic that the role carried out by a supervisor (or supervisee) determines, or at least influences, the supervisee's (or supervisor's) counter-role at each juncture. If, for example, the supervisor assumes a teacher role, it seems that the supervisee is likely to play a student or learner role. Likewise, when the supervisor acts as facilitator or coach, you might assume that the supervisee would take the cue and respond in kind to the facilitating or coaching. And when the supervisor seeks to establish a collegial relationship, the supervisee is apt to become the supervisor's colleague. Or, if role determination and influence moves in the opposite direction, that is, from supervisee to supervisor, the same kinds of consequences would be expected in reverse order.

The reciprocal nature of a supervisor-supervisee association is recognized as inherent in the supervisory process. However, the outcomes suggested in these scenarios cannot be assumed. To foster a harmonious and productive working relationship, the supervisor or supervisee may indeed choose to balance the other's role, that is, to play what is perceived to be the role expected by the other person. Still, the role may not represent this individual's preference, thereby leading to personal discomfort and possible inner conflict. Or, either person may choose not to play the role expected by the other, resulting in outward, expressed conflict.

ROLE PERCEPTIONS

Studies have uncovered discrepancies between supervisors' and supervisees' role expectations and perceptions. For instance, Tihen (1984) found that supervisees may expect the supervisor to play a role other than the one being exhibited. To illustrate, a supervisor may persist in a modeling role, while the supervisee expects to function as a fully participating and decision-making colleague rather than as an observer of the supervisory model. Pickering (1987) has reported that student supervisees and their supervisors also have certain expectations, often unstated, that go beyond clinical and supervisory competencies; and, furthermore, that the intent of communication messages between these individuals is not always made clear.

These kinds of findings help us to understand why there are role miscues, hence misguided feelings and reactions. In view of the many individual differences in role perceptions and expectations, as well as the necessary shifting of roles by both parties throughout any given supervisory interaction, this matter requires focused attention. As Anderson (1988) points out, "If supervision is to be productive, participants should be aware of the role perceptions they have for themselves and each other and the expectations they bring into the supervisory interaction" (p. 70). Herein lies the dilemma of supervision: what roles are effective in which settings, at which times, and for which persons?

ELEMENTS OF SUPERVISION

Identifying and considering the matters that compose supervision bring additional meaning to supervisor and supervisee roles. Two views, each representing a dissection of CD supervision from a particular perspective, are summarized in this section.

SUPERVISION TASKS

As previously mentioned, the ASHA position statement on supervision (ASHA, 1985), which was adopted officially by the association's Legislative Council in November 1984, contains the supervision committee's delineation of supervision tasks. Aimed primarily at the clinical teaching aspects of supervision, yet relating to supervision at different levels and in various settings, the 13 tasks (and 81 associated competencies, not enumerated in this chapter) have been instrumental in meeting the committee's objectives. That is to say, their various applications since 1984 indicate that they embody a framework for the discussion, analysis, and study of supervision; they offer a base of reference for supervision research, especially that concerning validation and efficacy questions; and they provide guidelines for all CD persons engaged in some form of supervision as it relates to clinical and educational program responsibilities. The tasks are listed in Table 23–1. As the committee noted, individual tasks, when actually carried out, receive differing degrees of emphasis according to the level and setting of supervision and other situational factors.

SUPERVISION COMPONENTS

Anderson (1988) has brought to our field another important way of looking at supervi-

sion, adapted from methods used in supervising teachers (Cogan, 1973; Goldhammer, 1969). In this view, a collaborative style of supervision (see next section) incorporates five components that take place in the order: understanding, planning, observing, analyzing, integrating—then are repeated in cyclical fashion throughout the supervisory process. A brief description of each component follows.

Understanding the supervisory process, in this context, requires that both the supervisor and supervisee be prepared for their respective roles, that they share their perceptions of these roles and their corresponding expectations, and that this open communication be maintained throughout their supervisory affiliation. Planning the supervisory process goes beyond traditional clinical planning to include planning for the supervisor as well as planning for the supervisee, all of which is done jointly by the two parties.

Observing the supervisory process, according to this scheme, does not involve the usual watch—take notes—evaluate sequence, which is typically one-sided and subjective, but rather has both the supervisor and supervisee objectively collecting and recording data. Analyzing the supervisory process naturally follows. In this stage, the data, both clinical

TABLE 23–1. THE TASKS OF CD CLINICAL SUPERVISION.

1. Establishing and maintaining an effective working relationship with the supervisee
2. Assisting the supervisee in developing clinical goals and objectives
3. Assisting the supervisee in developing and refining assessment skills
4. Assisting the supervisee in developing and refining clinical management skills
5. Demonstrating for and participating with the supervisee in the clinical process
6. Assisting the supervisee in observing and analyzing assessment and treatment sessions
7. Assisting the supervisee in the development and maintenance of clinical and supervisory records
8. Interacting with the supervisee in planning, executing, and analyzing supervisory conferences
9. Assisting the supervisee in evaluation of clinical performance
10. Assisting the supervisee in developing skills of verbal reporting, writing, and editing
11. Sharing information regarding ethical, legal, regulatory, and reimbursement aspects of professional practice
12. Modeling and facilitating professional conduct
13. Demonstrating research skills in the clinical or supervisory processes

and supervisory, are reviewed and interpreted together. Finally, integration of all that has taken place in the first four components occurs when the supervisor and supervisee exchange ideas about what has transpired, then begin their joint planning for the next cycle.

SUPERVISORY PROCESS

Although the terms supervision and the supervisory process have been, and will continue to be, used interchangeably in this chapter, the title separates them into distinct terms. In essence, they are equivalent. The redundancy is used to underscore the point that supervision, albeit the more recognizable term, is indeed a process, as stated in its dictionary definition. The term, supervisory process, then, is more descriptive, portraying a clearer image of ongoing events and interactions, of development, growth, and continuous change. This process theme, already evident in the discussion of sequenced components, is even more apparent in the continuum feature of supervision.

CONTINUUM CONTEXT

By its very nature, supervision exists and operates within a continuum context. A supervision event does not occur in isolation, but rather takes place in a milieu of surrounding influences. These influences are determined by the relative position, in time and level, of the supervision event on a continuum. The schematic diagrams in Figure 23–1 illustrate, in their simplest form, three of the major continua that impact CD supervision. It should be noted that, even though all of these continuum sequences are progressive and developmental, the segments in each continuum do not necessarily correspond to those in another. At a given point in time, any single

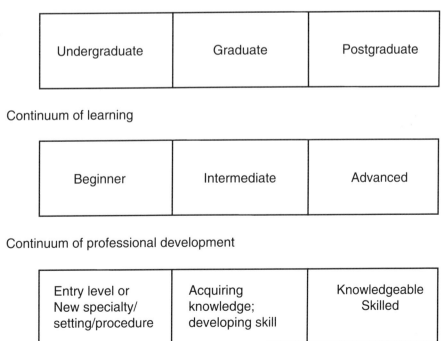

Figure 23–1. Continuum context for CD supervision.

supervision event could be represented at different places on the three tracks. For example, a postgraduate practitioner (third level, education) might know underlying theory and have related general experience in a particular area (second level, learning), yet not understand, or have specific skills for, the implementation of a new clinical procedure in that area (first level, professional development).

CONTINUUM OF SUPERVISION

In keeping with its surrounding continuum context, the process of supervision is implemented as a continuum. Serial consecutive steps in the process were recognized and described as levels (Rassi, 1978) and developmental stages (Hart, 1982) of supervision. Anderson (1988) later captured in her depiction of a supervision continuum the combination of these and other critical concepts and how they interface with one another. This is shown in Figure 23–2. Among the features illustrated in this continuum are: gradual, incremental change with increasing supervisee and decreasing supervisor participation in the supervised activity; continuous supervisee movement toward self-supervision; supervisor styles matched to correspond with

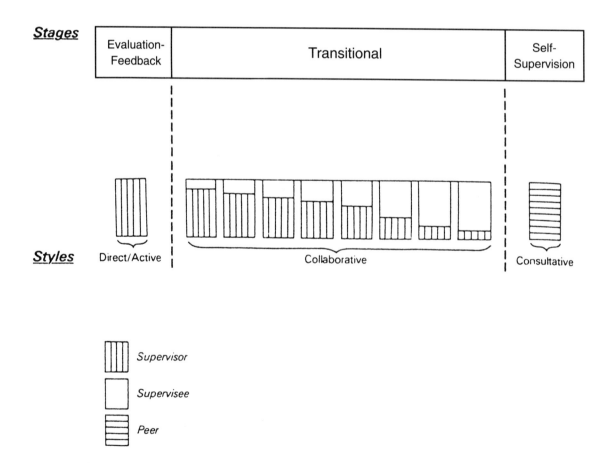

Figure 23–2. Anderson's continuum of supervision. (From *The Supervisory Process in Speech-Language Pathology and Audiology* (p. 62) by J. L. Anderson, 1988, Boston: College-Hill Press/Little, Brown and Company. Copyright 1988 by Pro-Ed. Reprinted by permission.

supervision stages; and the predominant collaborative supervisor style where the supervisor and supervisee work together in a mutually supportive manner. This view of supervision also emphasizes the need for situational adaptations, calling for shifts in direction and level along the continuum as required. The interconnection between the supervision continuum and its continuum context is thus apparent.

SUPERVISION RESEARCH

As indicated in this chapter's earlier account of the CD supervision movement, a body of research has emerged and grown. Many investigators have based their work on supervision ideas from such related disciplines as education, interpersonal communication, counseling psychology, social work, nursing, and medicine, as well as business management and industry. Although these resources continue to be used in CD supervision research design, a substantial database of our own has been generated through methodical data collection and analysis over the years.

Research designs in CD supervision have employed quantitative methods, including traditional and single-subject experiments, as well as qualitative, descriptive methods. Data have been obtained from supervisors and supervisees before, during, and after their interactions. A variety of data-gathering tools have been used, for example, questionnaires, rating scales, journals, audiotaped and videotaped proceedings, and observation analysis instruments. Conferences between supervisors and supervisees have served as the primary place and focus for CD supervision research.

The bulk of supervision research in the field has addressed preprofessional student supervision rather than professional or staff supervision; university-based practicum rather than practicum in other settings; clinical service tasks rather than other types of tasks; and supervision in speech-language pathology rather than supervision in audiology. Thus, although we have gained considerable insight on certain aspects of the process, more research questions need to be posed in these other dimensions. For detailed accounts of what our research has told us, what we ought to ask next, and how to go about doing it, you are referred to these book chapters on the topic: Doehring (1987), Strike and Gillam (1988), and Dowling (1989).

FUTURE DIRECTIONS IN CD SUPERVISION

The need for extensive educational and health care reform is recognized by professionals and the public alike. Substantial changes have already taken place within these systems and more are imminent. The impact on supervision in communicative disorders is clear. As personnel roles are redefined and programs restructured, supervision must undergo its own transformation in order to keep pace. Indeed, visionary supervisors can become the instruments of their own change, influencing supervision's form and direction in the years ahead. Discussed in this section are several avenues for exploring growth and change.

PREPARATION AND STUDY

Preparation of CD supervisors and supervisees for their roles, now conducted through preprofessional course work, doctoral study, continuing education workshops and seminars, and books and articles for self-study (Anderson et al., 1989), is typically optional rather than required. In addition, the information may not be readily available to some, or even known to exist by others. As a consequence, participation in these learning endeavors by individuals and by programs is disproportionately small.

In the years ahead, advocates of formal supervisor preparation will be working to convince professional organizations, institutions, and individuals in the field that preparation and study are important. Eventual inclusion of supervision course work and practicum in certification, accreditation, and continuing education requirements is a likely goal. Such issues as specialty certification, scopes of professional practice, and quality improvement will be pivotal in determining this supervision direction.

RESEARCH AND EXPERIMENTATION

If the field is to be persuaded that preparation and study contribute to effective supervision, data to support this view must be provided (Dowling, 1992a). Inquiry about the effectiveness of supervision itself represents the ultimate, yet most fundamental, set of supervision research questions: Does clinical supervision change supervisee behaviors such that these behaviors, in turn, change client behaviors? What are the outcomes, the effects of supervision at various levels? If there is resultant change, is the change desirable? Does change translate into learning and professional growth? These kinds of questions are beginning to be answered (Gillam, Strike Roussos, & Anderson, 1990; Shapiro & Anderson, 1989), but the quest has barely begun. Because (clinical) supervision efficacy is inextricably linked with clinical efficacy, the unraveling process is complex.

Experimentation in the use of innovative supervision methodologies is being dictated by our changing educational and health care systems. In university educational programs and their practicum field sites, as well as in the professional work settings where CD specialists supervise and are supervised, more efficient and effective ways to get the job done must and will be found. Continued examination of approaches used in allied disciplines and professions will help CD supervisors to adapt others' ideas and develop new ones. For example, *problem-based learning*, adapted from medical and nursing education, might be implemented at the level of preprofessional education (Rassi & McElroy, 1992a); *total quality management (TQM)*, adapted from industry, might be incorporated into the supervisory process at any level (Bess, 1992; Frattali, 1992); and *mentorship*, adapted from a wide range of fields, might be brought into the process at any point along the professional development continuum (Gavett, 1987; Rassi & McElroy, 1992a).

Adding computer applications to our repertoire in the supervisory process will continue to challenge innovators (Cochran & Bull, 1992; Rushakoff & Farmer, 1989). The possibilities seem to be limitless and, without question, quite necessary in this era of increasing demands on the time and energy of supervisors and supervisees. But, as technology further encroaches on our work environments, whether they are clinical, supervisory, or both, the need for improving interpersonal communication skills is likely to become even greater in the years ahead. Meanwhile, if the goals of efficiency and effectivess are to be attained, self-supervision strategies (Casey et al., 1988) must be cultivated at all levels.

SUMMARY

This chapter has provided you with an overview of CD supervision and the supervisory process. An integral educational and administrative function, supervision is multifaceted, encompassing a broad range of roles and activities that further professional growth and development at all levels in every work setting. Supervision is viewed as an ongoing process that contains certain elements and proceeds as a series of changing events along a continuum. Supervisors and supervisees assume various roles as the process unfolds.

Because of its basic importance to professional preparation and practice, supervision has developed as an area of interest and study in the field, involving individuals and organizations in collecting data, conducting research, disseminating information, and teaching others about the topic. As our discipline and professions continue to undergo substantial, rapid change, there is an ever-increasing need for analysis of the supervisory process and refinement of supervisory practice. Those who supervise and the quality of their supervision will shape, to a great extent, our professional future.

DISCUSSION QUESTIONS

1. Identify five supervisory activities that you have experienced, either directly or indirectly, in CD academic, service, and other work settings. Compare and discuss the differences and similarities in supervisory approach.
2. In your view, what have been the most significant developments in the CD supervision movement and what impact have they had on our field?
3. Discuss the concepts of role diversity, role interdependence, and role perception as they relate to your past supervision experiences and your expectations for future supervision experiences.
4. Select several of the 13 tasks of CD clinical supervision (ASHA, 1985) and suggest specific ways in which each might be discussed between a supervisor and supervisee during the understanding and planning stages (Anderson, 1988).
5. Visualize yourself in a supervisor or supervisee role, carrying out a specific, real or hypothetical work activity. Where appropriate, identify your place in these continuum tracks—education, learning, and professional development, as well as supervision (Anderson, 1988). Discuss the supervisory implications.

REFERENCES

American Speech and Hearing Association. (1972). Task Force on Supervision in the Schools. Supervision and continuing professional education. *Language, Speech, and Hearing Services in Schools, 3*(3), 3–17.

American Speech and Hearing Association. (1975a). News and announcements: Schools, hospitals, and clinics. *Asha, 17,* 238.

American Speech and Hearing Association. (1975b). Report of the legislative council: Supervision in speech pathology and audiology. *Asha, 17,* 175–176.

American Speech-Language-Hearing Association. (1978). Committee on Supervision in Speech-Language Pathology and Audiology. Current status of supervision of speech-language pathology and audiology. *Asha, 20,* 478–486.

American Speech-Language-Hearing Association. (1980). *Standards for accreditation by the Education and Training Board.* Rockville, MD: Author.

American Speech-Language-Hearing Association. (1981). Requirements for the certificates of clinical competence. *Asha, 23*(4), 287–291.

American Speech-Language-Hearing Association. (1983). New standards for accreditation by the Professional Services Board. *Asha, 25*(6), 51–58.

American Speech-Language-Hearing Association. (1985). Committee on Supervision in Speech-Language Pathology and Audiology. Clinical supervision in speech-language pathology and audiology. A position statement. *Asha, 27*(6), 57–60.

American Speech-Language-Hearing Association. (1990a). *Clinical supervision across settings: Communication and collaboration. Proceedings of the 1989 ASHA Workshop on Supervision.* Rockville, MD: Author.

American Speech-Language-Hearing Association. (1990b). A plan for special interest divisions and study sections. *Asha, 32*(2), 59–61.

American Speech-Language-Hearing Association. (1991). Related professional organizations (RPOs). *Asha, 33*(6/7), 11–12.

American Speech-Language-Hearing Association. (1992). *ASHA membership and certification handbook* (rev.). Rockville, MD: Author.

Anderson, J. L. (Ed.). (1970). *Conference on supervision of speech and hearing programs in the schools.* Bloomington, IN: Indiana University.

Anderson, J. L. (Ed.). (1980). *Proceedings of the Conference on Training in the Supervisory Process in Speech-Language Pathology and Audiology.* Bloomington: Indiana University.

Anderson, J. L. (1981). Training of supervisors in speech-language pathology and audiology. *Asha, 23,* 77–82.

Anderson, J. L. (1988). *The supervisory process in speech-language pathology and audiology.* Boston: College-Hill Press/Little, Brown.

Anderson, J. L., Brasseur, J. A., Casey, P. L., Hunt-Thompson, J., Laccinole, M. D., McCrea, E., Rassi, J. A., Smith, K. J., & Ulrich, S. R. (1989). Preparation models for the supervisory process in speech-language pathology and audiology. *Asha, 31*(3), 97–106.

Anderson, J. L., & Kirtley, D. (Eds.). (1966). *Institute on supervision of speech and hearing programs in the public schools.* Indianapolis: Department of Public Instruction.

Bernthal, J. E. (Ed.). (1985). *Proceedings of the Sixth Annual Conference on Graduate Education.* Council of Graduate Programs in Communication Sciences and Disorders. Lincoln: University of Nebraska.

Bess, F. H. (1992). Total quality management (TQM): Philosophy, rationale, principles, benefits, outcomes. In S. Dowling (Ed.), *Total quality supervision: Effecting optimal performance. Proceedings of a National Conference on Supervision* (pp. 17–26). Houston: University of Houston.

Brasseur, J. A. (1987). Preparation of supervisees for the supervisory process. In S. S. Farmer (Ed.), *Clinical Supervision: A coming of age. Proceedings of a National Conference on Supervision* (pp. 144–163). Las Cruces: New Mexico State University.

Casey, P. L., Smith, K. J., & Ulrich, S. R. (1988). *Self-supervision: A career tool for audiologists and speech-language pathologists.* (Clinical Series 10). Rockville, MD: National Student Speech Language Hearing Association.

Cochran, P. S., & Bull, G. L. (1992). Computer-assisted learning and instruction. In J.A. Rassi & M.D. McElroy (Eds.), *The education of audiologists and speech-language pathologists* (pp. 363–386). Timonium, MD: York Press.

Cogan, M. L. (1973). *Clinical supervision.* Boston: Houghton Mifflin.

Conture, E. (1973). *Special study institute: Management and supervision of programs for speech and hearing handicapped.* Syracuse, NY: Syracuse University.

Crago, M. B., & Pickering, M. (Eds.). (1987). *Supervision in human communication disorders: Perspectives on a process.* Boston: College-Hill Press/Little, Brown.

Darley, F. (Ed.). (1961). Public school speech and hearing services. *Journal of Speech and Hearing Disorders: Monograph Supplement, 8.* Washington, DC: American Speech and Hearing Association.

Doehring, D. G. (1987). Research on human communication disorders supervision. In M. B. Crago & M. Pickering (Eds.), *Supervision in human communication disorders: Perspectives on a process* (pp. 81–106). Boston: College-Hill Pres/Little, Brown.

Dowling, S. (1989). Research: Past, present, future. In S. S. Farmer & J. L. Farmer (Eds.), *Supervision in communication disorders* (pp. 314–350). Columbus, OH: Merrill.

Dowling, S. (1992a). Impact of supervisor training upon the development of supervisory philosophies. In S. Dowling (Ed.), *Total quality supervision: Effecting optimal performance. Proceedings of a national conference on supervision* (pp. 106–110). Houston: University of Houston.

Dowling, S. (1992b). *Implementing the supervisory process. Theory and practice.* Englewood Cliffs, NJ: Prentice-Hall.

Dowling, S. (Ed.). (1992c). *Total quality supervision: Effecting optimal performance. Proceedings of a national conference on supervision.* Houston: University of Houston.

Farmer, S. S. (Ed.). (1987). *Clinical supervision: A coming of age. Proceedings of a national conference on supervision.* Las Cruces: New Mexico State University.

Farmer, S. S. (1989a). Supervision in communication disorders: Evolution of a profession. In S. S. Farmer & J. L. Farmer (Eds.), *Supervision in communication disorders* (pp. 2–13). Columbus, OH: Merrill.

Farmer, S. S. (1989b). The trigonal model of communication disorders supervision: Constituents. In S. S. Farmer & J. L. Farmer (Eds.), *Supervision in communication disorders* (pp. 16–52). Columbus, OH: Merrill.

Farmer, S. S., & Farmer, J. L. (1989). *Supervision in communication disorders.* Columbus, OH: Merrill.

Frattali, C. M. (1992). TQM: Applications to clinical supervision. In S. Dowling (Ed.), *Total quality supervision: Effecting optimal performance. Proceedings of a national conference on supervision* (pp. 27–31). Houston: University of Houston.

Gavett, E. (1987). Career development: An issue for the master's degree supervisor. In M. B. Crago & M. Pickering (Eds.), *Supervision in human communication disorders: Perspectives on a process* (pp. 55–78). Boston: College-Hill Press/Little, Brown.

Gillam, R .B., Strike Roussos, C., & Anderson, J. L. (1990). Facilitating changes in supervisees' clinical behaviors: An experimental investigation of supervisory effectiveness. *Journal of Speech and Hearing Disorders, 55,* 729–739.

Godden, A. (1990–1991). Canadian supervisors report. *SUPERvision, 15*(1), 17–18.

Goldhammer, R. (1969). *Clinical supervision.* New York: Holt, Rinehart and Winston.

Hagler, P. (1991, November). *Constructs, principles, and practices: A 'different' view of clinical education.* Miniseminar presented at the annual convention of the American Speech-Language-Hearing Association, Atlanta.

Halfond, M. (1964). Clinical supervision—Stepchild in training. *Asha, 6,* 441–444.

Hart, G. M. (1982). *The process of clinical supervision.* Baltimore: University Park Press.

Kirtley, D. (Ed.). (1967). *Supervision of student teaching in speech and hearing therapy.* Indianapolis: Indiana Department of Public Instruction.

Kleffner, F. (Ed.). (1964). *Seminar on Guidelines for the Internship Year.* Washington, DC: American Speech and Hearing Association.

Larson, L. (1982). Perceived supervisory needs and expectations of experienced vs. inexperienced student clinicians. *Dissertation Abstracts International, 42*, 4758B. (University Microfilms No. 82–11, 183)

Leith, W. R., McNiece, E. M., & Fusilier, B. B. (1989). *Handbook of supervision: A cognitive behavioral system.* Boston: College-Hill Press/Little, Brown.

McCready, V., Runyan, S. E., Farmer, S. S., Rassi, J. A., Ringwalt, S. S., & Ulrich, S. R. (1989). CFY supervision: A supervisors' exchange. *SUPERvision 13*(3), 15–18.

Miner, A. (Ed.). (1967). A symposium. Improving supervision of clinical practicum. *Asha, 9*, 471–481.

Oratio, A. R. (1977.). *Supervision in speech pathology. A handbook for supervisors and clinicians.* Baltimore: University Park Press.

Peaper, R. (1991). Research Net Report. *SUPERvision, 15*(2), 5–6.

Pickering, M. (1987). Expectation and intent in the supervisory process. *The Clinical Supervisor, 5*(4), 43–57.

Rassi, J. A. (1978). *Supervision in audiology.* Baltimore: University Park Press.

Rassi, J. A., & McElroy, M. D. (1992a). Education in the clinic. In J. A. Rassi & M. D. McElroy (Eds.), *The education of audiologists and speech-language pathologists* (pp. 175–196). Timonium, MD: York Press.

Rassi, J. A., & McElroy, M. D. (Eds.). (1992b). *The education of audiologists and speech-language pathologists.* Timonium, MD: York Press.

Rushakoff, G. E., & Farmer, S. S. (1989). Supervision applications of microcomputer technology. In S. S. Farmer & J. L. Farmer (Eds.), *Supervision in communication disorders* (pp. 250–272). Columbus, OH: Merrill.

Schubert, G. W. (1978). *Introduction to clinical supervision in speech pathology.* St. Louis, MO: Warren H. Green, Inc.

Shapiro, D. A. (Ed.). (1989). *Supervision: Innovations. Proceedings of a National Conference on Supervision.* Council of Supervisors in Speech-Language Pathology and Audiology.

Shapiro, D. A., & Anderson, J. L. (1989). One measure of supervisory effectiveness in speech-language pathology and audiology. *Journal of Speech and Hearing Disorders, 54*, 549–557.

Staff. (1975). Welcome to CUSPSPA. *Newsletter of Council of University Supervisors of Practicum in Speech Pathology and Audiology*, p. 3.

Staff. (1982). CUSPSPA SUPERNET: Goals and Coordinators. *SUPERvision, 6*(1), 11–15.

Staff. (1991–1992). Minutes of the Executive Board of the Council of Supervisors in Speech-Language Pathology and Audiology. *SUPERvision, 16*(1), 4–8.

Strike, C., & Gillam, R. (1988). Toward practical research in supervision. In J. L. Anderson (Ed.), *The supervisory process in speech-language pathology and audiology* (pp. 273–298). Boston: College-Hill Press/Little, Brown.

Tihen, L. (1984). Expectations of student speech/language clinicians during their clinical practicum. *Dissertation Abstracts International, 44*, 3048B. (University Microfilms No. 84-01, 620)

Turton, L. J. (Ed.). (1973). *Proceedings of a Workshop on Supervision in Speech Pathology.* Ann Arbor: University of Michigan, Institute for the Study of Mental Retardation and Related Disabilities.

Ulrich, S. R. (1987). A developing specialty. In M.B. Crago & M. Pickering (Eds.), *Supervision in human communication disorders: Perspectives on a process* (pp. 3–29). Boston: College-Hill Press/Little, Brown.

Villareal, J. J. (Ed.). (1964). *Seminar on Guidelines for Supervision of Clinical Practicum in Programs of Training for Speech Pathologists and Audiologists.* Washington, DC: American Speech and Hearing Association.

Webster's ninth new collegiate dictionary (1990). Springfield, MA: Merriam-Webster.

CHAPTER 24

Functional Assessment

■ CAROL FRATTALI, Ph.D. ■

SCOPE OF CHAPTER

Functional assessment encompasses an aspect of clinical evaluation that measures a person's ability to perform daily life activities. Although recognized and used as a clinical tool since the early 1960s (e.g., Katz, Ford, Moskowitz, Jackson, & Jaffee, 1963; Mahoney & Barthel, 1965; Sarno, 1965), functional assessment has gained prominence only recently as both clinical and policymaking tools (e.g., Frattali, 1992, 1993; Hosek et al., 1986; Kane, 1987; Wilkerson, Batavia, & DeJong, 1992). It is distinguished from more traditional diagnostic assessment that describes the type, nature, and severity of specific impairments. Rather, functional assessment measures the level of disability that can result from an impairment. Described simply, it measures the functional consequences of an impairment.

Cast in the domain of speech-language pathology and audiology, functional assessment describes a person's ability to communicate despite the presence of impairments such as aphasia, dysarthria, or hearing loss. It is important to recognize that a one-to-one relationship between the level of impairment and level of disability may not exist. For example, a person with moderate aphasia may be quite proficient in communication, whereas a person with mild aphasia may be less proficient, depending on the ability to compensate for specific language deficits. Furthermore, two individuals with comparable levels of impairment may have disparate levels of disability. If disability is measured in terms of an individual's ability to return to work, a speech disorder may, for example, be far more disabling for a radio announcer than for a professional dancer. Therefore, functional assessment adds a dimension to evaluation that not only enhances clinical decision making and care planning at the level of the individual, but holds considerable weight in shaping public policy at state and national levels. Today, functional outcome measures have gained widespread recognition among service providers, payers, accreditation agencies, and government regulators as instruments that can yield objective data to determine candidacy for treatment, the cost/benefit of treatment, payment rates, discharge destination, and the quality of care.

The purposes of this chapter are threefold. First, functional assessment is defined and its uses described from policy making and clinical perspectives. Second, a sample of currently available measures will be introduced and reviewed. Finally, the limitations of these measures will be summarized as will current activities underway to refine them in attempts to attain greater sensitivity, reliability, validity, and usability. It is hoped that, as a result of this review, you will gain an appreciation for the value of functional assessment from both clinical and policy making points of view. You also will be steered in directions for future activities if you wish to advance this area of client assessment.

FUNCTIONAL
ASSESSMENT DEFINED

As mentioned above, functional assessment encompasses the measurement of a person's ability to perform daily life activities (e.g., walking, eating, toileting, dressing, communicating) despite the presence of a disease, disorder, or impairment. Before a definition can be formulated, however, you must appreciate the underlying conceptual framework within which such assessment fits. The World Health Organization (WHO) International Classification of Impairments, Disabilities, and Handicaps (World Health Organization, 1980) is recognized widely as a typology that sequences the possible consequences of a disease or disorder and, thus, suggests different types of assessment at each point along the continuum. The WHO classifications are described as follows:

Impairment is an abnormality of psychological, physiological, or anatomical structure or function at the organ level. Examples of impairment include paralysis; amputation; cognitive disorders; speech, swallowing or language disorders; and hearing loss.

Disability is a restriction or lack of ability manifested in the performance of daily tasks. A disability, then, is the functional consequence of an impairment. Examples of disability include difficulties in dressing, toileting, feeding, money management, and communication.

Handicap is a social, economic, or environmental disadvantage resulting from an impairment or disability. A handicap is defined, in large measure, by societal attitudes about individuals with disabilities. Examples of handicap are joblessness, dependency, and social isolation.

Batavia (1992) concisely summarizes the WHO typology: Impairment involves an aberration from the norm occurring at the organ level; disability involves a functional limitation occurring at the individual level; handicap involves a social disadvantage resulting from the relationship between the individual's disability and that person's environment. Consider, for example, a person with cerebral vascular disease who sustains a stroke. Stroke can result in aphasia (impairment), which, in turn, can result in communication difficulties (disability) and, thus, social isolation and joblessness (handicap). In the context of prevention, Batavia states, "with appropriate rehabilitative interventions, an impairment does not necessarily result in a disability. Similarly, with appropriate social and environmental interventions, a disability does not necessarily result in a handicap" (p. 3).

Another conceptual framework is proposed by Nagi (1965). Nagi's taxonomy of disability includes the elements of active pathology, impairment, functional limitation, and disability, which are described as:

Active pathology: Interruption or interference with normal processes and efforts of the organism to regain normal state.

Impairment: Anatomical, physiological, mental, or emotional abnormalities or loss.

Functional limitation: Restriction or lack of ability to perform an action or activity in the manner or within the range considered normal that results from impairment.

Disability: Inability or limitation in performing socially defined activities or roles expected of individuals within a sociocultural and physical environment.

If these two typologies are compared, Nagi's (1965) definition of functional limitation coincides with the WHO's (1980) definition of disability, and his definition of disability coincides with the WHO's definition of handicap.

The professions of speech-language pathology and audiology historically have focused clinical evaluation procedures at the level of impairment. A plethora of traditional diagnostic tests and instrumental procedures attest to the almost exclusive focus on measurement of specific physiological and behavioral deficits. These instruments have been designed for differential diagnosis and detailed description of such specific impairments as hearing loss, aphasia, dysarthria, voice or fluency disorders, apraxia, language delay, and dysphagia.

If you proceed along the continuum of the consequences of a disease or disorder, the next level of measurement would be that of functional assessment. Functional assessment is recognized widely as a measure of disability; thus, it measures the impact of impairment. Until recently, far less attention has been devoted to this level of measurement, and as a result, far fewer instruments are available.

The measurement parameters of handicap are the least well defined, with some asserting that functional assessment should capture level of handicap as well as disability (Batavia, 1992). Others believe that handicap is best measured by so-called quality of life measures, or handicap inventories. These measures examine more individually defined dimensions or expressions of life's experiences (e.g., perceived health status, mood, emotional control, return to work, learning and education, and leisure activities) (Flanagan, 1982). Thus, they are considered to be the most subjective of measures, usually designed as interviews or self-administered questionnaires (National Institute on Disability and Rehabilitation Research, 1990).

Within the framework of the WHO typology, as well as the discipline of human com-

munication sciences and disorders, the concepts of functional communication and functional assessment of communication can be defined. An advisory panel of the American Speech-Language-Hearing Association (ASHA), appointed to make recommendations for refinement of ASHA's Functional Communication Measures (ASHA, 1990), offered the following definition: "Functional communication is the ability to receive or convey a message, regardless of the mode, to communicate effectively and independently in a given environment" (p. 2).

The definition reflects a more holistic concept of communication, rather than one that compartmentalizes communication into its specific behavioral processes of, for example, speech intelligibility, verbal expression, auditory comprehension, and use of gestures. A more global description of communication is also offered by Sarno (1983). According to Sarno, communication effectiveness is "the total of the myriad of factors which contribute to the transmission of information" (p. 77). Consistent with the distinguishing features of impairment and disability, Sarno elaborates:

The impact of a verbal impairment on interpersonal interactions, on the use of verbal activities for leisure (i.e., watching TV), on the ability to resume employment, on the overall effect on the quality of life, and on the patient's ability to compensate and/or circumvent the deficits all play a part in the patient's effectiveness as a communicator. (p. 77)

With consensus on a definition of functional communication, the ASHA Advisory Panel (ASHA, 1990) proceeded to define functional assessment of communication as:

Measurement of the extent of ability to communicate with others in a variety of contexts, considering environmental modifications, adaptive equipment, time required to communicate, and listener familiarity with the client. Special accommodations of the communicative partner to either receive or enhance reception must be considered. (p. 2)

Once defined and framed conceptually, you can look with a more critical eye at the various functional communication instruments currently available. You can also determine the appropriateness of instrument use.

USES OF FUNCTIONAL ASSESSMENT

You should be aware that functional assessment has several intended uses. From a clinical practice perspective, functional assessment can provide vital information about a person's level of disability resulting from an impairment, Thus, it can aid in treatment and discharge planning as well as client and family counseling. From a clinical research perspective, reliable and valid functional assessment can provide information about treatment outcome and, thus, can aid in building scientific evidence of treatment efficacy, effectiveness, and efficiency. From a policy making perspective, functional assessment can provide information about a person's candidacy for treatment and the cost/benefit of treatment. Thus, for patient populations, functional assessment can help to shape public policy (e.g., by defining service eligibility criteria, setting payment rates, and judging the quality of care). The ensuing discussion will serve to broaden your perspective by presenting information from two vantage points: that of the policymaker and the clinician.

POLICYMAKERS' VIEWS

In the United States, the notion of functional assessment as a means for setting payment rates for rehabilitative services emerged after Medicare's Prospective Payment System was instituted in 1983. At that time Medicare, the federal health program for the elderly, restructured its payment system for inpatient hospital care in an effort to prevent bankruptcy from spiraling health care costs. The Medicare system now pays hospitals a predetermined fee for the average length of stay and range of hospital services for patients who are categorized into diagnosis related groups (DRGs). If hospital costs exceed the flat payment, hospitals absorb the loss; if costs fall below the flat payment, they keep the difference. Clearly, the new payment system provides strong incentives to curtail services and provide more cost efficient care. Inpatient rehabilitation units and outpatient services have been exempt (however subject to other payment limits) from the prospective payment system. But, as these exempt services grew at unprecedented rates, they too became earmarked for development of a prospective payment methodology.

The first major study to investigate the feasibility of a prospective payment system for rehabilitation was conducted in 1986 (Hosek et al., 1986). This study identified functional assessment as a means to develop a payment methodology for inpatient rehabilitative services by testing the hypothesis that functional status, rather than diagnosis, determines the cost of a hospital rehabilitative stay (Hosek et al., 1986). Hosek and her colleagues found a strong relationship between charges for rehabilitative care and functional status. In contrast, diagnosis did not prove to be a good predictor of charges. The investigators concluded that a prospective payment system for rehabilitation should be based on functional status, rather than diagnosis.

This study led a trail of others in attempts to develop a new payment system for rehabilitation (e.g., Kane, in progress; McGinnis et al., 1987; National Association of Rehabilitation Facilities, 1985; Wilkerson, Batavia, & DeJong, 1992). Yet, to date, a new payment methodology has not been proposed. It is speculated that the difficulty lies, in large part, with the lack of reliable and valid functional status measures available in the field.

Nevertheless, new federal laws and regulations, as well as national accreditation standards and payer guidelines, proceeded to emphasize the value of functional assessment by identifying it as a means of defining service eligibility criteria, justifying continuation of treatment, and judging the quality of care. For example, the Joint Commission on Accreditation of Healthcare Organizations (1994) requires that, on referral for rehabilitation services, a functional assessment is performed by a qualified professional. In addition, Medicare outpatient guidelines (Health Care

Financing Administration, 1989b) require speech-language pathologists to document the initial and present functional communication status of the client. The Medicare guidelines direct claims reviewers to pay a claim only if there is reasonable expectation that significant improvement in the client's overall functional ability will occur.

Particularly troublesome to clinicians and researchers is the move to rely solely on functional assessment data to make broad policy decisions about who receives what services and how these services will be reimbursed. Such activities are viewed as premature in light of the reported shortcomings of available instruments. Policymakers, on the other hand, have disputed this position, arguing that tools need not be overly sophisticated during a time of urgency for health care reform.

CLINICIANS' VIEWS

Despite the pressures of recent and impending public policy, which places considerable weight on functional assessment as a powerful measurement tool, functional assessment continues to lag behind the use of impairment measures. The trend is beginning to shift, however, as clinicians realize that functional outcome data can justify treatment and its reimbursement for individuals with communication and related disabilities. The trend, although recent, has long been supported by several experts in the field who have provided clear justification for incorporating functional assessment into routine clinical evaluation procedures. Thus, it would be a supplement to, not replacement of, traditional measures.

Sarno (1965) was among the first investigators in the field to recognize a distinction between an assessment of language and communication—although more traditional clinical tests are designed to discover what residuals a client may have in each language modality, functional tests assess what the client does in attempts to circumvent the language impairment. In this sense, Sarno believes that clinical tests are more often a measure of potential than actual language use. Other investigators have found that an assessment of impairment does not coincide with an assessment of disability (e.g., Aten, 1986; Bess, Logan, Lichtenstein, & Burger, 1989; Sarno, 1965). In fact, an inverse relationship between the findings of language impairment and communication disability is not unusual. This inverse relationship is described by Aten (1986): "Speaking fluently is not necessarily communicative, as patients with Wernicke's aphasia so vividly demonstrate. Conversely, the essentially mute patient, labeled mixed or Broca's type, may communicate a great deal in his or her animated, head nodding, nonlinguistic way" (p. 266). Bess and colleagues (1989) describe the same inverse relationship as it relates to hearing: "Some individuals with a mild hearing loss may experience a substantial disability and handicap, whereas others with a moderate hearing loss may not exhibit any form of disability or handicap" (p. 795). Finally, Murray, Marquardt, Richardson, and Nalty (1984) tested the hypothesis that patients with Alzheimer's disease appear to have more communicative competence than they actually do, given their ability to talk fluently until the later stages of the disease, and that patients with aphasia appear to have less communicative competence than they actually do, given their impaired language abilities. These investigators administered the *Communicative Abilities in Daily Living* (CADL) (Holland, 1980) to assess communication skills, and the *Porch Index of Communicative Abilities* (PICA) (Porch, 1971) to assess the speech and language skills of 10 individuals with aphasia and 10 individuals with dementia. Findings showed that the dementia group scored significantly better than the aphasia group on the PICA, and the aphasia group scored significantly better than the dementia group on the CADL. These findings, thus, confirmed the hypothesized inverse relationship between communication and language skills.

If assessment of speech, language, or hearing does not coincide with assessment of communication, it would seem reasonable that functional assessment of communication be incorporated routinely into the speech-language pathologist's and audiologist's standard battery of tests, not as a replacement but as a supplement to traditional diagnostic measures. Certainly, from the client's point of view, this level of assessment would be more meaningful because it is framed in terms of daily life activities. Furthermore, functional assessment is more meaningful to referral sources, such as physicians and teachers, who wish to know how specific impairments will affect an individual's ability to communicate basic needs, express thoughts and ideas, and converse with others, and, in turn, live independently, return to work or learn in school, and engage in social activities. Nevertheless, clinicians have not routinely incorporated functional assessment into their standard evaluation procedures. But increasingly, the reason lies less with a preoccupation on measurement of impairment than with the perceived lack of sufficient functional assessment instruments from which to choose. Most clinicians will agree that there are good clinical reasons for assessing the functional communication of clients. They acknowledge that formal asessment alone is likely to miss the often very effective strategies and resources used by the client (Sacchett & Marshall, 1992). This clinical perspective extends beyond the geographic boundaries of the United States and is shared by colleagues in other countries. In the clinical aphasiology world, Worrall (1992) reports that functional communication is viewed as important. Nevertheless, many clinicians are not using any of the available instruments. In a recent audit of client files in Brisbane, Australia, it was noted that no published functional communication assessments were used (Smith-Worrall & Burtenshaw, 1990). Similarly, a survey of British clinicians (Smith & Parr, 1986) found that most viewed functional communication as a very important goal of therapy, but available instruments fell short of their needs. The two major reasons for limited assessment of functional communication offered by the Australian clinicians were the perceived inadequacy of existing instruments and the clinicians' preference for informal observational assessments.

Given these perspectives on functional assessment, as well as an appreciation for its several intended uses, you can evaluate available instruments in terms of their sensitivity, validity, reliability, and usability. You should, however, approach this review with caution. Although all the viewpoints above are justifiable, you may never find a single tool that will suit all needs. In fact, all viewpoints may never converge to design a universally accepted tool. States Carey (1990):

It would, of course, be ideal to have a single instrument that would serve as the perfect clinical assessment tool, the perfect program evaluation tool, and the perfect management information system. It would also be ideal if someone could invent a vehicle that would have the luxury of a big car, the fuel efficiency of a small car, and the flexibility of a truck designed for hauling farm machinery. It is unlikely that such a vehicle will appear in the near future. (p. 234)

With Carey's (1990) words in mind, the following review identifies three categories of functional assessment instruments, each of which address functional communication: global instruments, rehabilitation-focused instruments, and communication-focused instruments.

A REVIEW OF SELECT MEASURES

As explained in earlier articles (Frattali, 1992, 1993), which included reviews of functional status measures, the design of an assessment tool is determined by the purposes for which it was developed. Thus, the scope (the range of functions measured) and precision (the sensitivity of the instrument to capturing gradations of change for particular functions) of available measures vary widely.

This variation is dependent on several factors including the user (e.g., clinician, researcher, policymaker), the setting in which used (e.g., hospital, rehabilitation facility, speech and hearing clinic), and intended uses (e.g., care planning, outcome evaluation, screening for referral, and resource allocation). If, for example, the tool is to be used as a screening instrument across the broad range of disabilities for purposes of referral, a more global and less sensitive instrument will fit the need. If, on the other hand, a tool is to be used for more in-depth assessment of specific disabilities for purposes of care and discharge planning or treatment outcome determinations, a more focused tool with sufficient sensitivity to capture functionally important change over time should be used.

In terms of setting, you will find that more global tools will be used in nursing facilities or hospitals to capture a broad range of disability for a larger mix of clients, and more focused tools will be used in speech and hearing clinics for a smaller mix of clients, namely, those with communication and related disabilities. The basic characteristics of select instruments, applicable for adult populations and in more widespread use in the field, are summarized in Tables 24–1 and 24–2.

GLOBAL INSTRUMENTS

Global instruments are those that measure the broadest range of disabilities, usually at a relatively low level of precision. They often are used to determine an individual's level of need as well as the need for referral to other specialists.

Two global instruments of current interest are those recently developed as a result of federal mandates, the Omnibus Budget Reconciliation Act of 1986 that mandated the development of a uniform needs assessment for hospital discharge planning, and the Omnibus Budget Reconciliation Act of 1987 that mandated the development of an assessment for residents in nursing facilities.

The *Assessment of Needs for Continuing Care* (ANCC) (Health Care Financing Administration, 1989a) includes an assessment of such areas as health status, functional status, family and community support, and environmental factors in postdischarge care. This instrument addresses communication in a separate section, which is rated on a 4-point scale of independence. Another global mea-

sure, the *Minimum Data Set for Nursing Home Resident Assessment and Care Screening* (Morris et al., 1991), is used for screening purposes in nursing facilities. Assessment domains include, in part, cognitive patterns, vision patterns, physical functioning and structural problems, continence, and psychosocial well-being. Communication and hearing patterns are addressed as a separate subsection of the instrument and are rated on a 4-point scale. This level of measurement is appropriate for screening, referral, and need determinations but does not provide sufficient information needed for more detailed care planning.

At the time of this writing, the MDS was undergoing further reliability and validity testing and the ANCC had yet to be field tested. Thus, any conclusive statements about the tools' psychometric properties remain premature. Communication assessment, as addressed by both tools, is characterized by a receptive-expressive dichotomy. Other modes of communication, however, are recognized. In addition, the MDS includes an assessment of hearing.

REHABILITATION-FOCUSED INSTRUMENTS

In general, rehabilitation-focused instruments are more limited in scope, yet more precise in their level of measurement when compared to global instruments. These instruments address functions commonly addressed by the multidisciplinary field of rehabilitation. They include, for example, mobility, dressing, feeding, communication, cognitive function, and psychosocial adjustment. Most of these instruments are designed as rating scales and a 5- to 7-point scale is common. The increase in levels, when compared to the global measures, is thought to increase measurement sensitivity and, thus, to capture more functional change.

Attempts at increasing a tool's sensitivity often are found in the number of modalities measured. In the case of rehabilitation-focused measures, communication is now segmented into additional component processes, including hearing, reading, production of written language, speech production, and use of assistive communication devices.

Many of the rehabilitation-focused instruments are criticized for their incomplete documentation of reliability and validity. Often the tools' psychometric properties are based on unpublished data. Of greater concern, however, is the conceptual framework in which such tools were developed, particularly as it relates to assessment of communication. As evidenced by this review, many of the rehabilitation-focused instruments measure communication at the level of impairment, rather than disability, because they measure communication by its component processes. If you refer to the previous definitions of functional communication and functional communication assessment, you may agree that these rehabilitation-focused instruments do not reflect an integrative concept of communication. This conceptual issue, however, is one that developers of functional communication instruments have addressed.

COMMUNICATION-FOCUSED INSTRUMENTS

As would be expected, the communication-focused instruments offer the most in-depth assessment of functional communication when compared to global and rehabilitation-focused instruments. These instruments, developed within the discipline of human communication sciences and disorders, are used primarily by speech-language pathologists and audiologists for the purposes of planning care, counseling clients and their families, providing information to other professionals involved in the care of the client, and documenting the outcome of treatment.

It was Martha Taylor Sarno (1965) who introduced the concept of functional communication assessment in the field, and Audrey Holland (1980) who introduced a more integrative conceptual framework for functional communication instruments. For example,

rather than assessing communication by its specific modalities (e.g., auditory comprehension, verbal expression, use of gestures, speech intelligibility), a more integrative framework was devised that allowed measurement of communication in various contexts (e.g., communication of basic needs, and conversation with a partner).

Sarno's (1965) *Functional Communication Profile* (FCP), although adhering to a modality-specific framework, consists of 45 integrated communication behaviors considered common language functions of everyday life, classified into five modalities: movement (e.g., gesture), speaking, understanding, reading, and miscellaneous (e.g., writing, calculation). The FCP uses a 9-point rating scale. In contrast, Holland's (1980) *Communicative Abilities in Daily Living* (CADL) is based on a more holistic communication model. It assesses functional communication in three areas: content/form (i.e., production and comprehension), cognition (e.g., appreciation for humor, untangling cause-effect relationships), and use (i.e., role playing and speech acts such as explaining and requesting). The CADL has 68 items, rated on a 3-point scale, incorporating everyday language activities.

Two more recent tools of interest are the *Communicative Effectiveness Index* (Lomas et al., 1989), and the *Revised Edinburgh Functional Communication Profile* (Wirz, Skinner, & Dean, 1990). Both instruments borrow from Holland's theoretical construct by addressing communication in a more integrative manner. The CETI assesses communication for social needs (e.g., dinner table conversation), life skills (e.g., use of telephone, understanding traffic symbols), basic needs (e.g., communication of basic needs such as toileting, eating), and health threats (e.g., calling for help after falling). The *Revised Edinburgh Functional Communication Profile* measures the communication functions of greetings, acknowledging, responding, requesting, and initiating.

Two measures that exclusively assess hearing include the *Hearing Handicap Inventory for the Elderly* (Ventry & Weinstein, 1982) and the

TABLE 24–1. CHARACTERISTICS OF SELECTED FUNCTIONAL STATUS MEASURES.

Instrument	Instrument Class	Domains	Assessment — Aspects of Communication Addressed	Method	Reliability/Validity
Functional Independence Measure (FIM) Version 4.0 (State University of New York at Buffalo, 1993)	Rehabilitation-focused	Self-care, sphincter control, mobility, locomotion, communication, social cognition.	Comprehension (auditory), expression (verbal), comprehension (visual), expression (nonverbal).	7-level ordinal scale from least independent to most independent.	Inter-rater reliability ranges from .88 to .93 for FIM 3.0 domain scores; and .82 to .91 for item scores. For eligible subscribers who participate in the Uniform Data System (UDS), inter-rater reliability ranges from .96 to .98 for FIM 3.0 domain scores, and .91 to .98 for FIM 3.0 item scores. The FIM is reported to have face validity and predictive validity (for minutes of help per day).
Patient Evaluation and Conference System (PECS) (Harvey & Jellinek, 1979, 1981)	Rehabilitation-focused	Functions related to rehabilitation medicine, rehabilitation nursing, physical mobility, ADL, communication, medications, nutrition, assistive devices, psychology, neuropsychology, social issues, vocational/educational activity, therapeutic recreation, pain, pulmonary rehabilitation, pastoral care.	Hearing, comprehension of spoken language, production of language, reading, production of written language, production of speech, swallowing, knowledge of assistive devices, skill with speaking with assistive communication devices, utilization of assistive communication devices, impairment in thought processing.	7-level ordinal scale from dependent to independent function.	Studies are ongoing. Preliminary studies found wide range of inter-rater reliability from .68 to .80. Content and construct validity are reported.
Level of Rehabilitation Scale-III (LORS III) (Carey & Posavac, 1982; Parkside Associates, 1986)	Rehabilitation-focused	ADL, mobility, communication, cognitive ability.	Auditory comprehension, oral expression, reading comprehension, written expression.	5-level interval scale	Inter-rater reliability for LORS IIB assessment domains ranges from .65 to .87. Inter-rater reliability for LORS III is conducted on an ongoing basis. Face validity for LORS III is reported.

314

Instrument	Focus	Domains assessed	Communication domains	Scale	Reliability/Validity
Rehabilitation Institute of Chicago Functional Assessment Scale-Version II (RIC-FAS II) (Heinemann, 1989)	Rehabilitation-focused	Functions related to the following services: nursing, physical therapy, occupational therapy, communicative disorders, psychology, social work, vocational rehabilitation, therapeutic recreation.	Hearing, auditory comprehension, oral expression, reading comprehension, written expression, speech production, chewing/swallowing, alternative/augmentative communication, money management.	7-level ordinal scale ranging from normal ability to severe disability.	Inter-rater reliability for RIC-FAS I ranged from .66 to 1 across item scores, with better than 75% to 100% agreement on most items. Studies on validity are underway.
Assessment of Needs for Continuing Care (ANCC) (HCFA, 1989)	Global	Health status, functional status (ADLs, IADLs), communication, environmental factors in postdischarge care, nursing and other care requirements, family and community support, patient/family goals and preferences, options for continuing care.	Comprehension, expression, usual mode(s) of communication.	4-level ordinal scale from independent to dependent function.	Information is not currently available.
Minimum Data Set for Nursing Home Resident Assessment and Care Screening (MDS) (Morris et al., 1991)	Global	Cognitive patterns, communication/hearing patterns, vision patterns, physical functioning and structural problems (including ADLs), continence, psychosocial well-being, mood and behavior patterns, activity pursuit patterns, disease diagnoses, health conditions, oral/nutritional status, oral/dental status, skin condition, medication use, special treatment and procedures.	Hearing, communication devices/techniques, modes of expression, making self understood, ability to understand others, change in communication/hearing.	4-level ordinal scale.	Based on published field test results, inter-rater reliability for key functional indicators in each assessment domain ranged from .47 to .91. Studies on validity are underway.

Source: Adapted from "Perspectives on Functional Assessment: Its Use for Policymaking" by C. Frattali, 1993, *Disability and Rehabilitation, 15*, pp. 1–9. Copyright 1993 by Taylor & Francis. Adapted by permission.

TABLE 24–2. CHARACTERISTICS OF SELECTED FUNCTIONAL COMMUNICATION INSTRUMENTS.

Instrument (reference)	Communication Components	Assessment Method	Applicable Populations	Reliability/Validity
Functional Communication Profile (FCP) (Sarno, 1969)	45 communication behaviors in the following areas: movement (e.g., gestures), speaking, understanding, reading, miscellaneous (e.g., writing, calculation).	9-point scale.	Adults with aphasia.	Concurrent and predictive validity (correlates with measures of auditory memory span and CADL); high inter-examiner reliability; test-retest reliability described as significant.
Communicative Abilities in Daily Living (CADL) (Holland, 1980)	68 items incorporating everyday language activities in the following areas: content/form (production, comprehension), cognition, use (role-playing, speech acts).	3-point scoring system (0= wrong, 1=adequate, 2=correct).	Adults with aphasia, mental retardation, or Alzheimer's disease; experienced users of hearing aids.	Concurrent validity [correlates with Boston Diagnostic Aphasia Examination (Goodglass & Kaplan, 1972), Porch Index of Communicative Ability (Porch, 1971, 1981), FCP, and direct observations of communication behavior]; high inter-examiner and test-retest reliability.
Hearing Handicap Inventory for the Elderly (HHIE) (Ventry & Weinstein, 1982)	25-item self-assessment questionnaire to identify perceived problems caused by hearing loss (i.e., emotional consequences and social and situational effects).	3-point scale (4=yes; 2=sometimes; 0=no).	Adults with hearing loss.	Reported reliability (by assessing internal consistency) as well as construct and content validity.
Self-Assessment of Communication (SAC) (Schow & Nerbonne, 1982)	10 self-assessment items addressing perceived difficulties in various communication situations, feelings about communication, and the reactions of others to one's hearing.	5-point scale (1=almost never/ never; 2=occasionally (about .25 of the time); 3=about half of the time; 4=frequently (about .75 time); 5=practically always/always.	Adults with hearing loss.	High test-retest and internal consistency, reliability, and is predictive of the extent of hearing impairment.
Communicative Effectiveness Index (CETI) (Lomas et al., 1989)	16 communication items categorized by social need, life skill, basic need, health threat.	10-cm visual analog scale from "not at all able" to "as able as before the stroke."	Adults with aphasia secondary to stroke.	On the basis of evaluation of 11 recovering and 11 stable aphasic patients, the tool appears to have good test-retest and inter-rater reliability; face and construct validity (correlates with global ratings of language and communication by spouses).
Revised Edinburgh Functional Communication Profile (EFCP) (Wirz, Skinner, & Dean, 1990)	Communication functions and modalities used: greetings, acknowledging, responding, requesting, initiating.	5-point effectiveness scale, and modality used is noted.	Adults with aphasia, developmental disorders, mental retardation, adults with cerebral palsy who use augmentative/alternative communication systems.	No concurrent validity; content validity evaluated by scoring 16 minute language samples and comparing with 10 exchanges; inter-rater reliability on 14 patients.

Source: Adapted from "Functional Assessment of Communication: Merging Public Policy with Clinical Views" by C. Frattali, 1992, *Aphasiology, 5,* 1, pp. 63–83. Copyright 1992 by Taylor & Francis. Adapted by permission. Adapted from *ASHA Functional Assessment of Communication Skills for Adults: Administration and Scoring Manual* (p. 10) by C. Frattali, C. Thompson, A. Holland, C. Wohl, and M. Ferketic, in progress, Rockville, MD: ASHA. Copyright 1994 by American-Speech-Language-Hearing Association. Adapted by permission.

Self-Assessment of Communication (Schow & Nerbonne, 1982). Although both instruments address measurement at the level of handicap (e.g., feelings of isolation, frustration, and dependency), they also provide important information on the perceived effect of a hearing impairment on daily function. The *Hearing Handicap Inventory for the Elderly* is fashioned as a self-administered questionnaire that requires a "yes," "no," or "sometimes" response to questions attempting to quantify the perceived emotional and social effects of hearing loss. The *Self-Assessment of Communication* is a 10-item questionnaire that samples the client's perception (using a 5-point scale) of the extent of the communication problems deriving from hearing loss.

LIMITATIONS OF AVAILABLE MEASURES

Despite the advances made in functional assessment, available instruments are deficient for various reasons. Many writers have judged that available functional communication instruments are incomplete in their documentation of psychometric properties (Skenes & McCauley, 1985), correlate poorly with observation of nonverbal communication (Behrmann & Penn, 1984), are not easy for the assessor to either administer or score (Houghton, Pettit, & Towey, 1982; Swisher, 1979), correlate so well with existing language measures that they probably are not measuring any separate dimension of communication (Holland, 1980), and have not been shown to be sufficiently sensitive to functionally important change over time.

If you were to summarize the limitations of available measures, you would conclude that available instruments have one or more of the following flaws. They are:

■ Limited in scope;
■ Conceptually flawed (i.e., assess at the level of impairment rather than disability; artificially tap functional communication behaviors)
■ Insufficiently sensitive to capturing functionally important change;

■ Weak in psychometric properties; (i.e., reliability and validity); and
■ Time-consuming to administer

By far, the most common problem identified among global and rehabilitation-focused measures is insufficient documentation of reliability and validity. Thus, the data derived from these measures are of questionable value and cannot be used, with any confidence, to make valid clinical or policy making decisions.

In summary, in the professions of speech-language pathology and audiology, there continues to be a need for functional communication instruments that are valid and reliable, easy to administer, and more sensitive to capturing functional communication changes. One project that is attempting to address these needs is underway by the American Speech-Language-Hearing Association (ASHA, 1993). ASHA's project, which is supported by a grant from the U.S. Department of Education's National Institute on Disability and Rehabilitation Research, is aimed at advancing the development of functional communication instruments by designing a valid and reliable tool that addresses communication in various natural contexts (e.g., communication of basic needs, social communication, daily planning). The project is tapping a broad level of expertise in the field, as well as in related fields of psychometrics and social psychology, to assist in this endeavor.

FUTURE DIRECTIONS

There is a clear need to advance the development of functional assessment instruments. The need becomes pressing in the wake of policy making that is relying heavily on functional outcome data to make weighty decisions about client care, and points to an area of research and development that is wide open to interested researchers and practitioners.

Acknowledging the reports of conceptual and technical deficiencies of available instruments, The American Congress of Rehabilitation Medicine appointed a Task Force on Measurement and Evaluation (Johnston, Keith, & Hinderer, 1992) to provide some direction to interested researchers and test developers in the multidisciplinary field of rehabilitation. The task force detailed general principles and technical standards that provide guidance in test development. Areas addressed include validity, reliability, norms and scaling, and technical manuals and guides. Also addressed are professional applications of measures including clinical applications, protecting the rights of persons being measured, program evaluation, and quality improvement.

These and other activities are directing researchers and test developers in the area of functional assessment. There is widespread recognition that collective and repeated contributions will be necessary to bring us closer to more accurate measurement of client needs in the context of daily life activities.

SUMMARY

Functional assessment carries considerable weight in deciding who will receive services, for how long, at what cost, and by whom. It becomes imperative, then, that available measures are sound in their design and psychometric properties. Once these tools are advanced to a point at which clinicians and policymakers can use them with confidence, better clinical and policy decisions will result. The next generation of functional communication instruments hopefully will solve the problems inherent in the tools currently available. Thus, there is much hope that you, as future clinicians and researchers, will successfully advance this area of assessment.

DISCUSSION QUESTIONS

1. Explain the difference between measures of impairment and disability; provide justification for why functional assessment cannot replace traditional diagnostic measures.

2. Describe the uses of functional assessment from both policy making and clinical perspectives.

3. Identify the limitations of available functional assessment measures.

4. Describe the desirable characteristics of a functional communication instrument.

5. Explain why two individuals with the same type and severity of impairment may have different levels of disability.

REFERENCES

American Speech-Language-Hearing Association. (1990). Functional communication scales for adults project: Advisory report. Rockville, MD: Author.

American Speech-Language-Hearing Association. (1993, Spring/Summer). Project Update, ASHA Functional Assessment of Communication Skills for Adults (ASHA FACS). Rockville, MD: Author.

Aten, J. L. (1986). Functional communication treatment. In R. Chapey (Ed.), *Language intervention strategies in adult aphasia* (2nd ed., pp. 266–276). Baltimore: Williams & Wilkins.

Batavia, A. I. (1992). Assessing the function of functional assessment: A consumer perspective. *Disability and Rehabilitation, 14*, 156–160.

Behrmann, M., & Penn, C. (1984). Non-verbal communication of aphasic patients. *British Journal of Disorders of Communication, 19*, 155–168.

Bess, F. H., Logan, S. A., Lichtenstein, M. J., & Burger, M. C. (1989). Comparing criteria of hearing impairment in the elderly: A functional approach. *Journal of Speech and Hearing Research, 32*, 795–802.

Carey, R. (1990). Advances in rehabilitation program evaluation. In M. R. Eisenberg & R. C. Grzesiak (Eds.), *Advances in clinical rehabilitation* (Vol. 3, pp. 217–250). New York: Springer.

Carey, R. G., & Posavac, E. J. (1982). Rehabilitation program evaluation using a revised Level of Rehabilitation Scale (LORS-II). *Archives of Physical Medicine and Rehabilitation, 63*, 367–376.

Flanagan, J. C. (1982). Measurement of quality of life: Current state of the art. *Archives of Physical Medicine and Rehabilitation, 63*, 56–59.

Frattali, C. M. (1992). Functional assessment of communication: Merging public policy with clinical views. *Aphasiology, 6*, 63–83.

Frattali, C. M. (1993). Perspectives on functional assessment: Its use for policymaking. *Disability and Rehabilitation, 15*, 1–9.

Harvey, R. F., & Jellinek, H. M. (1979). *PECS: Patient Evaluation Conference System*. Wheaton, IL: Marianjoy Rehabilitation Center.

Harvey, R. F., & Jellinek, H. M. (1981). Functional performance assessment: A program approach. *Archives of Physical Medicine and Rehabilitation, 63*, 43–52.

Health Care Financing Administration. (1989a). *Assessment of needs for continuing care* (Form HCFA-32; 10–89). Baltimore: Author.

Health Care Financing Administration. (1989b). *Medical outpatient therapy and comprehensive outpatient rehabilitation facility manual* (Section 502, Transmittal No. 87). Baltimore: Author.

Heinemann, A. W. (1989). *Rehabilitation Institute of Chicago—Functional Assessment Scale—Revised.* Chicago: Rehabilitation Institute of Chicago.

Holland, A. L. (1980). *Communicative Abilities in Daily Living: Manual.* Baltimore: University Park Press.

Hosek, S., Kane, R., Carney, M., Hartman, J., Reboussin, D., Serrato, C., & Melvin, J. (1986). *Charges and outcomes for rehabilitative care: Implications for the prospective payments system.* Santa Monica, CA: Rand.

Houghton, P. M., Pettit, J. M., & Towey, M. P. (1982). Measuring communication competence in global aphasia. In *Proceedings of the Clinical Aphasiology Conference* (pp. 28–39). Minneapolis, MN: Brookshire Publishers.

Johnston, M. V., Keith, R. A., & Hinderer, S. R. (1992). Measurement standards for interdisciplinary medical rehabilitation. *Archives of Physical Medicine and Rehabilitation, 73*, S3–S23.

Joint Commission on Accreditation of Healthcare Organizations. (1994). *Accreditation manual for hospitals.* Oakbrook Terrace, IL: Author.

Kane, R. (1991, May). *An update on functional assessment: Perspectives from consumers, practitioners, policymakers, and payers.* Presentation at the National Health Policy Forum Session, Washington, DC.

Kane, R. L. (1987). *PAC: A national study of post acute care: Proposal.* Baltimore: Health Care Financing Administration.

Kane, R. L. (in progress). *A national study of post acute care.* Minneapolis, MN: University of Minnesota School of Public Health.

Katz, S., Ford, A. B., Moskowitz, R. W., Jackson, B. A., & Jaffee, M. W. (1963). Studies of illness in the aged. The Index of ADL: A standardized measure of biological and psychological function. *Journal of the American Medical Association, 185*, 94–101.

Lincoln, N. B. (1982). The Speech Questionnaire: An assessment of functional language ability. *International Rehabilitation Medicine, 4*, 114–117.

Lomas, J., Pickard, L., Bester, S., Elbard, H., Finlayson, A., & Zoghaib, C. (1989). The Communicative Effectiveness Index: Development and psychometric evaluation of a functional communication for adult aphasia. *Journal of Speech and Hearing Disorders, 54*, 113–124.

Mahoney, F. I., & Barthel, D. W. (1965). Functional evaluation: The Barthel Index. *Maryland State Medical Journal, 14*, 61–68.

McGinnis, G. E., Osberg, J. S., DeJong, G., Mae, M., Seward, L., & Branch, L. E. (1987). Predicting charges for inpatient medical rehabilitation using severity, DRG, age, and function. *American Journal of Public Health, 77*, 826–829.

Morris, J. N., Hawes, C., Murphy, I., Nonemaker, S., Phillips, C., Fries, B. E., & Mor, V. (1991). *Minimum Data Set for Nursing Home Resident Assessment and Care Screening (MDS): Training manual and resource guide.* Natick, MA: Eliot Press.

Murray, J., Marquardt, T. P., Richardson, A., & Nalty, D. (1984). Differential diagnosis of aphasia and dementia from aphasia test battery scores. *Journal of Neurological Communication Disorders, 1*, 33–39.

Nagi, S. Z. (1965). Some conceptual issues in disability and rehabilitation. In M. B. Sussman (Ed.), *Sociology and rehabilitation* (pp. 100–113). Washington, DC: American Sociological Association.

National Association of Rehabilitation Facilities. (1985). *NARF position paper on a prospective payment system for inpatient medical rehabilitation services and a study regarding a prospective payment system for inpatient medical rehabilitation services: Final report.* Washington, DC: Author.

National Institute on Disability and Rehabilitation Research. (1990). Quality of life research in rehabilitation. *Rehab Brief, 11*, 1–4.

Parkside Associates, Inc. (1986). *Level of Rehabilitation Scale III.* Park Ridge, IL: Author.

Porch, B. E. (1971). *Porch Index of Communicative Ability.* Palo Alto, CA: Consulting Psychologists Press.

Sacchett, C., & Marshall, J. (1992). Functional assessment of communication: Implications for the rehabilitation of aphasic people: Reply to Carol Frattali. *Aphasiology, 6*, 95–100.

Sarno, M. T. (1965). A measurement of functional communication in aphasia. *Archives of Physical Medicine and Rehabilitation, 46*, 101–107.

Sarno, M. T. (1983). The functional assessment of verbal impairment. In G. Grimby (Ed.), *Recent advances in rehabilitation medicine* (pp. 75–81). Stockholm: Almquist & Wiksell.

Schow, R., & Nerbonne, M. (1982). Communication screening profile uses with elderly clients. *Ear and Hearing, 3*, 133–147.

Skenes, L. L., & McCauley, R. J. (1985). Psychometric review of nine aphasia tests. *Journal of Communication Disorders, 18*, 461–474.

Smith, L., & Parr, S. (1986). Therapists' assessment of functional communication in aphasia. *Bulletin of the College of Speech Therapists, 409*, 10–11.

Smith-Worrall, L., & Burtenshaw, E. J. (1990). Frequency of use and utility of aphasia tests. *Australian Journal of Human Communication Disorders, 18*, 53–67.

State University of New York at Buffalo, Research Foundation. (1993). *Guide for use of the Uniform Data Set for Medical Rehabilitation: Functional Independence Measure*. Buffalo: Author.

Swisher, L. (1979). Functional Communication Profile (FCP) (Review). In F. L. Darley (Ed.), *Evaluation of appraisal techniques in speech and language pathology* (pp. 205–207). Redding, MA: Addison Wesley.

Ventry, I. W., & Weinstein, B. E. (1982). The Hearing Handicap Inventory for the Elderly: A new tool. *Ear and Hearing, 3*, 128–134.

Wilkerson, D. L., Batavia, A. I., & DeJong, L. (1992). The use of functional status measures for payment of medical rehabilitation services. *Archives of Physical Medicine and Rehabilitation, 73*, 111–120.

Wirz, S. L., Skinner, C., & Dean, E. (1990). *Revised Edinburgh Functional Communication Profile*. Tucson, AZ: Communication Skill Builders.

World Health Organization. (1980). *International classification of impairments, disabilities, and handicaps*. Geneva: Author.

Worrall, L. (1992). Functional communication assessment: An Australian perspective. *Aphasiology, 6*(1), 105–110.

CHAPTER 25

Research Needs and Grantseeking

■ NANCY J. MINGHETTI, M.A. ■

SCOPE OF CHAPTER

Do many graduate students and novice researchers imagine being isolated with data pages, crumpled paper, worn-down pencils, and charts and graphs when presented with their first opportunity to do research? Absolutely! Research, however, is much more than data collection and statistical analysis. It is the opportunity to investigate an idea that has caught your interest or raised a question in your mind—a chance to pursue the "Why . . .?" or "What would happen if . . .?" Research can lead to discoveries and the acquisition of knowledge. It can be fascinating and even inspirational.

A look at research needs and grantseeking prompts the reader to consider two abilities: the skill to conduct research and the skill in writing plans for that research. These abilities shape the intent of graduate courses in research and form the prerequisites for becoming a researcher or a research consumer. This chapter sets the stage for learning these skills and provides a foundation for why research

is important to your work as an audiologist or speech-language pathologist.

This chapter will acquaint you with some basics of research, the research needs in the discipline of human communication sciences and disorders, and an understanding of the grantseeking process.

IS RESEARCH RELEVANT?

Have you ever seen a child with delayed language over the course of several treatment sessions and finally determined why a particular procedure did not work? Have you ever discovered a cueing technique that was particularly useful for an adult with aphasia? If so, then you have been thinking in a research mode. In one case, you were troubled about something and took steps to solve the problem; in the other, you found an approach that produced a desirable result, then acted to understand the strategy and generalize the behavior. The situations prompted you to investigate.

One colleague cleverly describes these motivators as "stone-in-the-shoe" and "light bulb" phenomena. In fact, research questions emerge from practical, logical, and accidental sources (Locke, Spirduso, & Silverman, 1987).

Considering that *Webster's New World Dictionary* defines research as "a careful, systematic study undertaken to discover or establish facts or principles" (1982), the above examples are oversimplified. The point is that research is relevant and can and does make a difference to what you do clinically.

UNDERSTANDING RESEARCH TYPES

There are many types of research. Traditionally, research in the discipline of human communication sciences and disorders has followed two paths, basic and applied. Olswang (1990), explaining that the boundaries between these research types are not always clear, cites the work of Ventry and Schiavetti (1986) highlighting their differences: "*Basic* research is described as scientific research 'directed toward the development of knowledge per se,' versus *applied* research, which is 'undertaken to solve some problem of immediate social or economic consequences' " (p. 45). For example, in our professions, some investigations look to define the underlying processes of a communication disorder; others focus on whether and how a clinical procedure works and if it is efficacious.

The beginning investigator should understand that research types have subcategories. For example, one type of applied research, clinical research, may be conducted to better understand the clinical processes of assessment and treatment of communication disorders. In turn, a particular type of clinical research, treatment efficacy research, may document how well treatment works (Olswang, 1990). Because methods for each research type may have both overlapping and unique features, it is important to become acquainted with the nuances of research types. No matter what type, all research begins with questions, defines data sources, and presents plans for analysis. (See Appendix 25A for "Basic Steps in the Planning and Conduct of Research.")

Research types should not be confused with the design and accompanying methods one uses to conduct research. The research design is the "plan of attack." This will vary depending on the purposes of the study, the nature of the problem, and ultimately, the specific research questions. Authorities in research differ in their design classification criteria (Isaac & Michael, 1983; Locke, Spirduso, & Silverman, 1987). To list distinct categories would be misleading because the categories are not always mutually exclusive, and there may be as many similarities as differences. For introductory purposes, the beginning researcher often learns about quantitative and qualitative research. Quantitative research (that which can be measured numerically) includes design alternatives such as experimental or quasi-experimental designs. Qualitative research (that which can be described through text, for example, interview transcripts and field observation) is interpretive and includes, for example, historical or ethnographic designs. Each of these research paradigms is used in our discipline. Their different perspectives allow for investigations that can address the richness of communication sciences and disorders. For example, a quantitative question might be, "does the frequency of misarticulated /r/ decrease with a specific method of intervention?" A qualitative question might be "how do parents' views about their children's communication impairments change with the introduction of treatment?" The reader is encouraged to examine more complete information in these areas and to compare the schemes presented in current textbooks exclusively devoted to research design and methodology.

ADDRESSING RESEARCH NEEDS

The subject of research needs is complex. It can refer to the particular scientific priorities of the discipline of human communication sciences and disorders and to specific research training needs. Discussions of research needs are constantly evolving. Newly acquired information and changes in the pool of research talent affect our ability to accurately assess progress in addressing research priorities and identifying further needs.

A discipline's scientific community drives research priorities. By the proposal applications submitted to various funding agencies, scientists send a message about what research studies are important. There are hundreds of priorities in all the scientific areas, and a corresponding number of individuals, institutions, and organizations may differ on the foremost scientific needs. Although recognizing that priorities change, the National Institute on Deafness and Other Communication Disorders (NIDCD) gathered consensus on research needs in 1989 by calling together a task force. For the first time in the history of the United States, 100 respected U.S. experts in basic and clinical science from a broad variety of specialties in deafness and other communication disorders met to identify short- and long-range research goals.

This task force agreed that, by combining basic and applied research with currently available technology, investigators should be able to solve many of the problems of otitis media, nerve deafness, balance disorders, language deficiency, and diseases of taste and smell. They identified research opportunities in the biomedical sciences that can lead to the prevention, cure, and amelioration of many communication disorders. However, they expressed concern that the achievement of many goals may have to await the implementation of new and expanded research training mechanisms. They recognized that the most critical need is the recruitment and education of scientists. The task force recommendations are published in *A Report of the Task Force on the National Strategic Research Plan* (National Institute on Deafness and Other Communication Disorders, 1989). The 350-page document delineates research priorities for basic and applied research in the following topic areas: deafness and hearing disorders; balance and the vestibular system; voice and voice disorders; speech and speech disorders; language and language disorders; smell, taste, and touch; and cross-cutting issues. Recognizing that the scientific priorities within a discipline change and may change rapidly, NIDCD has developed a process whereby elements of the plan are updated annually.

There are many important research questions yet to be resolved in hearing, speech, language, and related disorders. Trends in these inquiries will parallel the technological, social, economic, and environmental changes of our world. For example, a glimpse into hearing science shows us that emerging technologies will profoundly influence improvements in amplification. Among other things, studies will focus on efficacy of the use of cochlear implants and attitudes about the use of other sensory aids. Tremendous progress in brain and nervous system research, which led to the declaration of the 1990s as "The Decade of the Brain," has great promise for language intervention for individuals affected by neurological disorders.

Our society's changing demographics also illustrate research priorities. For example, a growing culturally diverse population underscores the need for more cross-cultural and cross-racial investigation in all areas of communication disorders, as reported by the NIDCD Working Group on Research and Research Training Needs of Minority Persons and Minority Health Issues (1992).

Much has been written about why we need scientific data. Minifie (1990) makes a case for scientific data as critical to the knowledge base of the discipline of human communication sciences and disorders. He states that the basic premise upon which this field was established was that knowledge gained through research should be the fundamental driver of clinical treatment. He further elaborates that, throughout the history of our professions, the "pendulum has swung between our commitments to doing everything we can to help the patient to having a primary commitment to advancing knowledge" (p. 240), often without balance between the two perspectives. Minifie expresses concern that the knowledge base for the discipline has softened and urges our leaders to renew their commitment to developing knowledge. Generation of new knowledge is essential to the livelihood of our professions. Only then can effective and predictable treatments be provided as part of the intervention process.

Jerger (1993) cautions that "research is not complete until its implications have been translated to practice" (p. 47). The theme of bridging science and practice has become a major, and sometimes controversial, professional issue in the research arena (Kent, 1989–1990). It is related to another issue—how the discipline develops individuals interested in conducting research. At a time when the number of scientists is decreasing in the membership of the American Speech-Language-Hearing Association (Shewan, 1993), there is concern that the development of productive and competitive researchers is diminishing. The ideal researcher, according to Jerger, "is an individual who combines a familiarity with the rigors of the scientific method with firsthand knowledge, based on patient contact, of what are the important questions to address" (p. 46). He emphasizes the need to train researchers who focus on substantive, clinically relevant issues and who are willing to collaborate with specialists in other disciplines to address broad questions raised by the present explosive growth of knowledge.

Kent (1993) states that research training should consider the need to prepare scientists for the development and conduct of programmatic research, that is, for studies that are thematically linked, often in a progressive investigation of a particular problem. He highlights the importance of preparing scientists for changes in research directions during an individual career and for participation in interdisciplinary research efforts. Further, he feels that students in educational programs not only need exposure to other disciplines, but also need instruction in integrating that knowledge.

At a landmark 1993 conference on Research Mentorship and Training (Minghetti, Cooper, Goldstein, Olswang, & Warren, 1993), co-sponsored by the American Speech-Language-Hearing Foundation and the National Institute on Deafness and Other Communication Disorders, scientific leaders recognized that no single model of research training will be uniformly successful across institutions and individual research careers. Conference presenters reinforced the concept that research careers will be enhanced substantially by encouraging exchange of information among scientists and stimulating innovative and collaborative research training opportunities, with the hope that funding agencies will recognize the application of unique research skills to clinically relevant questions.

In summary, data derived from scientific investigations will keep us focused on addressing the substantive issues—and ultimately translating the results into effective services. Research data are crucial to developing new knowledge and formulating guidelines that establish best practice patterns. Only then can we improve the quality of service delivery nationwide (Goldberg, 1991). As we approach the turn of the century, pragmatic issues reinforce these thoughts. Our work is affected by rising health and education costs, increased clinical specialization, the diversity of populations served, and rapid technological and scientific advances (Minghetti & Frattali, 1993). We are increasingly being called on to prove that what we do makes a difference. Payers, administrators, policy makers, and consumers, alike, demand accountability. Quality research and research training are necessary to ensure our competitive position in the workforce.

MOVING BEYOND THE MYTHS AND BARRIERS

Myth or reality?: Research has no connection to what I do in my clinical environment.

> *I must be committed to a full-time research position in a laboratory to conduct successful research.*

Students can participate in research only if they are in a doctoral degree program.

Clinical settings do not provide the time and resources necessary to support research efforts.

Through my work as a developer and administrator of funding programs, I have had extensive discussions with novice investigators. Conducting research seems formidable for a number of reasons. Among their perspectives:

■ Exposure to research is mostly in theory, rather than practical application.
■ Research is discussed on a grand scale; it seems out of reach and insurmountable.
■ Availability of role models and research mentors may be limited; beginning researchers often feel that they are on their own or their requests for help are regarded as an imposition.
■ Instruction in research methodology is inadequate.
■ Insufficient time is spent on learning how to interpret research results.
■ Access to populations for study may be limited.
■ At the student level, research is often discussed as supplemental, rather than integral to coursework; research projects compete with other requirements such as clinical hours, thesis, comps.
■ Research is not for everyone; making it a requirement may not be the most effective approach.
■ A "research culture" is missing in academic programs; that is, the environment to inspire and motivate students to be involved in research often exists only for those who have committed to full-time research careers.
■ Students often do not receive credit for their part in research efforts.

These barriers are related, in part, to how our academic programs and professional settings do or do not support research efforts. However, beginning investigators also must take respon-

sibility for accelerating their success. Students can look to undergraduate and graduate clinical experiences for "light-bulb" opportunities. Observations and ideas at this level can set the stage for more vigorous inquiries.

If you decide to enter the world of research, know that small research projects are valuable. Research questions do not have to be novel; they can validate findings or address new insights to existing research. Think about your question. Does it anticipate or fill a need? Perhaps you are finding a need to fill or building on earlier research efforts.

Mentors can help you move beyond the "I wonder if. . . ." to the research question. Success in aligning yourself with experienced researchers to shape your investigation depends on your commitment and willingness to listen and learn. The "match" should meet your mutual interests. Compatibility is essential to effective collaboration.

It is desirable to seek a mentor who is publishing in your domain of interest. Competent mentoring, however, is so important that beginning researchers may have to adjust their interest to accommodate work somewhat peripheral to their long-range goals, rather than selecting a topic with which the mentor is not familiar. As long as the topic remains within the novice's broad areas of interests, it is possible to gain essential experience in formulating questions, designing studies, and applying the methods germane to the research domain.

Associating with mentors who have research expertise and are actively formulating questions is the best way to learn the current status of a research area. "Conversing with peers, listening to professorial discussions, assisting in research projects, attending lectures and conferences, exchanging papers, corresponding with students and faculty at other institutions are all ways to capture the elusive state of the art" (Locke et al., 1987, p. 41). Informal situations present opportunities to ask questions, raise critical points, and encourage a potential mentor to take interest in your idea.

The 1993 Conference on Research Mentorship and Training revealed that mentors also are seeking how best to maximize the mentoring relationship. Haring (1993) proposes that the traditional, hierarchical model of mentoring has not been effective in meeting the challenge of encouraging larger numbers of professionals in audiology and speech-language pathology to become researchers. A traditional model emphasizes a dyad in which benefits flow one way from a more senior mentor to a less experienced person. She discusses the developmental process of mentoring and explores alternative mentoring models and how these relate to hierarchy, power, and the status quo. She further explains that one alternative, a networking mentoring model, encourages new perspectives and empowerment, and may help the discipline address its research needs more effectively. This model is based on reciprocal exchange of benefits among groups of people. Published proceedings from this conference will orient the interested reader to the complexity of issues in this area (Minghetti et al., 1993). Attention to this topic and a transformation of mentoring practices will serve the discipline well in training the next generation of researchers.

GRANTSEEKING: A BLUEPRINT FOR ACTION

Assume that factors are in place for you to do research. Whether or not you seek funding, you must know how to write a research plan. Think of your plan as a blueprint for action.

Because internal funding for research may be minimal, most investigators seek additional funds to complete a proposed project. Thus, a major part of research training involves grantseeking. Your research plan forms the basis for any proposal submitted for grant funding. If you have an opportunity as a graduate student or beginning investigator to work on funded research projects, you usually have exposure to grant requirements and procedures and may even share in writing responsibilities. This is an excellent way, and may be the best way, to learn the process.

Good research proposals and successful grantseeking have always depended on sound organization (Gelatt, 1988). Consider the words of Locke and colleagues (1987) from the book *Proposals That Work:*

It is obvious that the probability of funding will rest mostly on the selection of a target for inquiry and the competence displayed in designing and justifying the study. A deceptively large contribution toward funding, however, is made by the clarity and style of writing in the proposal. (p. 9)

Before you get started, give yourself what I call the OPT of thinking clearly—the One Page Test. Identify in simple, lay language your question(s), objectives, and strategies by writing them on a single page. This self-assessment will help you focus and will provide direction for the actual writing process.

Proposal writing is not a linear process from beginning to end. That is, you will have to do many things simultaneously to meet proposal submission timelines: seek sources of funds, complete applications, obtain institutional approval, develop proposal materials, and so on. A novice is advised to make a chart of these sequenced events with responsibilities and deadlines (see Appendix 25B).

Read *all* instructions for submission of a proposal to a funding agency, keeping in mind that you will shape your proposal according to the grant competition. Although application requirements may vary from one funding source to another, all have common elements. They include

1. An Abstract: This summary concisely describes the project's specific aims, methodology, and long-term objectives. It should refer to the project need and impact. A good abstract is important, because it is often the first part read by reviewers and should provide a glimpse into the soundness and creativity of your study.
2. The Research Plan: This is the main part of your proposal. Major components include
   a. Objectives: Presents the problem or issue to be addressed with the specific objectives of the study.
   b. Significance: Outlines the precise need and the importance of the study.

c. Methods, Procedures, Evaluation: Provides a description and justification of the project design. Describes how the subjects will be identified, selected, used, and protected. Identifies the type(s) of evaluation to be used, including measurement techniques, instrumentation, data analysis, and the rationale for their use. This section should provide sufficient detail for reviewers to make informed judgments about the technical soundness of the research procedures.

d. Personnel, Facilities, Resources: Delineates who will be involved with the management of the project. The interests, training, and experience of the investigator(s) should be directly related to the project objectives. Describes the roles and responsibilities of personnel in relation to the project tasks. Biographical sketches and/or curricula vitae may be required. Time commitments should be given for staff and, if applicable, consultants or members of advisory groups. Also describes the available facilities, equipment, supplies, and resources that will ensure the likelihood of the project's success.

3. Management Plan: This outlines the ordered tasks that will accomplish the project objectives. Includes timelines for activities. These data are often displayed in a flowchart for ease of understanding.

4. Budget: All expenses should be documented with care, including a justification for each item. Be aware that some funding agencies may not cover certain types of expenditures according to their rules of application.

5. Letters of Endorsement or Confirmation: Letters of support from respected experts in the field of proposed study may be useful in demonstrating that the project is worthy and the investigator is competent. Another type of letter is one that confirms the participation or support of organizations or individuals essential to the study. These letters are usually included in an appendix.

6. Dissemination of Results: Many funding sources ask how the results of the study will be disseminated to the intended audiences. Be specific about which results will be reported and include plans beyond the requisite published article or conference presentation.

7. Appended Material: The funding source will provide guidelines as to what can be included. If you are unclear about the requirements, contact the funder.

Two excellent references for suggestions on writing these sections are *Proposals That Work* (Locke et al., 1987) and *Getting Funded: A Complete Guide to Proposal Writing* (Hall, 1988).

PREVENTING PROPOSAL REJECTIONS

There are common reasons why proposals are rejected for funding. For example, in grant competitions at the American Speech-Language-Hearing Foundation over the last 6 years, a representative sample of errors included the following:

- Guidelines for the proposal content and format were not followed *exactly.*
- The project design and methodology were not described thoroughly or did not correlate with the type of research proposed.
- Proposed activities were unrealistic within the alloted time frame.
- The proposed study did not match the competition's funding priority.
- The review of literature to support the need was incomplete.
- The effects of the study beyond the proposed project were not addressed.
- The proposal was poorly written.
- The budget was either unrealistic or unjustified.
- Proposal page limitations were not followed.
- Letters of support were missing or not submitted on time.
- Deadline for submission was not met.

Paying attention to details pays off. Addressing perpectives of both funders and reviewers is critical to your success in writing a proposal. Become familiar with funding agencies' competition priorities and requirements. Be versed on the criteria and mechanics for evaluation. Ask a colleague who has not been through the development of your proposal to read your submission with a re- viewer's mind and eye. Remember that proposal writing always takes longer than you expect. A good rule is to have your final draft completed 1 month in advance of the submission deadline. This will allow time for proofreading, refinements, and completion of missing elements.

Keep one final thought in mind. Valuable, sound, and well-written proposals are subject to rejection for funding. Competition for dollars is high. Reviewers must make hard decisions when faced with strong contenders. At times, there may not be a clear reason why a proposal is rejected or why one proposal had more appeal to a review panel. Learn as much as you can from the evaluation process and resubmit your proposal. Proposal writing improves with each experience.

SEARCHING FOR KING MIDAS

Now that you have a well-conceptualized plan, the only thing you need is funding. Unlike the mythological King Midas who could instantly turn everything into gold by a single touch, finding the most appropriate funding source is a time-intensive procedure.

The ratio of proposals funded to those rejected is about 6 to 100 (Locke et al., 1987). It is wise, then, to use careful thought and efficiency when you approach the task of sending proposals through the right channels. A good first step is to assemble a list of potential sources based on matching interests. Your search should take multiple routes. Faculty and research staff often maintain information on sources in their area of expertise and communicate periodically with key persons in granting agencies. Many universities have a grant library or database identifying agencies and foundations. Standard reference publica-

tions, such as those found in Appendix 25C, provide a profile of funding sources.

The Foundation Center in New York publishes *The Foundation Directory, Foundation Grants Index, Source Book Profiles, National Directory of Corporate Giving, Foundation News* and operates three regional reference centers and a computerized information service of nongovernmental funding sources.

Computerized information searches may also help you identify funding opportunities and learn about other funded projects on topics related to your proposal. Computer Retrieval of Information on Scientific Projects (CRISP) contains data on the research programs supported by the U.S. Public Health Service. When you indicate the topic(s) and year(s) in which you are interested, CRISP will generate a computer printout of funded projects. There is no charge for this service. Dialog Information Services, Inc. (DIALOG) has over 300 individual databases in a broad scope of subject areas. For a fee, it can access records that range from a bibliographic reference with an abstract to a directory entry for an organization. Its databases have information on public- and private-sector funding and private funding histories.

Once you have narrowed your list of potential sources, most agencies will send you their specific funding information at no or minimal cost. Examples include the National Institutes of Health's (NIH) *Guide for Grants and Contracts*, the National Science Foundation's *Bulletin*, and the American Speech-Language-Hearing Association's *Research Bulletin*.

The National Institute on Deafness and Other Communication Disorders (NIDCD) created a clearinghouse in 1991 to disseminate information and facilitate a network among organizations and individuals who have an interest in deafness and other communication disorders. The clearinghouse publication, *Directory, Associations and Organizations with an Interest in Deafness and Other Communication Disorders*, will help you locate sources that sponsor funding opportunities for research. The Program Planning and Health Reports Branch of NIDCD publishes*The Research and*

Development Mechanisms of the National Institute on Deafness and Other Communication Disorders. It lists sources of support (within and outside of NIH) for research and research training. This reference is useful for investigators from the pre- and postdoctoral levels to the senior investigator level. The NIH Office of Grants Inquiries publishes *Helpful Hints on Preparing a Research Grant Application to the National Institutes of Health. Research in Human Communication*, an annual report from the NIDCD Advisory Board, details the institute's major accomplishments and funding initiatives. All of these publications are distributed through the clearinghouse.

The American Speech-Language-Hearing Association (ASHA) has a Research Division that provides services and products to individuals interested in obtaining research funding information. Its *Research Bulletin* lists grants available for research in communication sciences and disorders. The division maintains a computerized database of current grants awarded for field research by federal and nonfederal agencies and organizations. It also produces a *Grants Directory*, a publication with more detailed information about individual grants and investigators. The Research Information Service (RIS) is a computerized database with information on doctoral and postdoctoral communication sciences and disorders programs in the United States and Canada. ASHA members may request the Division to conduct a DIALOG search for potential funding sources in communication sciences and disorders.

The American Speech-Language-Hearing Foundation sponsors research funding opportunities for student researchers and new investigators as part of several program initiatives. These grants often spearhead pilot studies and provide leverage for larger federal and nonfederal grants, in addition to giving novices a vote of confidence in their early research efforts.

Appendix 25D in this chapter provides mailing and contact information for selected information sources.

SUMMARY

The discussion continues nationwide about health care and education reform. It is anybody's best guess how the decade of the '90s will be viewed in retrospect. However, it is a fact that we, as knowledge experts and service providers, are part of the big picture. We must be proactive in serving children and adults with communication disorders. The programs and policies that emerge as part of our global society need to be based on information, not bias, not intuition (Carney, 1991). Research leads to that information. Research helps us continually invent new ways to diagnose and treat people and improve the quality of care.

"Only those who can see the invisible can do the impossible" (Wright, 1990). Look with new eyes. Turn your curiosity into discovery. You can generate big results by participating in research efforts. You can help ensure that the discipline of human communication sciences and disorders will continue to grow and thrive.

DISCUSSION QUESTIONS

1. Discuss the research needs in the discipline of human communication sciences and disorders.
2. Distinguish between research types and research designs.
3. Describe the essential elements of a grant proposal.
4. How might you proceed from a research idea to a funded project?

REFERENCES

Carney, P. J. (1991). Research: Our path to the frontier. *Asha, 33*, 5–6.

Gelatt, J. P. (1988). The business of grantseeking. *Asha, 30*, 43–45.

Goldberg, B. (1991). Digging for truth. *Asha, 33* , 37–48.

Hall, M. (1988). *Getting funded: A complete guide to proposal writing.* Portland, OR: Continuing Education Publications.

Haring, M. J. (1993). Mentoring for research: Examining alternative models. In N. J. Minghetti, J. A. Cooper, H. Goldstein, L. B. Olswang, & S. F. Warren. (Eds.), *Research mentorship and training in communication sciences and disorders: Proceedings of a national conference* (pp. 117–125). Rockville, MD: American Speech-Language-Hearing Foundation.

Isaac, S., & Michael, W. (1983). *Handbook in research and evaluation* (2nd ed.). San Diego: EdITS Publishers.

Jerger, J. (1993). Research training and mentorship in hearing disorders. In N. J. Minghetti , J. A. Cooper, H. Goldstein, L. B. Olswang, & S. F. Warren (Eds.), *Research mentorship and training in communication sciences and disorders: Proceedings of a national conference* (pp. 41–48). Rockville, MD: American Speech-Language-Hearing Foundation.

Kent, R. D. (1989–1990). Fragmentation of cinical service and clinical science in communication disorders. *National Student Speech Language Hearing Association Journal, 17*, 4–16.

Kent, R. D. (1993). Research training and mentorship in voice/speech/language disorders. In N. J. Minghetti, J. A. Cooper, H. Goldstein, L. B. Olswang, & S. F. Warren (Eds.), *Research mentorship and training in communication sciences and disorders: Proceedings of a national conference* (pp. 31–39). Rockville, MD: American Speech-Language-Hearing Foundation.

Locke, L. F., Spirduso, W. W., & Silverman, S. J. (1987). *Proposals that work.* Newbury Park, CA: Sage Publications.

Minghetti, N. J., Cooper, J. A., Goldstein, H., Olswang, L.B., & Warren, S. F. (Eds.). (1993). *Research mentorship and training in communication sciences and disorders: Proceedings of a national conference.* Rockville, MD. American Speech-Language-Hearing Foundation.

Minghetti, N. J., & Frattali, C. M. (1993, October). Networks: *Making connections. Newsletter of Society of Hospital Directors of Communicative Disorders Programs,* pp. 3–6.

Minifie, F. D. (1990). Research in treatment efficacy: Where is the profession? In L. B. Olswang, C. K. Thompson, S. F. Warren, & N. J. Minghetti (Eds.), *Treatment efficacy research in communication disorders* (pp. 239–243). Rockville, MD: American Speech-Language-Hearing Foundation.

National Institute on Deafness and Other Communication Disorders. (1989). *A report of the national task force on the national strategic research plan.* Bethesda, MD: Author.

National Institute on Deafness and Other Communication Disorders. (1992, April). NIDCD Working Group on Research and Research Training Needs of Minority Persons and Minority Health Issues. Report presented at the meeting of the NIDCD Working Group, Bethesda, MD.

Olswang, L. B., (1990). Treatment efficacy research: A path to quality assurance. *Asha, 32,* 45–47.

Shewan, C. M. (1993). Research training and research project funding in communication sciences and disorders. In N. J. Minghetti, J. A. Cooper, H. Goldstein, L. B. Olswang, & S. F. Warren (Eds.), *Research mentorship and training in communication sciences and disorders: Proceedings of a national conference* (pp. 11–29). Rockville, MD: American Speech-Language-Hearing Foundation.

Siegel, G. M. (1993). Research: A natural bridge. *Asha, 35, 36*–37.

Ventry, I., & Schiavetti, N. (1986). *Evaluating research in speech pathology and audiology.* New York: Macmillan.

Webster's new world dictionary, second college edition. (1982). New York: Simon & Schuster.

Wright, M. S. (1990). *Poster inscription.* Jefferston, VA: Perelandra.

APPENDIX 25A: Basic Steps in the Planning and Conduct of Research

1. Identify the problem area.
2. Survey the related literature.
3. Define the actual problem for investigation in clear, specific terms.
4. Formulate testable hypotheses and define the basic concepts and variables.
5. State the underlying assumptions that govern the interpretation of the results.

6. Construct the research design to maximize internal and external validity.
   a. Selection of subjects
   b. Control and/or manipulation of relevant variables
   c. Establishment of criteria to evaluate outcomes

   d. Instrumentation—selection or development of the criterion measures
7. Specify data collection procedures.
8. Select the data analysis methodology.
9. Execute the research plan.
10. Evaluate the results and draw conclusions.

Source: From *Handbook in research and evaluation* (2nd ed.) (p. 16) by S. Isaac and W. Michael, 1983, San Diego: EdITS Publishers. Copyright 1983 by Robert R. Knapp. Reprinted by permission.

APPENDIX 25B: Sample Flowchart

"Once a problem has been defined and an appropriate funding agency identified, the following items can be supplemented as required by local circumstance"

TIME FRAME

First response to the request for proposals

Preproposal or letter of intent deadline

Deadline for submission to Human Subjects Review Committee

Deadline for obtaining administrative signatures

Deadline for submission to typist

Deadline for submission of proposal

Award announcement date

MAJOR DEVELOPMENT STEPS

Obtain guidelines

Contact program officer at funding agency

Select primary authors of proposal

Prepare abstract or prospectus and submit

letter of intent

Contact units for support or collaboration

Obtain initial administrative approval

Complete review of the literature

Determine study design

Prepare first draft of proposal

Prepare abstract of proposal

Initiate human subjects review

Initiate internal peer review

Prepare budget

Revise proposal based on feedback

Collect vitae

Obtain letters of endorsement

Obtain written assurances from support sources

Complete institutional forms

Type final document

Obtain administrative signatures

Duplicate proposal

Submit proposal

Source: From *Proposals That Work* (p. 133–134) by L. F. Locke, W. W. Spirduso, and S. J. Silverman, 1987, Newbury Park, CA: Sage Publications. Copyright 1987 by Sage Publications, Inc. Reprinted by permission.

APPENDIX 25C: Standard Reference Publications for Funding Sources

Catalog of Federal Domestic Assistance (CDFA) lists federal agencies with appropriate interests, as well as support programs within those agencies. It is published annually with updates twice a year. Many states publish a similar catalog of state assistance. Washington, DC: U.S. Government Printing Office.

Directory of Grants for Organizations Serving People with Disabilities lists foundation and federal project funding according to disability areas. Research Grant Guides, Inc., P. O. Box 1214, Loxahatchee, FL 33470.

Grants Register includes sources listed in CDFA but has much additional information and wider coverage, for example, equipment use programs and foreign exchange opportu-

nities for research personnel. St. Martin's Press, Inc., 175 Fifth Ave., New York, NY 10010.

National Directory of Corporate Giving provides application information, giving priorities, and financial data on over 2,300 corporate foundations and corporate giving programs. The Foundation Center, 70 Fifth Ave., New York, NY 10003.

The Foundation Directory identifies non-governmental sources by categorizing nearly 3,000 of the largest foundations. It includes both application information and number and kind of grants available from each source. The Foundation Center, 70 Fifth Ave., New York, NY 10003.

APPENDIX 25D: Sources of Research Funding Information

American Speech-Language-Hearing Association
Research Division
10801 Rockville Pike
Rockville, MD 20852
(301) 897-5700

American-Speech-Language-Hearing Foundation
10801 Rockville Pike
Rockville, MD 20852
(301) 897-5700

Computer Retrieval of Information on Scientific Projects (CRISP)
Research Documentation Section
Information Systems Branch
Division of Research Grants
National Institutes of Health
Westwood Building, Room 148
Bethesda, MD
(301) 594-7267

Dialog Information Services, Inc. (DIALOG)
3460 Hillview Avenue
Palo Alto, CA 94304
(800) 334-2564

Grantsearch CFDA
Capitol Publications Inc.
P. O. Box 1453
Alexandria, VA 22314-2053
(800) 847-7772

National Institutes of Health
Grants and Contracts Guide Distribution Center
Building 31, Room B3BEOM
Bethesda, MD 20892
(301) 496-1789

National Institute on Deafness and Other
Communication Disorders Clearinghouse
National Institutes of Health
P.O. Box 37777
Washington, DC 20013-7777
(800) 241-1044

National Science Foundation
Language, Cognition, and Social Behavior Program
1800 G Street, NW
Washington, DC 20550
(202) 357-9859

National Science Foundation
Science and Technology Information Systems (STIS)
Office of Information Systems
1800 G Street, NW, Room 401
Washington, DC 20550
(202) 357-7555

U.S. Department of Education
National Institute on Disability and Rehabilitation Research
400 Maryland Ave. SW
Washington, DC 20202
(202) 205-8134

U.S. Department of Education
Office of Special Education Programs
330 C Street
Switzer Building
Washington, DC 20202
(202) 205-5507

Veterans Administration Audiology and Speech Pathology Service
Medical Center
50 Irving Street, NW
Washington, DC 20422
(202) 745-8270

CHAPTER 26

Professional Autonomy and Collaboration

■ CAROL FRATTALI, Ph.D. ■

SCOPE OF CHAPTER

The title of this chapter may sound like an oxymoron. How can you be at once autonomous and interdependent? As the health care and education systems continue to evolve, however, the term "professional autonomy" departs from the notion of independence in its traditional sense.

Throughout the history of the discipline of human communication sciences and disorders, speech-language pathologists and audiologists have aggressively pursued an identity that is unique and separate from others. They believed this was their professional right. But today this right is regarded, at its extreme, as a liability for many professionals who work in isolation and resist current realities that require collaboration with other professionals to provide quality of care to those they serve.

Any system in which you work is interdependent; that is, the quality of and access to your services often are dependent on the actions or services of others. Consider, for example, the hospital patient. During the course of a 4-day hospital stay, the patient may have interacted with 60 different employees, many of whom are specialists. Their work, in turn, depends on the work of multiple technicians and support staff. To answer basic questions posed by the patient (i.e., What is wrong with me? Will I get better? What kind of treatment will help me?), these 60 individuals must collaborate to assemble that patient's medical profile and plan of care. As the human services have experienced rapid division of labor, hospitals today can now boast about 350 different job classifications (Lathrop, 1992). What has resulted, in the absence of professional collaboration, is care that is complex, compartmentalized, and fragmented. Collaboration, however, is not antithetical to autonomy. Rather, collaboration is synonymous with professional growth. On most scales of professional maturity or psychosocial development, you move from independence to interdependence.

Throughout this chapter, professional autonomy is defined, evidence of autonomy in the field is provided, and issues surrounding efforts to achieve autonomy are presented. The need to regard autonomous professions as interdependent is justified. The chapter closes with a discussion of team approaches to clinical management and the pros and cons associated with professional collaboration.

PROFESSIONAL AUTONOMY DEFINED

Autonomy means self-government or independence. It is distinguished from the term hegemony, meaning the domination of one state or group by another (ASHA, 1986). The former Ad Hoc Committee on Professional Autonomy of the American Speech-Language-Hearing Association (ASHA) applied the term "autonomy" to the professions of speech-language pathology and audiology, and adjusted the dictionary definition with some special connotations: "An autonomous profession is one in which the practitioner has the qualifications, responsibility, and authority for the provision of services which fall within its scope of practice" (ASHA, 1986, p. 53).

The Ad Hoc Committee on Professional Autonomy recognized, in formulating its definition, that autonomy does not mean complete freedom. This is particularly true from the perspective of regulation:

> Even the most entrenched professions are closely scrutinized and their practices repeatedly reviewed by bodies established by federal and state statutes, by accreditation agencies, by consumer groups, and by peers in the same profession. With the growing involvement of governmental agencies and corporations in underwriting the costs of human services, and with the growing trend for challenging professional competence through litigation, there is an ever-increasing abridgement of the independence of all professions. (p. 53)

Implied in the definition of professional autonomy, then, is the responsibility for formulating standards for preparation for autonomous practice, defining the scope and standards of practice, and developing individual and institutional standards for the delivery of services to individuals with communication and related disorders.

PROFESSIONAL QUALIFICATIONS AS EVIDENCE OF AUTONOMY

The qualifications of speech-language pathologists and audiologists are defined primarily through certification and state licensure. ASHA's Certificates of Clinical Competence are issued to individuals who present evidence of their ability to provide "independent clinical services to persons who have disorders of communication" (ASHA, 1993b, p. 76). Individuals who meet the standards specified by ASHA's Council on Professional Standards may be awarded a Certificate of Clinical Competence in Speech-Language Pathology (CCC-SLP) or a Certificate of Clinical Competence in Audiology (CCC-A). Individuals who meet the standards in both professional areas may be awarded both certificates. The standards for certification form the basis for definitions of qualifications in state licensure laws.

At the time of this writing, 43 states licensed speech-language pathologists and/or audiologists. Not one of these licensure laws requires that services be under the supervision or control of any other person or limits referrals to particular sources. These licensing laws authorize qualified practitioners to evaluate and treat all persons with communication disorders, as defined within their scopes of practice.

Licensure and certification, as indicators of professional autonomy, are also reflected in national accreditation standards. For example, the hospital accreditation standards of the Joint Commission on Accreditation of Healthcare Organizations (Joint Commission on Accreditation of Healthcare Organizations, 1994) describes the requirements for providing rehabilitation services to clients:

RH.1.1.5.1 There is evidence that each individual who provides physical rehabilitation services meets all applicable licensure, certification, or registration requirement. (p. 168)

Although it is important to recognize that certification and licensure qualify individual practitioners to deliver all services that may fall within the scope of practice, the Ad Hoc Committee on Professional Autonomy offers a caveat (ASHA, 1986). Providing specific diagnostic and treatment services for which the practitioner is not otherwise qualified shows inadequate concern for clients' best interests and may result in exposure to liability. Members of the professions, therefore, are bound by the ASHA Code of Ethics (ASHA, 1993a), which states: "Individuals shall engage in only those aspects of the professions that are within the scope of their competence, considering their level of education, training and experience" (p. 17). Otherwise stated, professionals whose services fall clearly within their scopes of practice, but who cannot demonstrate competence to provide these services, are well advised to seek preparation beyond that entailed in satisfying the requirements for CCC and state licensure.

Technological, clinical, and scientific advances in the field will continue at a rapid pace. In just one year's time, ASHA approved and published new policies that expanded the scopes of practice of speech-language pathologists and audiologists. These advanced areas of practice include: external auditory canal examination and cerumen management, electrical stimulation for cochlear implant selection and rehabilitation, neurophysiologic intraoperative monitoring, balance system assessment, vocal tract visualization and imaging, instrumental diagnostic procedures for swallowing, and management for tracheoesophageal puncture/fistulization (ASHA, 1992). Professionals must remain current if they are to preserve their autonomy. It is not enough to have completed the requirements for certification and licensure. The professional must make a commitment to lifelong learning. Through continuing education activities, and membership in related professional organizations and special interest divisions, practitioners can remain abreast of developments in the field, and can continually acquire new competencies. Our Code of Ethics (ASHA, 1993a) also includes a proscription that individuals shall continue their professional development throughout their careers. This commitment to lifelong learning is rooted in our obligation to protect the consumers we serve (Cherow, 1992). (See Chapter 3 by Battle on Certification and Licensure and Chapter 5 by Madell on Professional Standards.)

FEDERAL REGULATIONS AND AUTONOMY

The Ad Hoc Committee on Professional Autonomy (ASHA, 1986) and ASHA's Health Care Financing Division (ASHA, 1993c) document well the speech-language pathologist's and audiologist's autonomy as reflected in federal regulations. Within the context of federal regulations, speech-language pathologists and audiologists relate to physicians on an equal basis, rather than subordinate basis that requires prescription or supervision. The U.S. Department of Health and Human Services' Office of Family Assistance recognizes this professional relationship: "Services for individuals with speech, hearing, and language disorders means diagnostic, screening, preventive or corrective services provided by or under the supervision of a speech [-language] pathologist or audiologist, for which a patient is referred by a physician" (42 *Code of Federal Regulations*, 440.110[c]). This relationship also has been described by such federal agencies as the Maternal and Child Health Service, the Veterans Administration, and the Health Care Financing Administration (HCFA) (ASHA, 1993c). Further, The Ad Hoc Committee on Professional Autonomy (ASHA, 1986) states that, under the Hearing Conservation Amendment of the Occupational Safety and Health Administration, programs designed to determine hearing loss among American workers must be supervised by either a physician or an audiologist (29 *Code of*

Federal Regulations, 1910.95[g][3]). In addition, under the Longshoremen's and Harbor Worker's Compensation Act (P.L. 98-426), audiograms for the purpose of evaluating hearing loss among workers may be administered by a licensed or certified audiologist or by an otolaryngologist.

Medicare regulations for speech-language pathology also describe clearly the autonomy of outpatient speech-language pathology services. The regulations specify that a speech-language pathologist can establish the written plan of care (42 *Code of Federal Regulations,* 405.1717[a]). Staff from ASHA's Health Care Financing Division (ASHA, 1993c) point out that, as early as 1977, speech-language pathology services were exempt from physician referral for non-Medicare patients. The Institutional Services Provider Branch of HCFA notified ASHA that, "Rehabilitation agencies as providers of outpatient speech [-language] pathology services will be permitted to accept referral from normal sources. . ." (HCFA, personal correspondence, March 17, 1977). "Normal" here means any individual who suspects the presence of a communication disorder.

Finally, the U.S. Department of Health and Human Services (1979), in its descriptions of health professions in *A Report on Allied Health Personnel,* recognized the autonomous nature of speech-language pathology and audiology:

> Speech [-language] pathology and audiology focus on disorders in the production, reception and perception of speech and language. In clinical practice, the speech pathologist (or speech-language pathologist) and audiologist identify individuals who have such disorders and to determine the etiology, history, and severity of specific disorders through interviews and special tests. These health professionals plan and facilitate optimal treatment through remedial procedures, counseling, and guidance. They also make appropriate referrals for medical or other professional attention. (p. xiv-1)

If you were to consider, in its totality, the evidence of professional autonomy in certification standards, state licensure laws, federal regulations, and accreditation agency requirements, you would have sufficient

information to conclude that speech-language pathology and audiology are, in fact, autonomous professions. Speech-language pathologists and audiologists can diagnose communication and related disorders, accept referrals from any source, refer to other professionals, and develop or modify plans of care. That said, it is important to restate that our professions are far from the full autonomous state to which we aspire, because of third-party payer and other federal and state regulatory restrictions. Speech-language pathologists, for example, are still not recognized under the Medicare program as independent providers (unless they establish status as a rehabilitation agency). Furthermore, audiologists cannot receive Medicare reimbursement for audiologic evaluations that are performed for the purposes of a hearing aid (see Chapter 28 by Loavenbruck for further discussion about autonomy and the professional doctorate in audiology).

As autonomous professionals practice in today's complex, compartmentalized, and fragmented health care and educational systems, they must recognize a basic responsibility to work in collaboration with others in order to render a cohesive model of service to an increasingly diverse client population.

INTERDEPENDENCE: THE TIES THAT BIND US

Sherman Grinnell (1989), in his reflections on autonomy and independence for health professionals, states, "Since the days of the American revolution and Declaration of Independence, we Americans have focused on achieving and maintaining personal independence" (p. 115). Thus, Grinnell maintains that professionals have always held to the ideal of independent work. Grinnell (1989) contrasts the ideal for autonomy with the realities of the health care system. In the early days, when professionals were few in number, communities were small, and expertise was limited, the individual professional could function in a highly independent manner. As society grew in size and complexity, however, the model of the independent professional became less viable and increasingly became part of larger bureaucratic structures. Today, states Grinnell, complexity is at an all-time high, with additional factors of advanced technologies, more medically complex patients, and more areas of specialized knowledge contributing to that complexity. In addition, these professionals are subject to policy and administrative restrictions (e.g., third-party payer and managed health care limitations), making autonomy difficult, if not impossible.

As education and health care reforms become imminent in this country, we can dispel any traditional notions about autonomy. As the general education movement takes place, school-based speech-language pathology and audiology services are changing dramatically. For example, many schools are forming site-based teams, comprising staff speech-language pathologists or audiologists, to address the issues of dropout rates, crime and violence, illiteracy, poor math scores, and other system-wide issues (Boyer, 1983). To reduce fragmentation when students are pulled out of class for therapy, speech-language pathologists and audiologists are providing more intervention services in the classroom. Thus, they are collaborating with teachers and other educators to integrate therapy into on-line classroom performance. New terms, suggesting team models of service delivery, include collaborative consultation, literature-based therapy, inclusive education, coteaching, and meaning-based instruction. Each model implies interdependent relationships with other education professionals (see Chapter 17 by Montgomery for further discussion of new school-based models).

Within the context of health care, large purchasers will be more interested in contracting with cohesive networks of providers, rather than with individual providers. Interdependent relationships with other professionals, such as physicians, physical therapists, optometrists, psychologists, and occupational therapists, will be key to successful contract negotiations. Managed health care systems will want to contract with providers who can integrate their services along interdisciplinary and programmatic lines (e.g., a stroke rehabilitation program, a hearing health care program). Many hospitals already are managing by product line, thus integrating all services related to a "product," such as head injury rehabilitation, under one program. In doing so, departmental lines of operation are erased as clinicians form interdisciplinary teams, develop integrated plans of treatment, and cotreat the client (see Chapter 15 by Sutherland Cornett for further discussion of new service delivery models in health care). The ease with which speech-language pathologists and audiologists can make the transition to team models of service will depend largely on individual notions of autonomy.

Grinnell (1989) identifies four operative modes when interacting with other professionals. These modes are based on a framework of psychosocial development (Harvey, Hunt, & Schroeder, 1961) and can be used to trace the evolution of autonomy. They are (with corresponding modes of psychosocial development):

1. Collaboration by command (dependence)
2. Collaboration by specialist division of labor (mutuality)
3. Competitive cold war (negative independence)
4. Collegial collaboration (autonomous interdependence)

The modes are arranged in order of positive psychosocial development, with dependence being the least developed level and autonomous interdependence the most developed level.

COLLABORATION BY COMMAND—DEPENDENCE

This mode defines the traditional superior/subordinate hierarchy of bureaucratic organizations. This mode is successful when an educated elite is in charge of an army of less educated people. It is particularly outmoded when tasks are complex and changeable and when the people doing the work are highly educated and skilled—conditions common in education and health care systems. Except in the simplest of settings, no one individual can possess enough knowledge and skills to play the role of superior. In addition, highly educated professionals who possess the needed knowledge and skills cannot demonstrate their competence in the role of subordinates. Using this mode of operation, autonomy is very limited except as allowed by the person in charge.

SPECIALIST DIVISION OF LABOR—MUTUALITY

This mode has been used widely for organizing technical and scientific specialists, especially in research, development, and high technology organizations. This mode works well as long as professionals work within their scopes of practice, and the scopes of practice of others do not overlap. The mode works well when change is relatively predictable and slow. Once overlap occurs and the professional practice boundaries are blurred, you often enter the next mode—competitive cold war.

COMPETITIVE COLD WAR— NEGATIVE INDEPENDENCE

This mode of operation is chosen willfully by few; it is an unintended consequence of a breakdown in the operation of either the command or specialist division of labor modes. This mode is likely when one profession is dominant and other professions are fighting to gain autonomy. It also erupts during times of rapid change when scopes of practice overlap and professionals begin fighting for their "turf." Autonomy is always limited and at-risk, needing constant vigilance and defense. Those who do not compete effectively will have little autonomy. Whatever autonomy one does have may have little to do with competence and quality of work. States Grinnell (1989),

> In this mode both the quality and cost of health care suffer. The health care consumer is the big

loser. Too much energy goes into engaging in, and managing, the competitive conflict. The focus is on outdoing other professionals rather than delivering high-value care to the consumer. Unless health care professionals are individually and collectively able to work out their issues of interdependence, this mode is likely to be quite prevalent in the health care system of the future. What is most needed in order to escape this predicament is improved interpersonal communications to develop improved working relationships. Unfortunately, many professionals do not put a high value on this skill or support the need for high-quality working relationships. (p. 119)

The next mode relies heavily on interpersonal communication to achieve collegial collaboration.

COLLEGIAL COLLABORATION— AUTONOMOUS INTERDEPENDENCE

Grinnell (1989) believes this mode of operation is less prevalent than need would warrant. Most professionals have not taken the opportunity to develop ways of working with others. Yet, in work environments in which the knowledge and skills possessed by professionals are complex, where client needs are multiple and diverse, and where high value care is in demand, this may be the only mode that can result in adequate performance. This mode is often associated with high performance systems. Rather than compromising autonomy, this mode enhances autonomy. There is a high degree of autonomy in areas of expertise as well as growing autonomy in areas that represent interdisciplinary activities and advancements. Grinnell (1989) states,

> In terms of its ability to focus on the needs of the consumer first and to use the full range of capabilities of the professionals in its system, this mode is most likely to provide comprehensive and high quality care, especially for complex . . . needs. It has the greatest capacity to adapt to rapid change in either professional practice or consumer needs. It depends primarily on the abililty of professionals to develop open, two-way communication among all participants in order to sustain collegial working relationships. The development of these communication processes

in turn depends on the existence of attitudes of mutual respect, trust, and interdependence among professionals. (p. 120)

Today, very few professionals can work with full autonomy and independence. Thus, autonomy must be found in other ways. Clearly, states Grinnell (1989), "the modes of collaboration by command and competitive cold war do not allow this. Only the commander in the former model has much autonomy, and everyone is on shaky ground with the latter" (p. 120). That leaves two options: specialist division of labor and collegial collaboration. The former, however, is successful only when scopes of practice do not overlap, which does not reflect current realities. As professions continue to advance, their scopes of practice will expand. Thus, professional boundaries begin to overlap. It appears that the most viable mode in which to operate today is collegial collaboration. But a major commitment must first be made for effective interdependence.

As mentioned above, team approaches to service delivery have finally gained due recognition in education and health care. Witzel (1993) reminds us, however, that a team approach to clinical management in the discipline of human communication sciences and disorders has been in place since the 1940s. The cleft lip and palate teams were early models of interdisciplinary cooperation. In 1943, the Academy of Cleft Palate Prosthesis was formed to encourage cooperation among other specialties of the health arts group. This association, now the American Cleft Palate-Craniofacial Association, retained its original purpose: "communication and cooperation among professionals from all disciplines interested in craniofacial anomalies" (American Cleft Palate-Craniofacial Association, 1992, p. xii).

In view of the long-standing nature of teaming in the field, you may be versed in team models of care. Today, the terms multidisciplinary, interdisciplinary, and transdisciplinary care are used often and sometimes inaccurately. How are they similar? How do they differ? And what are the advantages and disadvantages of each?

TEAM APPROACHES TO CLIENT CARE

Today, it is considered parochial to regard service provision within the narrow boundaries of a discipline. Clearly, speech-language pathologists and audiologists have established themselves as the experts in the scientific study and clinical management of com- munication disorders. Yet, the area of communication is widely shared as a professional interest in such diverse areas as medicine, nursing, psychology, linguistics, rehabilitation engineering, and expressive arts. We should welcome, rather than discourage the interest of others. States Griffin (1990),

The mindsets of the profession[s] must turn to one of collaboration with other practitioners rather than competition about who will provide the service. Professional survival cannot depend on who gets to provide the service at the expense of the job of another practitioner. Instead, a shared vision of patient outcomes must drive the service delivery system, while mutual respect, trust and cooperation must be the working foundation among the professions. (p. 34)

It is vital to make this mental shift for teaming to be successful. With this orientation as a backdrop, the different team approaches to care can be discussed. The following information is taken, in large part, from an earlier publication (Frattali, 1993).

THE MULTIDISCIPLINARY APPROACH

A multidisciplinary approach to service delivery means that persons from several disciplines are involved in the delivery of service. The approach, however, is discipline-oriented with each team member responsible only for the activities related to his or her own discipline (Halper, 1992). Each discipline formulates separate goals for the client. Therefore, your knowledge base and skills need only be limited to your particular discipline. For example, in educational settings, a student might receive separate services from a speech-language pathologist, reading specialist, psychologist, and occupational therapist. In health care, the multidisciplines could, for example, include the physician, physical therapist, occupational therapist, and social worker. Using a multidisciplinary approach, there is no attempt to integrate services into a cohesive plan. Communication across disciplines often is absent and can be sensed by a client. A lack of coordinated care could result in overlap or fragmentation of service that increases costs and compromises quality. The major disadvantage of the multidisciplinary model is that it addresses the client's individual needs separately, and risks losing sight of how these needs, considered together, can affect the person as a whole (Nevlud, 1990).

THE INTERDISCIPLINARY APPROACH

Similar to the multidisciplinary approach, the interdisciplinary approach involves persons from several disciplines. Their activities, however, are performed to achieve a common goal. Now, these professionals have the added responsibility of a group effort on behalf of the client (Rothberg, 1992). According to Melvin (1980),

> This effort requires the skills necessary for effective group interaction and the knowledge of how to transfer integrated group activities into a result which is greater than the simple sum of the activities of each individual discipline. The group activity of an interdisciplinary program is synergistic, producing more than each could accomplish individually and separately. (pp. 379-380)

Using the interdisciplinary approach, each practitioner addresses first the integrated plan of care during treatment, rather than a specific or isolated need of the client. For example, if the plan includes work on sitting balance, physical therapy may coordinate this aspect of treatment, nursing staff may carry out the plan on the hospital unit, and the prescribed techniques would be used during speech-language pathology services and occupational therapy. Sharing of therapeutic approaches is encouraged. The goals of this approach are to increase learning/performance trials, thereby resulting in less chance for the client to forget or lose important skills,

and to more firmly instill and generalize target behaviors (Nevlud, 1990).

Cotreatment often is part of an interdisciplinary approach. This is a treatment method in which two professionals work simultaneously with the client to achieve the goals as detailed in the care plan. Dysphagia management offers a good example of cotreatment, in which the occupational therapist and speech-language pathologist work together to improve a client's feeding (e.g., through the use of adapted utensils) and swallowing (e.g.,through the use of compensatory techniques) abilities.

THE TRANSDISCIPLINARY APPROACH

Many variations on the meaning of the transdisciplinary approach exist. From the perspective of school-based services, Catlett (1992) describes this approach as follows:

> In the transdisciplinary/collaborative model, it is assumed that "no one person or profession has an adequate knowledge base or sufficient expertise to execute all functions (assessment, planning, and intervention) associated with providing educational services for students" (ASHA, 1991). Thus all team members contribute to the coordinated approach . . . designed for each [client] and family, although each team member's responsibility for implementation may vary. . . .
>
> For example, if a child with a communication disorder needs to be provided with simple directions in the classroom, the speech-language pathologist can assist the classroom teacher in implementing specific techniques and strategies. Similarly, an audiologist might work with a classroom teacher to coordinate seating and environmental modifications for a child with a hearing loss. (p. 3)

This definition coincides with the above definition of the interdisciplinary approach. The concept of cotreatment is derived from this interpretation. Another definition of the transdisciplinary approach comes from the field of health care. It is based on the premise that one person can perform several professionals' roles by providing services to the client under the supervision of individuals from the other disciplines involved (Halper, 1992). According to Halper:

Representatives of various disciplines work together in the initial evaluation and care plan, but only one or two team members actually provide the services. . . . It should be noted that regardless of who is providing the service, professionals are still accountable for areas related to their specific discipline and for training the team member who is delivering the service. (p. 2)

Using this definition, the transdisciplinary approach, which is the most controversial of the three approaches, represents the concept of the multiskilled health practitioner. The multiskilled health practitioner is one who is cross-trained to provide more than one function, often in more than one discipline (Bamberg & Blayney, 1992). This concept is threatening to many practitioners, who fear their responsibilities will shift to practitioners with lesser training and competency. Thus, the approach presents a serious risk to ensuring quality of care, particularly in a climate of cost containment and staff shortages.

THE PROS AND CONS OF TEAMWORK

Teamwork has many obvious advantages, but its disadvantages must also be acknowledged. Two proponents of the interdisciplinary team approach, Catlett and Halper (1992), although espousing its benefits, provide a realistic account of its shortcomings. These benefits and shortcomings are listed in Table 26–1.

Perhaps the most positive benefit of teamwork is that the client is treated as a "whole person," rather than as a "collection of parts." The latter concept results from a high degree of specialization, in which practitioners focus on clinical aspects of functioning germane to their discipline (e.g., speech, hearing, mobility, respiration) while losing sight of the total person being treated. Thus, a team approach fosters a more humane approach to care, as well as integrated, not isolated interventions. Further, a team ap- proach results in better communication among professionals, as well as with clients and their families. Information conveyed to clients by multiple service providers can now be synthesized and, thus, better understood. Teamwork can also result in quicker decision making by bringing together diverse knowledge and skills and reducing or eliminating duplication or fragmentation of effort. Finally, integration of clinical management results in a more cohesive regimen of treatment, thus reducing the likelihood of unnecessary care and increasing the likelihood of better client outcomes.

On the negative side, however, teamwork takes time. This is perhaps the biggest barrier, particularly in view of current realities as practitioners are pressured to increase their caseloads, productivity, and thus, the bottom line. Nevertheless, time is needed for team meetings, planning and developing care plans, educating others, agreeing and disagreeing, negotiating and compromising, and coming to consensus. This can result in a decrease in productivity, which often conflicts with the efficiency goals of the organization (whether written or unwritten) to remain viable in the marketplace.

Many practitioners also perceive a loss of autonomy as a result of teamwork; thus, a territorial spirit can surface. There may be a lack of confidence or trust in the opinions and decisions of others. Recall Grinnell's (1989) and Griffin's (1990) suggestion for a shift in mental models. This shift is necessary for professional collaboration. The perceived loss of autonomy results when practitioners sense a loss of independence. Often, the team, rather than individual practitioners, is given recognition. A perceived loss of autonomy results in mistrust. Confidence levels drop, professional roles clash, territorialism surfaces, and team members may undermine the team effort.

Fortunately, most disadvantages of teamwork can be overcome with an open attitude and feelings of mutual respect and trust. When professionals can look beyond their own provincial concerns to those of the client, many barriers to professional collaboration can be overcome.

TABLE 26–1. IMPACT OF THE INTERDISCIPLINARY TEAM APPROACH

Positive Impact	Negative Impact
Patient treated as a "whole person"	Additional time needed for communication and negotiation
Integrated, rather than isolated interventions	Decrease in productivity
Easier communication with a cohesive team, from patient's point of view, resulting from synthesis of information	Loss of autonomy
Results in quicker decision making by bringing together diverse knowledge and skills	Lack of confidence/trust in opinions/ decisions of others
Duplication or fragmentation of service is reduced or eliminated	Team members' perceptions of roles may clash
	Territorialism

Source: Adapted from Team Approaches: Working Together to Improve Quality by C. Catlett and A. Halper, 1992, Summer, *Quality Improvement Digest.* Copyright American Speech-Language-Hearing Association. Adapted by permission.

SUMMARY

Professional autonomy today embraces the notion of interdependence rather than independence. Our complex and dynamic health care and education systems, coupled with diverse client needs and rapid technological and scientific advances, force us to discard our more traditional notions of autonomy. Sibbet and O'Hara-Devereaux (1991) suggest that no single individual, profession, or institution has enough information or know-how to make decisions. A team rather than an individual approach is, thus, the preferred approach. Together, team members should have sufficient wisdom and experience to envision the right direction and to draw the proper "clinical maps" for clients.

The professions of speech-language pathology and audiology have made great strides in their pursuit of autonomy. This pursuit continues with movements toward the professional doctorate, specialty certification, and status as point of entry into the health care system (i.e., entering the system without referral from other professionals). As part of these pursuits, you are well advised to look beyond the world of your own discipline and integrate within the broader and multidisciplinary health care and education systems.

DISCUSSION QUESTIONS

1. Define professional autonomy in both its traditional and more contemporary aspects.
2. Provide evidence of autonomy in professional qualifications and federal regulations.
3. Describe the multidisciplinary, interdisciplinary, and transdisciplinary team approaches. Which is the preferred approach? State your rationale.
4. How might you envision professional autonomy in the year 2000? In the year 2020?

REFERENCES

American Cleft Palate-Craniofacial Association. (1991). Constitution of the American Cleft Palate-Craniofacial Association. Pittsburgh, PA: Author.
American Speech-Language-Hearing Association. (1986). The autonomy of speech-language pathol-

ogy and audiology (Report by the Ad Hoc Committee on Professional Autonomy). *Asha, 28*, 53–56.

American Speech-Language-Hearing Association. (1991). A model for collaborative service delivery for students with language-learning disorders in the public schools. *Asha, 33*(Suppl. 5), 44–50.

American Speech-Language-Hearing Association. (1992, March). Guidelines, position statements, report. *Asha, 34*(Suppl. 7), 9–40.

American Speech-Language-Hearing Association. (1993a). Code of ethics. *Asha, 35*, 17–18.

American Speech-Language-Hearing Association. (1993b). Implementation procedures for the standards for the certificate of clinical competence (Report by the Clinical Certification Board). *Asha, 35*, 76–83.

American Speech-Language-Hearing Association. (1993c). Technical assistance packet on professional autonomy. (ASHA document from the Health Care Financing Division). Rockville, MD: Author.

Bamberg, R., & Blayney, K. D. (1992). The history and current status of multiskilled health practitioners. In E. D. Blayney (Ed.), *Healing hands: Customizing your health team for institutional survival* (pp. 25–38). Battle Creek, MI: W. K. Kellogg Foundation.

Boyer, E. (1983). *A nation at risk*. Princeton, NJ: Carnegie Foundation for Education.

Catlett, C. (1992, Summer). Team approaches in education settings. *Quality Improvement Digest* (pp. 3–6). Rockville, MD: American Speech-Language-Hearing Association.

Catlett, C., & Halper, A. (1992, Summer). Team approaches: Working together to improve quality. *Quality Improvement Digest*. Rockville, MD: American Speech-Language-Hearing Association.

Cherow, E. (1992). Professional practices perspective on choice and independence. *Asha, 34*, 18.

Frattali, C. M. (1993). Professional collaboration: A team approach to health care. Clinical Series #11.

National Student Speech-Language-Hearing Association. Rockville, MD: National Student Speech Language Hearing Association.

Griffin, K. (1990). Interdisciplinary collaboration means professional viability. *Texas Journal of Audiology and Speech Pathology, 16*, 33–35.

Grinnell, S. K. (1989). Autonomy and independence for health professionals? *Journal of Allied Health, 18*, 115–121.

Halper, A. (1992). Team approaches in healthcare settings. *Quality Improvement Digest* (pp. 3–6). Rockville, MD: American Speech-Language-Hearing Association.

Harvey, O., Hunt, D., & Schroeder, H. (1961). *Stages of psychosocial development*. New York: John Wiley and Sons.

Joint Commission on Accreditation of Healthcare Organizations. (1994). *Accreditation manual for hospitals*, Oakbrook Terrace, IL: Author.

Lathrop, J. P. (1992). The patient-focused hospital. *Healthcare Forum Journal, 35*, 76–78.

Melvin, J. L. (1980). Interdisciplinary and multidisciplinary activities and the ACRM. *Archives of Physical Medicine & Rehabilitation, 70*, 379–380.

Nevlud, G. N. (1990). The team approach: Curent trends and issues in rehabilitation. *Texas Journal of Audiology and Speech Pathology, 16*, 21–23.

Rothberg, J. S. (1992). Knowledge of disciplines, roles, and functions of team members. In American Congress of Rehabilitation Medicine (Ed.), *Guide to interdisciplinary practice in rehabilitation settings* (pp. 44–71). Skokie, IL: American Congress of Rehabilitation Medicine.

Sibbet, J. J., & O'Hara-Devereaux, M. (1991). The language of teamwork. *Healthcare Forum Journal, 34*, 27–30.

U.S. Department of Health and Human Services, Public Health Service, Health Resources Administration. (1979). *A report on allied health personnel*. Washington, DC: Author.

Witzel, M. A. (1993). Cleft lip and palate and craniofacial treatment. *Asha, 35*, 42–43.

■ CHAPTER 27 ■

Burnout

■ ROSEMARY LUBINSKI, Ed.D. ■

Ever since Claire Smith (pseudonym) was a little girl, she wanted to be a teacher. At 4 years old she would arrange her books and supplies on a make-shift desk and pretend to be both teacher and student. In high school, when asked to choose a setting for her career day field trip, she decided to visit the school for the deaf where her cousin attended. This visit led Claire on a path of becoming a speech-language pathologist. Thirteen years later, when she drove past the school for the deaf , she cursed the day she had ever visited there. " I probably should have been an accountant. I really thought I could do everything for my clients, but what I'm doing really doesn't mean anything, and no one really cares if I do it. They're all turkeys, everyone of them."

In the intervening 13 years, Claire earned a master's degree with honors and had been working as a speech-language pathologist for 7 years in a large residential rehabilitation center for neurologically impaired teenagers and adults. Claire's caseload consisted of severely impaired brain injured patients and stroke patients. Many of the patients were nonverbal, severely physically impaired, and had limited support or contact with family. From her first day on the job, Claire suspected that her supervisor was incompetent. He did the minimum to promote the program within the center, despite the talent and motivation of the staff of four speech-language pathologists and one audiologist. Despite the fact that the program could accommodate at least one other speech-language pathologist, nothing was done to enlarge the program. Suggestions from the staff for enhancing the program were discouraged, and continuing education was minimally supported. Claire had suggested that the staff needed inservice and consultation on new developments in assistive communication devices, but her supervisor suggested that she "read about it." A new executive director of the center recently indicated that staff cuts were imminent, although no one knew where they would be or when.

Claire's distress regarding the bleak outlook within her department was compounded by her recent divorce from her husband. She was faced with increased role responsibilities for caring for her 2-year-old son, finding more affordable housing, and maintaining her position at the center. In addition, her father had died 6 months ago after a lengthy illness necessitating that Claire assume more direct care for her mother who has multiple sclerosis. She felt concerned that her mother's needs were becoming too great and that long-term care might be necessary for her. Her only brother lived too far away to help on a daily basis and suggested that Claire make any arrangements she thought best for their mother.

Claire began to experience serious physical symptoms immediately after the death of her father. Medical examination and testing revealed that, in addition to chronic insominia, her blood pressure had increased abnormally, and she had a stomach ulcer. Her physician prescribed a tranquilizer and ulcer medication, both of which Claire took sporadically—afraid to develop a dependency on "pill popping." Claire chronically felt tired , irritable, and "down." She had recently resumed smoking, a habit which she had quit for 7 years, and had lost 15 pounds. Her personal philosophy was that "everyone has problems; I really should be able to deal with all this."

SCOPE OF CHAPTER

Claire's case illustrates that professionals in communication disorders are not immune to "burnout." Although most professionals experience some fatigue, frustration, and stress related to professional life, some professionals will experience such depleting stress from one or a variety of sources that they may be candidates for burnout. As the best antidote for burnout is prevention, this chapter is presented to introduce students and professionals to this potential problem, provide strategies for self-identification, and suggestions for both prevention and management. Maslach (1982) says "The risk of burnout is less likely to become reality if you get a head start on it" (p. 131). Academic and clinical training programs as well as professional agencies and organizations have a responsibility to concentrate on knowledge and skills but also on how to become and remain a "totally healthy" professional. Additional beneficiaries of this humanistic approach are clients, co-workers, and families.

DEFINITIONS AND SYMPTOMOTOLOGY

STRESS

Although there are many definitions of stress, one definition that appears both comprehensive and applicable to professionals in communicative disorders is given by Monet and Lazarus (1977). They state that stress "consists of any event in which environmental demands, internal demands or both tax or exceed the adaptive resources of an individual, social system, or tissue system" (p. 3). Thus, stress may emanate from some combination of professional and/or personal events of our environment, our own personal makeup to cope with stressors and their effects, and our individual perception of the situation.

Each of us usually is able to cope with life's demands. For any number of reasons, however, one's internal and external coping resources may become so strained at certain times that adaptation is ineffective to meet the problem. In the case of acute stress, the individual is thrown off balance for a short period of time before stability returns. For example, when preparing for a final examination, a student may focus only on studying for that test for a week, while neglecting other academic and personal pursuits. After the test, the student resumes a regular daily routine. In contrast, chronic stress occurs when a person is challenged over a long period of time by mild to severe stressors. Persistent stress tends to result in a "snowball" or "pile-up" effect. Individuals may not even be completely conscious of the nature or severity of the stressors affecting them or of the numerous serious effects. They may be aware, however, that their ability to cope effectively is diminished.

Chronic stress, in particular, takes an insidious and viscious physical and psychological toll on an individual. Physical effects of stress can range from mild to extreme. Such effects include fatigue, insomnia, headaches, gastrointestinal disorders, dermatological disorders, susceptibility to infection, hypertension, and heart disease (Farmer, Monahan, & Hekeler, 1984). Psychologically, the person may feel some degree of anxiety or depression. How the person perceives and eventually copes with chronic stress may in itself cause further problems. For example, skipping nutritious meals may lead to unnecessary weight loss; use of drugs may lead to a dependency; and social withdrawal may lead to a feeling of even greater despair.

BURNOUT DEFINITION

A special effect of chronic stress is burnout. Maslach (1982) defines burnout as a "syndrome of emotional exhaustion, depersonalization, and reduced personal accomplishment that can occur among individuals who do 'people work' of some type" (p. 3). Burnout is a unique process rather than an event (Farber, 1983). Maslach believes that burnout is rooted in the relationship between caregiver and care receiver. Many clients with communication disorders and their families may have such a multitude of serious and complicated problems, that trying to meet their needs may tax a professional's internal and external resources. In some clinical situations, the caseloads may be so high that there is a lack of adequate time to provide the counseling and support needed to enhance traditional therapy. In yet other clinical situations, clients may have little support from family or significant others and depend even more on the speech-language pathologist or audiologist for that sustenance. Some clients are unmotivated and noncompliant, other clients and famlies may provide little or no obvious appreciation for professional skill and support.

Burnout can emanate from many other sources as well. Table 27–1 lists sources of burnout adapted from research by Macinick and Macinick (1990), Maslach (1982), Scheller (1990), and Tschudin (1990). Unreasonable demands of the professional position, inadequacy on the part of co-workers and supervisors, and the policies and procedures governing the agency may individually or in combination contribute to burnout. In some clinical positions, there will be a lack of autonomy and opportunity for self-actualization. For example, if a clinician such as Claire has little opportunity to create innovative programs and receives little reinforcement from her supervisor, this may contribute to burnout. Job insecurity and low pay, combined with increased financial pressures, may also be critical. Discrimination based on age, race, or gender lead to stress. Inadequate supervision, unclear criteria for performance evaluation, and evaluations that focus only on "what you could do better" are all detrimental. Finally, negative relationships with co-workers or supervisors create a hostile situation where burnout is likely to occur.

A professional's own personality characteristics may be a source of burnout. Maslach (1982) uses adjectives such as submissive, anxious, fearful, passive, impatient, insecure, and intolerant to describe the personality pro-

TABLE 27–1. SOURCES OF BURNOUT IN HELPING RELATIONSHIP PROFESSIONS.

Client factors
Overly demanding clients and/or families
Complicated, serious problems of clients and/or families
Lack of client/family responsiveness
Lack of client/family appreciation

Professional situation factors
Size of caseload
Too many responsibilities
Lack of autonomy
Little opportunity for self-actualization
Low pay; few salary increases
Job insecurity
Little opportunity for continuing education
Tedium
Excessive paperwork and inadequate time to complete it
Inadequate working conditions and/or resources
Discrimination: sexism, ageism, racism
Inadequate supervision
Unclear criteria for professional evaluation
Evaluation based on negative factors only
Co-worker competition or incompetence
Lack of co-worker support
Interdisciplinary conflict or competition
Unprofessional attitudes on part of supervisor or co-workers
Rigid or unrealistic institutional policies

Personal factors
Unrealistic expectations; perfectionism; need to do it "all"
Not being able to say "no"
Not being able to delegate work to others
Lack of confidence
Need for approval from others
Hostility
Impatience
Personal and/or family health problems
Family pressures
Competing demands of job and family

Source: Adapted from "Strategies for Burnout Prevention in the Mental Health Setting" by C. Macinick and J. Macinick, 1990. *International Nursing Review, 37*, 247–250.

file of a burnout candidate. Maslach cautions, however, that *all* individuals, given the right (or wrong) degree of stressful circumstances may be ripe for burnout. Burnout may occur in the strongest of personalities when stresses are prolonged, intense, or unresolved. In Claire's case there are numerous familial pressures coexisting with the pressures inherent in her professional situation.

The issue of competing demands from job and family deserves special attention because the profession of speech-language pathology, in particular, is dominated by women. It should be remembered, however, that many professional men do share in caregiving and homemaking duties and thus also experience difficulties in balancing competing demands of professional and family life. Shewan and

Blake (1991) in a recent study of caregiving needs of our professions found that while the median number of dependents for affiliates of the American Speech-Language-Hearing Association (ASHA) was only one, caregiving duties consumed 20 hours per week. Full time speech-language pathogists spent more time than did audiologists; women spent more time than did men in caregiving duties.

Bonnar (1991) states that caregiving is not valued in our society and is perceived as "invisible work." Caregiving involves other than "housework duties," and tends to be considered within the female domain of responsibilities. The recipients of caregiving are children and the elderly. The U.S. Department of Labor (1990) reports that 65% of women who had children under 18 years of age were employed. Scharlach and Boyd (1989) found that 23% of employees had some caregiving duties for elderly parents. Stone and Short (1989) reported that close to 1 million working women were faced with caregiving responsibilities for both children and adults. These statistics are likely to have implications for benefits from individual employers as well as for federal policy and legislation affecting maternity, parental, or family leave (McGovern & Matter, 1992).

Several themes emerge from this discussion of sources of burnout. The sources of burnout are individual, diverse, and multiple. The stressors can range from mild to severe. Given the proper combination of circumstances, everyone in a helping profession such as speech-language pathology or audiology is a candidate for burnout. What appears critical is self-perception of stressors and an individual's internal and external resources for coping successfully with them.

STAGES OF BURNOUT

Cherniss (1980) postulates that there are three stages during the process of burnout for those in helping professions. In Stage 1 there is an imbalance between the demands and resources to deal with job stress. There are too few personal or institutional resources to equalize increasing demands. This leads to Stage 2 when the individual reacts to this strain with feelings of anxiety, tension, fatigue, and exhaustion. Finally, in Stage 3, defensive coping emerges characterized by emotional detachment, withdrawal, cynicism, and rigidity. A vicious and insidious cycle emerges: The greater the demands placed on the professional, the greater need for resources. Resources, however require energy that, unfortunately, has become depleted.

EFFECTS OF BURNOUT

The effects of burnout are as numerous and complex as are the causes. Table 27–2 divides the effects of burnout into four major catetories: professional effects, psychological effects, physiological effects, and effects on significant others. Maslach (1982) says that one of the most obvious signs of burnout is the sense of *emotional exhaustion* in which the professional feels frustrated, physically exhausted, and emotionally depleted. The individual feels hopeless and as though there is "no more to give." The natural strategy to cope with such emotional exhaustion is to try to distance oneself from work. The professional perceives that with self-withdrawal from the source(s) of the problem, particulary the persons involved, stability will be recovered. Unfortunately, this response leads to *depersonalization* in which the professional resents and denigrates the clients, co-workers, or others who are perceived as the root of the problem. Maslach adds that such a negative perception eventually leads to a sense of *personal inadequacy*. In this state one feels a deep sense of failure and inability to accomplish one's goals. All of these feelings blend and lead to poor quality and quantity of work performance as well as depression. Consequently, some individuals may change careers or job positions, reduce work load, and/or seek counseling.

TABLE 27–2. EFFECTS OF BURNOUT.

Professional effects
Detachment
Depersonalization
Sense of inadequacy
Irritated with clients
Do less work
Work performance deteriorates

Psychological effects
Sadness
Anger
Frustration
Tension
Anxiety
Depression
Forgetful
Suspicious
Paranoid

Physiological effects
Feeling of exhaustion and chronic fatigue
Increased susceptibility to illness and infection
Poor eating habits
Frequent headaches
Insomnia
Gastrointestinal disorders
Dermatological disorders (e.g., hives, exema)
Back and neck disorders
Hypertension
Heart attack
Stroke

Effects on significant others
Marital conflict
Family discord

The psychological effects are also apparent and range from feelings of sadness, anger, and frustration to depression, suspiciousness, and paranoia. Many conflicting feelings abound. Feelings such as being annoyed and frustrated lead to detachment; irritation and overload lead to depersonalization; reduced self-esteem leads to depression.

One of the most common physiological effects is a sense of chronic exhaustion. The persistent negative responses of emotional depletion, depersonalization, and sense of inadequacy combined with pervasive delete-rious psychological effects may lead to serious health problems. These health problems can take any individual or combination of forms such as headaches, susceptibility to infections, insomnia, gastrointestinal disorders, and hypertension. At the most serious end of the continuum, some individuals may suffer a heart attack or stroke. Numerous other obvious health problems may also occur such as poor eating habits, alchohol abuse, smoking, and overuse of or dependency on tranquilizers or other drugs.

The effects of burnout may reach to co-workers and family. For example, a professional who is experiencing burnout may withdraw from co-workers, view them in a suspicious manner, or become dependent on them for completing a job. When burnout is rampant within an agency, a negative climate may pervade the institution, and job satisfaction and morale are likely to be low (Cherniss, 1980). Frequent job turnover is also a result and has economic and quality improvement implications.

Family members are likely to bear some of the brunt of professional burnout. Marital conflict and family discord are well documented by many professionals who feel burned out (e.g., Social Work: Siefert, Jayaratne, & Chess, 1991; Teaching: Sakharov & Farber, 1983; Medicine: Mawardi, 1983; Nursing: McLaughlin & Erdman, 1992; Day Care Workers: Maslach & Pines, 1977). Spouses and children may make comments such as "Dad's grumpy all the time," "I can't seem to do anything right for Mom any more," "Since you got that job you've not been the person I married." The professional may be unaware that the angry outbursts at home are a reflection of professional burnout. A professional who is emotionally and physically exhausted from stresses in the work place cannot magically leave them at the door when family time begins. In addition, the effects of stresses associated with marriage, family life, finances, and other outside issues complicate and magnify professional stresses and their effects. A vicious and insidious cycle of stress and maladaptive coping is likely to occur.

STRESS IN HUMAN
SERVICE PROFESSIONS

A logical question you might ask is why is burnout so common among human service professionals. A helping relationship involves an investment of knowledge and skill blended with facilitating interpersonal qualities to effect change in another individual. Individuals drawn into helping professions such as speech-language pathology and audiology tend to be oriented to people rather than things and to helping those in trouble (Pines, 1983). Other helping professions include, but are not limited to, those related to teaching, psychology, counseling and social work, medicine, and nursing. The fact that so many helping professions work in impersonal institutions further complicates the situation. Farmer et al., (1984) state that at least four factors inherent in helping professions that are inherently stressful: (a) the complexity of our clients and their needs; (b) the difficulty in evaluating "success" in the helping professions; (c) poor perception of helping relationships by others; and (d) the decision making process inherent in many helping relationship agencies. Maslach (1982) calls burnout the "cost of caring."

The fact that human services are frequently offered through governmental and institutional settings further complicates the situation. Caplan and Jones (1975) state that there are stresses particular to institutional settings, including role ambiguity, role conflict, and role overload. For example, in some institutional settings, there are unclear job definitions, discipline boundaries, and criteria for success. Role conflict emerges from inappropriate or unclear demands on the professional or disparity between individual and institutional ethics and values. Finally, role overload develops from caseloads that are too large or too demanding. The setting by its very nature may be insensitive to the demands on or needs of individual professionals. Farber (1983) cautions that this attitude may increase as economic resources to support human service programs decrease.

BURNOUT IN SPEECH-
LANGUAGE PATHOLOGY
AND AUDIOLOGY

Several studies have addressed the topic of burnout among speech-language pathologists (Miller & Potter, 1982; Potter & Rudensey,1982; Potter, Hellesto, Shute, & Dengerink, 1988). In Miller and Potter's study of speech-language pathologists, 43% of the respondents considered themselves to have experienced moderately severe burnout. Burnout appeared related to job dissatisfaction, job effectiveness, and lack of management and support services for coping. Interestingly, burnout was not related to setting, years of employment, caseload, client severity level, paperwork demands, or collegial relationships.

In a second study that investigated how speech-language pathologists coped with burnout, Potter and Rudensey (1984) found that 16% of their respondents were leaving the profession because of burnout. Effective coping strategies included adapting personal career goals to be more realistic, understanding motivations for being in a helping profession, increasing communication with administrators, and developing a self-change attitude. They also found that there were some effective strategies generated by agencies to reduce burnout among speech-language pathologists. These included systematic solicitation and implementation of employee suggestions, group discussions, flexible break times, released time for continuing education, and clear communication of current job expectations. Potter and Rudensey concluded that a team approach involving speech-language pathologists and administrators could be effective in improving the mental health of clinical staff.

Two studies have specifically addressed burnout among audiologists (Potter et al.,

1988). In the first study of 184 clinically certified audiologists, 40% of the respondents considered themselve as mildly burned out, 30% as moderately or severely burned out, and 29% as not experiencing burnout. Factors contributing to burnout included feelings of job ineffectiveness and dissatisfaction. In a follow-up survey of audiologists that explored causes and coping strategies related to burnout, the same authors found that 15% of their respondents were leaving the profession, and another 67% had considered this option. The authors concluded that strategies that might reduce burnout among audiologists include (a) having employees participate more in orgnizational policy setting, (b) reducing caseloads and paperwork, (c) inclusion of more uninterrupted flexible break time, (d) matching of supervisor's and employee's role expectations, (e) and accurate job descriptions (1988, p. 25).

SELF-IDENTIFICATION STRATEGIES

Perhaps in reading this chapter you have said "that's me" or asked "could that really happen to me?" At times, most professionals will have negative experiences associated with professional life. What is critical, however, is prolonged, excessive, and destructive experiences and perceptions that lead to professional burnout. Recognition of warning signs is the first step in prevention or recovery from burnout. Three inventories by Farmer, Monahan, and Hekeler (1984) focus on the sources of stress, the effects of stress, and the behaviors used to cope with stress in human services. Although there are many other well-established stress and burnout inventories available in the literature (e.g., Symptom Checklist 90—Revised [Derogatis, 1977]; Ways of Coping Checklist [Vitaliano, Russo, Carr, Maiuro, & Becker, 1985]), these inventories serve as good starting points for self-evaluation. Each of these inventories requires that you iden-

tify and/or rate sources of stress, effects of stress, and strategies you use to cope with per ceived difficulties.

A second method of identifying burnout is to talk with co-workers and family about your behaviors and reactions. These individuals may be well aware of changes in your attitude and behavior that may signal potential burnout. It should be noted, however, that many colleagues may be hesitant to comment spontaneously on another's behaviors even when concerned.

REMEDIATION OF BURNOUT

Both professionals and their employment settings have a vital interest in remediating or preventing burnout. Thus, changes that will reduce stress and foster productive coping strategies can emanate from professionals and/or your setting. There are two basic ways to approach this problem: (a) change yourself and your attitudes or (b) remove the cause(s) of the stress (Tschudin, 1990). Excellent sources for more in-depth reading on how to cope with burnout include works by Maslach (1982) and Pines, Aronson, and Kafry (1981). Numerous studies on the effects of stress-reducing programs tend to show positive outcomes for the professional and the setting (e.g., Lees & Ellis, 1989).

CHANGING YOURSELF AND YOUR ATTITUDES

Macinick and Macinick (1990) and Maslach (1982) are among many authors who suggest that at least some remediation of burnout stems from changing one's own attitudes. Systems rarely change, individuals do. Thus, remediation begins with understanding yourself and understanding, accepting, and working smart even within a flawed system.

Thus, professionals who feel burned out need to self-analyze goals, expectations, and value systems governing their professional lives. Changing one's own attitudes also involves development of problem-solving strategies that maximize inner strengths and accomplishments. Productive problem solving entails problem identification, presentation of alternative solutions and their potential benefits, and consideration of the costs involved in solving the problem.

An initial step in coping with burnout is to assess your strengths. Personal strengths may be ignored by a professional who feels stressed. Farmer, Monahan, and Hekeler (1984) suggest that you begin by listing what you consider your physical, emotional, social, intellectual, spiritual, and other strengths. Such analysis may lead you to affirm your positive qualities, cultivate a more positive self-image, and to call up these resources when stressed.

If you are feeling burned out professionally, you may need to analyze your own movitations influencing the practice of your job. Tschudin (1990) suggests that many professionals bring "personal luggage" to work such as carryover of childhood expectations to adulthood, guilt, vague resentments, perfectionism, inability to say no, overcaring for others, and lack of confidence. Tschudin states that "when you look at the stress produced from within yourself, you begin to see that the responsibility lies with you, and within you. But it takes a lot of personal strength to accept this, cope with it and use it positively" (p. 41). Some individuals can do this self-analysis and self-change alone; others need the help of a mentor or counselor.

Working Smarter

A second strategy that professionals may adopt to change themselves is to "work smarter." Professionals who feel burned out do not need to work harder but do need to make a more productive investment in their work life. Working smarter, according to Maslach (1982), involves changing your job to be less stressful and more efficient. This can be achieved by setting realistic goals, doing the same thing differently, improving time management, taking breaks, and taking things less personally.

Setting realistic goals stems from an analysis of what *really* needs to be done, resources for completion, and available time. "Setting realistic goals involves a recognition of your limitations as well as your abilities" (Maslach, 1982, p. 91). The value of changing how things are done is that you will feel more in control of the situation. This strategy begins with analysis of the steps involved in tasks and their eventual elimination or modification. For example, one clinician may want to begin the day at 7 AM with completion of paperwork from the previous day, although another would rather come in later and do this at the end of the day. Taking a planned break from work is also essential in remediating burnout. Some professionals need quiet times dispersed between clients; others need to "go out for lunch," and still others divert some of their professional time to less intense or stressful tasks. Finally, and perhaps most difficult, professionals need to perceive difficult situations as objectively as possible.

Decompression Activities

Taking care of yourself outside the work situation helps relieve burnout. Maslach (1982) states that "the demands of a caring profession necessitate that professionals take good care of their body and spirit" (p. 95). Examples of physical decompression activites include exercise, noncompetitive physical activities, a healthy diet, plenty of rest, and specific relaxation techniques.

Exercise, one of the most popular stress reduction techniques, helps to condition the cardiovascular system to withstand stress (e.g., Tatelbaum, 1989). Exercise activities such as walking, jogging, swimming, and other aerobics all result in direct medical, endurance, flexibility, and emotional benefits (Farmer, Monahan, & Hekeler, 1984). Relaxation activities include deep breathing, progressive muscle relaxation, autogenic training, biofeedback, yoga, imagery, and meditation (Peddicord, 1991). Listening to music also helps to naturally "tranquilize" people (Parachin, 1991). Many of these relaxation activities can be done throughout the work day.

Psychological dempression activities include participation in meaningful and enjoyable outside activities and "accentuation of the positive." Participation in recreation activities such as hobbies can help counterbalance a day of stress. Taking an occasional day off from work or going on a planned vacation can contribute to well-being. Unfortunately, because of demanding caseloads, financial needs, and competing demands from work and home, some professionals have or make little time available just for themselves. Maslach (1982) states that "frustrations and failures can be put into perspective when balanced by satisfactions and successes" (p.95). In order to help others effectively, you consistently need to fortify yourself physically and psychologically.

Continuing Education

Participation in continuing education programs offered through the work place or professional organizations is an excellent strategy for dealing with burnout. Continuing education helps you gain new skills to work more effectively and efficiently, stimulates creative thinking and problem solving, and opens networks with other professionals. Inservices offered through your employment setting might focus not only on assessment and intervention issues related to communication disorders but also on time management, conflict resolution, and stress management.

Attendance at regional, state, or national meetings provides an opportunity for many professionals to combine educational enhancement with the opportunity to "get away" from the stresses of both work and family. Generally, there are social activites at these events where you can initiate or renew professional and personal friendships. In order not to be disappointed with the continuing education program offered, you should be sure to carefully review announcements to determine if the stated objectives match your background and needs at the time. Finally, you may find yourself "recharged" when you are the presenter at a continuing education program. The challenge and intellectual stimulation inherent in the preparation as well as the positive feedback afterward may help relieve burnout.

Support and Counseling

Social support is defined as "information that leads individuals to believe that they are cared for and loved, esteemed, and valued and they participate in a network of communciation and mutual obligation" (Pines, 1983, p. 156). Cobb (1976) considers support an "immunization" against stress. A supportive individual is an active listener, and provides nonjudgmental emotional backup, assistance, insight, and feedback. The primary vehicles for offering support are open communication, active listening, and accessibility. Maslach (1982) adds that humor also is an important supportive coping technique. "Being able to joke and laugh about a stressful event reduces the tension and anxiety—it also seves to make the situation less serious and less overwhelming" (p. 60).

In many institutional settings, individual mentors are available to discuss technical and psychological aspects of the job. The Clinical Fellowship Year (CFY) supervisor may assume this role for the first year professional, with co-workers, formally or informally, possibly adopting this relationship. Pines, et al. (1981) suggest that even staff meetings can help reduce burnout if they focus on articulation of shared problems and staff development. Similarly, in some settings, particularly large institutional settings such as school districts or hospitals, work-setting support groups may be available. These groups focus on developing staff effectiveness and problem solving through free expression of feelings, offering of suggestions and feedback, and realistic goal setting (Scully,1983). There may be specific topic agendas such as techniques for stress management, methods of conflict management, development of self-esteem, and assertiveness (Tschudin, 1990).

Support offered by family and friends is also valuable although "bringing home" stressful topics may exaccerbate burnout rather than relieve it. Maslach (1982) states that family and friends tend to offer comfort, appreciation, and positive experiences. Her research has also identified the critical importance of a good marriage or intimate relationship in "counterbalancing" the stresses of a job. Some authors suggest that spirituality may sustain individuals through stressful times. Spirituality goes beyond participation in formal religious organizations and focuses on a person's perception of his or her place in the universe and the creation of a personal value system (Farmer et al., 1984).

CHANGING JOBS

There may be times in your professional life when, despite your concerted efforts to adapt to and cope with stresses, a change in employment may be the best alternative. Maslach (1982) cautions us to consider carefully what a change means and its expected outcome. "Change does not automatically guarantee success and happiness" (p. 107). Change may involve assuming another position in the same organization such as becoming a supervisor or administrator. Pines et al. (1981) describe this as "quitting upward." It may also mean changing employment settings but working in a comparable position or a new one. Finally, change may mean leaving the professions of speech-langauge pathology or audiology.

In considering a change, you need to assess whether the new position really results in a removal of current stressors. It is quite possible that a position in a new agency entails very similar stressors to your present position. Further, a new position may have unique or additional stressors with which you are not prepared to cope.

Before you change positions, remember that there is a certain degree of stress inherent in changing positions. For example, there may be unfamiliar duties and routines associated with the new position, philosophical differences in service delivery, and "great expectations" for performance. Should you be changing geographical areas, there is the added stress of relocation perhaps to an unfamiliar area that lacks a personal support system.

Notwithstanding these cautions, change can be invigorating and challenging. A new position may be a true antidote for burnout. This may be the perfect opportunity to use coping skills learned in a previous position. It may also be a chance to demonstrate heretofore unrecognized abilities and to fulfill personal career goals.

PREVENTION OF BURNOUT

Early identification of burnout is the most effective way to cope with burnout. As Maslach (1982) states, the key to prevention is early action. The risk of burnout is less likely to become reality if you are forewarned . Thus, students and professionals alike can benefit from an awareness of the presenting signs of burnout and the development of work and life styles that help prevent its emergence.

What are some practical ways to discourage burnout? Knowing the scope of your professional duties helps to define your job in realistic terms. If some of the duties are beyond your abilities, these should be discussed with your supervisor to determine how you might gain needed skills or how the duties might be reassigned. Discussion with your supervisor should also focus on how you will be evaluated in your position so that you have a clear conception of the agency's performance exectations. Unless you have this information, you may assume too many duties, assume duties for which you are unprepared, and work toward goals that are unrealistic or unappreciated.

A second strategy for preventing burnout is to enlist the help of a mentor who can provide objective feedback to you about your performance and with whom you can discuss potential and real problems. This person may be an excellent resource for helping you to work smarter and more effectively within your agency. Maslach (1982) states that colleagues may serve as an "early warning system" to each other when early burnout symptoms appear.

A third strategy for preventing burnout is to incorporate the burnout coping strategies into your life from your student days and your earliest professional employment. For example, you should periodically and objectively self-analyze your professional goals and motivation; participate in exercise, recreation, and continuing education programs; and seek support when needed.

NEEDED RESEARCH

The professions of audiology and speech-language pathology have undertaken little specific research in the area of professional burnout (e.g., Miller & Potter, 1982; Potter & Rudensey, 1984). There appears to be little reason to suspect that these professions are more immune to burnout than other helping professions such as social work, nursing, and education. Numerous national issues including changing demographics of our target populations; the focus on increasing costs of health care, education, and rehabilitation; demands for definition of efficacy of treatment; and technological advancements in our own professions mean that our professions are undergoing scrutiny and modification. The time is ripe for inclusion of the topic of burnout in our training programs to prepare future professionals to function effectively at an emotional and interpersonal level in their work settings. Finally, although burnout affects both genders, being female-dominated professions, we should be particularly sensitive to the competing demands and ensuant stress many women experience in balancing work and family life. Much can be gained from an exploration of not only the stressors but also the productive strategies women and men use to meet competing demands. Our professions and the individuals we serve would benefit from closer introspection into such professional issues.

SUMMARY

At some point in a professional career, audiologists and speech-language pathologists may incur prolonged stress that leads to burnout. Burnout is defined as emotional and physical exhaustion, a feeling of incompetence and depersonalization. Burnout arises from an intermingling of factors including the nature of our clients' problems, complex work setting factors, and our own personal makeup. It results in deterioration in work performance, psychological disorders, physiological changes, and changes in relationships with clients, co-workers, and significant others. Coping with burnout involves changing one's own attitudes about work and success; working smarter; incorporating excercise, recreation, and other decompression techniques into daily life; partipating in continuing education; and seeking peer, family, or professional support. The best antidote for burnout is prevention, which involves discussion of burnout etiology and symptoms during preprofessional training. Approaching employment with a self-monitoring attitude will also help prevent burnout. Speech-language pathologists and audiolgists who consider a holistic approach to professional life that focuses on balancing theoretical and technical knowledge with self-care will surely provide quality services to those who can benefit.

DISCUSSION QUESTIONS

1. What are some warning signs of burnout?
2. What would you do if one of your colleagues demonstrated signs of burnout?
3. Why may it be difficult to incorporate burnout coping strategies into your professional and personal life?
4. What personal strengths and resources can you develop to help you function effectively as a professional?
5. What societal factors do you believe contribute to burnout within human service professions?

REFERENCES

Bonnar, D. (1991). The place of caregiving work in contemporary societies. In J. Hyde, & M. Essex (Eds.), *Parental leave and child care*. Philadelphia: Temple University Press.

Caplan, R., & Jones, K. (1975). Effects of workload, role ambiguity, and type A personality or anxiety, depression, and heart rate. *Journal of Applied Psychology, 60*, 713–719.

Cherniss, C. (1980). *Staff burnout job stress in the human services*. Beverly Hills: Sage Publications.

Cobb, S. (1976). Social support at a moderator of life stress. *Psychosomatic Medicine, 38*, 300–314.

Derogatis, L. (1977). *SCL-90 Administration, Scoring and Procedures Manual*. Privately published by Author.

Farber, B. (1983). Dysfunctional aspects of the psychotherapeutic role. In B. Farber (Ed.), *Stress and burnout in the human services professions* (pp. 97–115). New York: Pegasus.

Farmer, R., Monahan, L., & Hekeler, R. (1984). *Stress management for human services*. Beverly Hills: Sage Publications.

Lees, S., & Ellis, N. (1990). The design of a stress-management program for nursing personnel. *Journal of Advanced Nursing, 15*, 946–961.

Macinick, C., & Macinick, J. (1990). Strategies for burnout prevention in the mental health setting. *International Nursing Review, 37*, 247–250.

Maslach, C. (1982). *Burnout: The cost of caring*. Englewood Cliffs, NJ: Prentice-Hall.

Maslach, C., & Pines, A. (1977). The "burnout" syndrome in day care settings. *Child Care Quarterly, 6*, 100–113.

Mawardi, B. (1983). Aspects of the impaired physician. In B. Farber (Ed.), *Stress and burnout in the human service professions* (pp. 119–128). New York: Pergamon Press.

McGovern, P., & Matter, D. (1992). Work and family coping demands affecting worker well being. *American Association of Occupational Health Nurses Journal, 40*, 24–35.

McLaughlin, A., & Erdman, J. (1992). Rehabilitation staff stress as it relates to patient acuity and diagnosis. *Brain Injury, 6*, 59–64.

Miller, M., & Potter, R. (1982). Professional burnout among speech-language pathologists. *Asha 24*, 177–180.

Monet, A., & Lazarus R. (Eds.). (1977). *Stress and coping*. New York: Columbia University Press.

Parachin, V. (1991). Pressure-proof your life: Creative ways to reduce stress. *Today's Nurse, 13*, 9–11.

Peddicord, K. (1991). Strategies for promoting stress reduction and relaxation. *Nursing Clinics of North America, 26*, 867–874.

Pines, A. (1983). On burnout and the buffering effects of social support. In B. Farber (Ed.), *Stress and burnout in the human service professions* (pp. 155–174). New York: Pergamon Press.

Pines, A., Aronson, E., & Kafry, D. (1981). *Burnout*. New York: The Free Press.

Potter, R., & Rudensey, K. (1984). Coping with burnout. *Asha, 26*, 35–37.

Potter, R., Hellesto, P., Shute, B., & Dengerink, J. (1988). Burnout among audiologists: Its incidence and causes. *The Hearing Journal, 41*, 18–25.

Sakharov, M., & Farber, B. (1983). A critical study of burnout in teachers. In B. Farber, (Ed.), *Stress and burnout in the human service professions*. New York: Pergamon Press.

Scharlach, A., & Boyd, S. (1989). Caregiving and employment: results of an employee survey. *The Gerontological Society of America, 29*, 382–387.

Scheller, M. (1990). *Building partnerships in hospital care*. Palo Alto, CA: Bull Publishing.

Scully, R. (1983). The work setting support group: A means of preventing burnout. In B. Farber (Ed.), *Stress and burnout in the human service professions*. New York: Pergamon Press.

Shewan, C., & Blake, A. (1991). Caregiving: A common role for ASHA members. *Asha, 35*, 35.

Siefert, K., Jayaratne, S., & Chess, W. (1991). Job satisfaction, burnout, and turnover in health care social workers. *Health and Social Work, 16*, 193–202.

Smith, F. (1991). 3 ways to manage stress. *Nursing, 21*, 131–132.

Stone, R., & Short, P. (1990). The competing demands of employment and informal caregiving to disabled elderly. *Medical Care, 28*, 513–526.

Tatelbaum, J. (1989). *You don't have to suffer: a handbook for moving beyond life's crises.* New York: Harper & Row.

Tschudin, V. (1990). Support yourself. *Nursing Times, 86,* 40–42.

United States Department of Labor, Women's Bureau. (1990, September). *20 facts on women workers* (Fact sheet No. 90-2). Washington, DC: Author.

Vitaliano, P., Russo, J., Carr, J., Maiuro, R., & Becker, J. (1985). The ways of coping checklist: revision and psychometric properties. *Multivariate Behavioral Research, 20,* 3–26.

CHAPTER 28

The Professional Doctorate in Audiology: the Au.D.

■ ANGELA LOAVENBRUCK, Ed.D. ■

SCOPE OF CHAPTER

The professional doctorate has been an issue of debate and discussion for the members of the American Speech-Language-Hearing Association (ASHA) for at least 25 years. Recent events, however, have coalesced and defined the discussion for the audiology profession. With the possible exception of the audiologist's role in hearing aid dispensing in the 1970s, few issues have been as controversial as the movement calling for the professional doctorate, the Au.D., as the entry level degree for the practice of audiology. The need for replacement of the master's degree with a professional doctorate (Au.D.) as the entry level degree has been supported by every major audiology association and by the majority of audiologists in a number of published surveys (Caccavo, 1992; Van Vliet, Berkey, Marion, & Robinson, 1992). For a variety of reasons, however, it does not have the complete support of academia or of the current governance of ASHA. The need for a professional doctorate has been discussed by academia in every educational conference since the Highland Park Conference in 1963. Each time, it has been rejected in favor of the master's degree and the notion that the academic doctorate could serve both as the producer of the scientists needed for research and scholarship and the producer of the large number of skilled practitioners needed to provide services to growing numbers of consumers.

Currently, academicians represent only about 7.5% of ASHA membership. Yet they constitute approximately 34% of Legislative Council membership (51 of 148) and 78% of the Executive Board (7 of 9 board members). (ASHA, 1993). With this kind of top-heavy representation of academia, a mandate for change in ASHA standards within our national organization can also be delayed. Clinical audiologists will always be outnumbered in these forums. Further, the present governance structure in ASHA necessitates convincing not only academicians of the wish of practitioners for change, but also convincing our speech-language pathology colleagues, to whom we are tied in a lockstep notion of educational and training needs of the need for and wisdom of such a change for the audiology profession. Although ASHA's long-range plan calls for the development of separate governance structures for audiology and speech-language pathology, it is difficult to evaluate how quickly such a development will take place. The institution of a Vice President for Professional Practice in Audiology on the Executive Board, scheduled to begin in 1995, may not be enough to counter the difficulties presented by audiology's minority position within the structure of ASHA.

In spite of these obstacles, however, in the short period of time from 1988 to 1992, a concept discussed since the earliest days of the audiology profession has been brought to the forefront as a change critical to the future of the field. In many ways, discussions of the Au.D. highlight the chasm of understanding between academics, often far removed from day-to-day practice, and practitioners whose professional lives are limited by the unwillingness of the academic community to take decisive action. There are three critical components that must be discussed: (a) scope of practice in audiology, (b) the adequacy of the master's degree and current Certificate of Clinical Competency (CCC) requirements to ensure competency and autonomy, and (c) the professional doctorate (Au.D.) as an approach to solving a number of problems faced by the profession of audiology.

SCOPE OF PRACTICE

In the 1960s, diagnostic audiology essentially consisted of basic pure tone and speech audiometric procedures and several differential diagnostic tests. Procedures such as acoustic immittance audiometry and auditory evoked potential testing were laboratory and research procedures. Hearing aid technology was relatively simple, and audiologists' involvement in hearing aid fitting was limited to comparative testing of a few stock hearing aids. The current landscape of our profession is vastly different. The rapid expansion of scope of practice is well documented (ASHA, 1990; ASHA, 1992a, 1992b, 1992c, 1992d, 1992e, 1992f), and reflects an increasing knowledge base and concomitant burgeoning of technology.

Currently, audiologists in most practice settings must be able to provide a wide array of diagnostic and remedial services in areas such as probe-tube assessments for measuring and fitting hearing aids, evaluation and fitting of complex amplification systems and assistive listening devices, diagnostic and rehabilitative services for cochlear implant recipients, and electrophysiological measurement of auditory and vestibular systems. Similar expansion has also occurred in areas such as cerumen management, intraoperative monitoring, industrial hearing care, and the provision of audiology services in school settings. The increasing complexity of hearing aid technology, diagnostic procedures and equipment, and new rehabilitative techniques demands technical and professional expertise that could not have been anticipated in the early 1960s.

Although it might be argued that the role of the audiologist in some practice settings does not include the broad scope of responsibility found in more comprehensive practice settings, it is axiomatic that academic and clinical training must prepare audiologists for a representative cross section of responsibilities that are not setting-specific. The existence of practice settings that severely limit the autonomy of audiologists ought to be a source of concern for the profession, not the foundation of our standard-setting mechanism. The education of audiologists cannot be linked to the lowest common denominator or to a notion of "basic competence" that became outdated in the 1960s.

The notion that the master's degree is good enough for some practice settings, notably schools and offices of otolaryngologists, should be examined with care (Fowler & Wilson, 1989). The granting of entry level degrees and ASHA certification (that are now tied together by Educational Standards Board [ESB] and Clinical Certification Board [CCB] requirements) must be designed to assure consumers that the audiologist has basic competencies that are current, as opposed to competencies that may have described our scope of practice 30 years ago. Consumers must be assured that our CCC represents competence, not a vague notion of "minimum" competence for some portion of our scope of practice. It would also be foolhardy to create a multiple certification system of "less and more" qualified practitioners. In addition, our certification credential must be portable, to allow the certified individual to practice in any setting. Most critically, regardless of the setting in which consumers seek the services of an ASHA-certified audiologist, they must have assurance that their needs can be met by the practitioner whom they see.

It also seems reasonable to question if the increasing limitations of the academic and practical training offered within the master's degree programs leads to the recruitment of students who will accept as reasonable the low pay, lack of autonomy, limited scope of practice, lack of input, and restricted upward mobility represented by some audiology work settings. We must recruit better prepared students into our graduate training programs by demanding more rigorous liberal arts, science, and math preparation at the undergraduate level. We must offer a professional preparation format that meets the demands of our scope of practice today and prepares us for a future that most certainly will be more demanding. Autonomy should be more than a figure of speech—it should be central to both the recruitment and training process.

INADEQUACY OF THE MASTER'S DEGREE MODEL

ASHA's recent activities with respect to the Au.D. were precipitated by a number of fac-

tors, but the central one is a widespread acknowledgment that our master's degree structure and CCC requirements can no longer produce competent audiology practitioners (Feldman, 1984; Lynn & Loavenbruck, 1991; Miller & Deutsch, 1983). This central factor affects our ability as a profession to provide competent diagnostic and rehabilitation services to our patients. It affects our autonomy. It affects the students we recruit into our profession. It affects our ability to interact as peers with other professions, and it affects our ability to obtain equitable and autonomous reimbursement for our services in the current and proposed changes in the health care delivery system.

ACADEMIC AND PRACTICUM PREPARATION IN THE MASTER'S DEGREE MODEL

In the ASHA CCC validation study (ASHA, 1987), panels of experts and a large, stratified random sample of practitioners delineated the tasks, knowledge areas, and skills essential for competent entry-level practice in the profession of audiology. The panels were asked to define the tasks that made up the practice of audiology and to identify the knowledge areas and skills needed to perform these tasks competently. Participants in the study were also asked to identify the point in time when each knowledge or skill should be acquired by a clinically competent audiologist. Finally, they were asked to judge the importance of each knowledge and skill area to consumer protection. The overwhelming majority of audiology participants indicated that virtually all of the knowledge and skill areas should be acquired prior to completion of the CCC requirements, *not* as part of continuing education or on-the-job training.

Knowledge or skill areas judged to be important for consumer protection were also classified as areas needing to be mastered prior to the completion of certification requirements. In addition, respondents to the Clinical Inventory Survey conducted as part of this study indicated that professional coursework was underrepresented for audiology and that practicum hours should be increased (Lingwall, 1988a). Although this study was not conducted to determine the need for a professional doctorate, it is clear that the breadth of knowledge and skill areas considered essential to competent and ethical practice of audiology cannot be mastered in a 2-year time frame. In discussing the task faced by academia, Decker (1990) discussed the impossibility of preparing competent students and the need to "brush over" complex topics because of the confines of the master's degree time frame.

Additional evidence of the inadequacy of graduate school education in audiology was provided by a survey conducted by Oyler and Matkin (1987). The authors were interested in certified audiologists' perceptions of the adequacy of graduate education in pediatric audiology. They sent parallel questionnaires to 200 audiologists who had received their CCC as of 1984 and to the program directors of 94 ESB-accredited audiology programs. In assessing their findings, Oyler and Matkin (1987) state that program directors overestimate the adequacy of their programs and that a finding of serious concern is that about 60% of the audiologists acquired less than 15 hours in assessment of children 2 years old and younger. In addition, Oyler and Matkin (1987) note that over 40% of both groups stated that the CCC requirements were insufficient to prepare audiologists to provide pediatric habilitation services. The authors state that, "it seems inappropriate that one-fourth of audiologists could provide habilitation to a population they have never encountered during their supervised experience" (p. 30).

Two cornerstones of the master's degree model are the notions that: (a) graduate programs cannot provide all of the 375 clock hours of practicum required for the CCC, therefore externship experiences are essential; and (b) practicum skills that cannot be obtained in the 375-hour graduate practicum requirement will somehow be obtained in the Clinical Fellowship Year (CFY), and that consumers will be further protected by ASHA's Code of Ethics, which states that members

shall not provide services for which they are not qualified. Few defenders of the adequacy of these mechanisms can be found.

The externship issue has become one of significant concern. Not only are externships in various aspects of audiology difficult to find, but the financial responsibility for the externship is also in question. Ehrlich, Merton, Sweetman, and Arnold (1983) identified a number of conflicting attitudes between clinic administrators and university personnel in the Denver area. Clinic administrators asked the universities for reimbursement for the training costs incurred by the clinics serving as externship sites. Clinic personnel noted that training costs were real and that those costs should be borne by the university or the student. They stated that they were "baffled by the contradiction that universities should be reimbursed for training but hospitals or other clinical organizations should not" (p. 26). The universities refused, stating that: "We believe that it is fair and reasonable to expect professionals in voluntary externship settings to accept this [responsibility] and then to convince their administrators to underwrite the cost of this professional contribution" (p. 27). The universities' position was that, even though the externship experience was required for a degree, neither students nor the university should be required to pay externship settings for the supervised experience. Rather, it was the clinics' "obligation to make a contribution to higher learning and to the training of graduate students" (p. 27). University personnel also underestimated the amount and intensity of supervision their students required. Clinic personnel stated that, in settings where consumers expect and are purchasing professional service, student externs are not able to provide professional quality because of their limited experience. These factors often limit the nature of supervised practicum experiences students are able to receive.

The CFY concept is also troublesome. Richard Flower (1987) has stated: "At one time in our professional fantasy life, we envisioned the CFY as a formal, closely supervised internship experience, completed in an approved clinical setting. With each year that has passed, this fantasy is farther from reality" (p. 32). The vagueries of the CFY as a vehicle for ensuring clinical competence are increasingly troublesome. As currently structured, CFY candidates are left, with widely varying success, to search the marketplace for a suitable paid supervised experience. When compared to the more controlled internship and residency experiences required in other professions, the CFY does not measure up. University settings produce an admittedly unfinished product in master's degree programs and leave the responsibility of completion up to those in practice and to the student. Flower also points out the difficulty in finding CFY employment because of employers' unwillingness to accept responsibility for the extensive supervision needed and the possibility that third-party payers will refuse reimbursement for services provided by clinical fellows.

It is also important to discuss the students we are currently attracting. Statistics for 1989 indicate that the verbal and quantitative Graduate Record Examination scores of incoming audiology students ranked close to the bottom of the 98 disciplines represented (Speaks, 1989). Similarly, our profession has seen an increasing rate of failures on the National Teachers Examination. Lovrinic (1992) states: "We face some real dilemmas—how to prepare students who are not at the top academically to work in a field that is changing in dramatic and exciting ways with faculty who are not always the most up to date in their own knowledge in all the areas covered by the profession" (p. 15). An important question to ask is: Why would we choose to continue to do so?

AUTONOMY

The need for a professional doctorate to replace the master's degree as the entry level degree can also be viewed in terms of professional stature and autonomy. In a 1985 keynote address to the Council of Graduate Programs in Communication Sciences and Disorders, Flower (1985) stated: "There is no first rank human services profession in this nation that does not require doctoral level entry. Therefore our profession will probably never achieve that status so long as it merely requires Master's level entry" (p. 4). Curtis (1984) observed that individuals with master's degrees were assigned minor roles in the management of patients, whereas those who hold doctoral degrees were full partners in making diagnostic decisions. Carhart (1976) stated that "the person who has achieved certification in audiology from ASHA has emerged as a professional whose recognized competency is defined by the master's degree and a moderate amount of supervised clinical experience. . . . As long as either ASHA or clinical audiology are satisfied to accept only this definition as describing competence in clinical audiology, [we] cannot expect to be recognized as equal to professionals who hold the doctorate as one of their inviolate requirements" (p. xxxvi). Although ASHA states that audiologists are "autonomous" professionals, many would agree that our notions of our own autonomy are illusory. Feldman (1981) summarized many of the barriers to autonomy : "We are rarely autonomous practitioners. Our independence, as well as our identity, is shielded from the public by our institutional image. . . . Our existence is a dependent one. . . . Our autonomy is contingent upon a shift in training orientation" (pp. 942–943).

Feldman (1984) calls for emphasis on preparation for employment in the private sector and for a professional doctorate. Lynn and Loavenbruck (1991) note that employment interviews of young master's level clinicians indicate that many complete their degrees feeling competent to provide only the most basic services to adult, cooperating patients. Counseling of any kind, hearing aid fitting and dispensing, real ear testing, evaluating and fitting digital instruments or other state-of-the-art equipment, diagnostic testing such as ABR or ENG, pediatric audiology— all are typically beyond the capability of newly graduated and even newly certified audiologists. It is difficult to see how either consumers or other health professionals could believe that such clinicians are autonomous professionals.

Our lack of autonomy is probably most noticeable in many otolaryngology-based practices. In such settings, audiologists seldom take case histories, often administer only the tests specified by the physician, do not interpret results to patients, or counsel them about the communication implications of the loss noted, and do not write a report that they sign. With rare exception, the audiologists in these office settings are "on-call" for the physician, and their job is defined as the ability to obtain audiometric data quickly so that the flow of patients in the office is unimpeded. If the flow of patients slows down, audiologists may be expected to "help out" in the front office by answering the telephone, scheduling patients, filing and providing general office help—roles that do not enhance our professional image.

INCOME LEVEL

The income level of audiologists does not compare favorably to that of other master's level health care practitioners. Engleman (1992) gathered salary data from a number of sources indicating that the salaries of audiologists and speech-language pathologists are at the bottom of the range paid to master's level professionals. For example, the mean income of audiologists in 1992 was $36,496, while that for physical therapists was $54,898. Engleman's data also illustrate that audiologists with Ph.D.s also do not fare as well when their incomes are compared to those of other doctoral degree professions. The mean salary of Ph.D. level audiologists was $49,000, while that of other professions ranged from $71,400 for optometrists to $107,006 for osteopaths. Engleman notes that less than 10% of audiologists hold doctoral degrees, and their incomes are almost 50% greater than those with master's degrees. Engleman summarizes that, historically, audiologists have aligned themselves academically and economically with allied health professionals. A recent ASHA Data article (Blake & Slater, 1993) supports Engleman's findings. Of the 17 national associations surveyed by ASHA, only two reported mean salaries lower than those for speech-language pathology and only

four were lower than those for audiology. If audiologists want more for their profession economically, concerns about upgrading educational requirements must be met by aligning the audiology profession with other professional doctorates, not by reorganizing the bachelor's-master's format we now have.

Some have expressed concern that doctoral entry level standards will price audiologists out of some otolaryngology and hospital/clinic-based practices, and also that school districts will not meet the increased salary expectations of doctoral level professionals. It might be hypothesized, however, that many audiologists in practice settings that limit their role have little information about the financial value of the services they provide. In fact, the procedures administered by audiologists in a typical otolaryngology practice account for thousands of dollars in billing. There are examples of otolaryngology-audiology partnerships that acknowledge the unique contribution of each to a successful practice. In addition, hospital settings may offer possibilities for financial arrangements other than salaried positions. For example, in many hospital-based otolaryngology practices, physicians are paid salaries for certain aspects of their work, but then are permitted to use the facilities of the hospital for their own private practice. Some audiologists have already delineated a similar role for themselves. The call for national health reform represents a unique opportunity for audiologists to present themselves as cost-effective providers of hearing health services and as capable of serving as a point of entry into the hearing health system. One would expect that doctoral level professional education would both attract and prepare audiologists, not only with more extensive education, skill, and information, but also with a level of assertiveness that would improve the profession's position in health care reform.

HISTORY OF DISCUSSIONS OF THE PROFESSIONAL DOCTORATE

In our struggle to make the bold changes needed to move audiology into the 21st century, it is important to carefully examine our credentialing history. In the early 1960s, ASHA was struggling to revise credentialing requirements from an undergraduate degree and multiple layers of certification to the academic master's degree and single level certification as entry level requirements for both speech-language pathology and audiology. Early discussions of doctoral education centered around whether there was need for a professional doctorate in addition to the traditional academic Ph.D. as an advanced degree or was the academic doctorate (Ph.D.) "robust" enough to encompass the educational needs of the scientist as well as those of the **advanced** practitioner. In 1963, academic participants of the Highland Park Conference on Graduate Education (ASHA, 1963) rejected the professional doctorate and instead expressed support for development of a "clinical" Ph.D. and a "research" Ph.D., a contradictory dichotomy which has continued to be debated. As early as 1969, Darley was critical of the amount of time available in master's programs to develop clinical skills necessary for practice.

It is important to remember that these early discussions were held mainly among academics. The profession of audiology was in its early stages and was represented by a small number of practitioners. It is not surprising, then, that ASHA's professional certification involved standards mainly determined by academicians to fit into the circumscribed time frame of an academic master's degree, with degree titles determined by the departments that housed our programs (Master of Arts, Master of Science, Master of Education, etc.). The lockstep notion began at that point that exactly the same number of course credits, practicum hours, and post-graduation experience were needed for speech-language pathologists and audiologists, following the standard academic model. In 1963, the standards developed for the CCC were based on the notion that the CCCs ensured the public "that the bearer has minimum competence to practice the profession." The 1965 standards have been subjected to limited changes (mainly in the area of undergraduate preparation) which became effective in 1993. In the face of signifi-

cant increases in the scope of practice in audiology, the widely acknowledged inadequacy of the revised CCC requirements has been one of the primary reasons for the renewed and organized effort to replace the master's degree with doctoral-level entry requirements for the audiology profession.

A 1976 conference held by the Big Ten University programs in audiology and speech-language pathology considered the need for a professional doctoral program, including benefits, problems, and strategies for establishing these programs. A draft curriculum was created, but no action was ever taken to establish any professional doctoral programs. The robust Ph.D. argument was reaffirmed by the participants at the 1983 St. Paul Conference on Graduate and Undergraduate Education. The arguments made by several practitioners (Loavenbruck, 1983) that the master's degree in audiology needed to be replaced by doctoral level entry requirements were rejected in favor of the academics' support of traditional models. However, calls for a professional doctorate in audiology continued.

In 1986, a Task Force on Audiology was appointed by ASHA's Executive Board (EB) to recommend direction for ASHA activity in relation to audiology practice. The EB resolution acknowledged that, in the 10 years since the first Task Force on Audiology met, technological changes, federal and state regulations and legislation, changes in the Code of Ethics, and changes in national health care delivery systems had a "synergistic effect on the scope of audiology practice and models for service delivery." The task force was asked to prioritize key issues of concern and strategies for action. Twenty recommendations were made (ASHA, 1988) and prioritized in order of importance. Recommendations 2, 3, 4, and 6 are pertinent to the discussion of doctoral-level entry requirements. The task force recommended that ASHA address the quality of undergraduate, graduate, and continuing audiology education; address the issue of raising standards, including making the CFY a residency program as part of a professional doctorate; promote the autonomy of the audiology profession; and develop a plan to promote professional education at the doctoral level. The task force recommended that the professional doctorate should be post-bachelor's, not post-master's, and that the professional doctorate should become the entry level by 1998.

In response to growing dissatisfaction among audiologists with the ongoing degree and training structure, the Academy of Dispensing Audiologists (ADA) convened a Conference on Professional Education in October, 1988. Conference participants recommended a specific professional doctorate, a specific degree title (Au.D.), and model curricular content and further recommended that the Au.D. should be the entry-level degree for audiology practice and that a plan be devised for existing practitioners to upgrade their credentials to the doctoral level (Academy of Dispensing Audiology [ADA], 1988). The ADA's call for a professional doctorate as the entry level degree for the practice of Audiology has been supported by virtually every major audiology organization, including the American Academy of Audiology, The Academy of Rehabilitative Audiology, The American Academy of Private Practice in Speech-Language Pathology and Audiology, numerous state speech-language and hearing associations and state audiology organizations. Support has also been expressed by the Veteran's Administration—a major employer of audiologists throughout the country (Beck, 1991).

Also in 1988, the American Academy of Audiology was formed. Its central theme was the transformation of audiology into a doctoral level profession. Membership in this organization has skyrocketed in its 5-year history and it now boasts representation of more than half of the certified audiologists in the country. The proliferation of professional audiology associations throughout the country is in many ways the culmination of years of dissatisfaction with the responsiveness of ASHA and the state associations to the needs and aspirations of audiologists. In 1988, however, ASHA's Legislative Council created the Committee on Doctoral Preparation to examine issues pertinent to research and "clinically oriented" doctoral programs. One of the recommendations of this committee was the formation of an Ad Hoc Committee on Professional Education in Audiology (ASHA, 1991a).

THE AD HOC COMMITTEE ON PROFESSIONAL EDUCATION

The Ad Hoc Committee on Professional Education met in 1991 and 1992. It examined a number of alternative professional education models, including: (a) expanding or restructuring the current master's degree; (b) incorporation of a "clinical track" or emphasis into existing Ph.D. degree programs; (c) the development of clinical Ph.D. programs; and (d) bolstering undergraduate coursework in audiology to allow more advanced coursework to be presented at the master's level. The ad hoc committee (ASHA, 1992e) recommended that:

1. ASHA support the professional doctorate degree, designated Doctor of Audiology (Au.D.), as the entry-level degree for the profession of audiology;
2. By January 1, 1996, the Council on Professional Standards in Speech-Language Pathology and Audiology disseminate revised standards for the CCC in audiology that are consistent with the Au.D. The year 2001 was recommended as the goal for implementation of the new standards;
3. ASHA reorganize its governance with separate representation for the two professions on all boards;
4. ASHA facilitate development and implementation of the Au.D., assist institutions of higher learning in implementing the Au.D. program, and serve as a clearinghouse for guidelines and information about the Au.D.;
5. ASHA develop guidelines and innovative mechanisms to assist practicing audiologists to upgrade their credentials if they choose; and
6. ASHA investigate grant support to institutions that wish to develop Au.D. programs.

Although all members of the ad hoc committee agreed that the master's degree could no longer produce competent practitioners and that transition to a doctoral-level profession was needed, a minority report was filed. The minority report did not support the recommendation that the Au.D. be the only degree for entry into the practice of audiology and disagreed with the year 2001 as the goal for implementation of the new requirement. The minority report recommended that institutions that did not or could not have Au.D. programs, but that could provide academic and clinical doctoral preparation equivalent to that of the professional doctorate in their existing doctorates, should be viable alternatives. These recommendations were rejected by the ad hoc committee for a number of reasons: (a) The committee believed that these recommendations were a blueprint for the use of the Ph.D. for professional education, rather than for research, and that this would further deteriorate the science base of our profession; (b) the minority recommendations would enable academic institutions to keep their master's programs intact, thus creating two groups of practitioners who could call themselves audiologists. Although the master's level individuals theoretically would no longer be eligible for ASHA certification, they would still be eligible for state licensure, thus jeopardizing the goal of transforming audiology into a doctoral level profession.

The ad hoc committee recommendations and the minority recommendations became LC resolutions 4A and 4B , respectively, and were presented to the Executive Board in August 1992 and to the Legislative Council in November 1992. The Executive Board of ASHA resoundingly defeated both resolutions and instead proposed its own resolution, LC 5. The Executive Board resolution called for support of the development of both professional and "clinical doctorates," but voted for the doctorate as only one of the entry-level degrees. In other words, nothing would change since the master's degree would continue to suffice for entry into the profession and for ASHA certification.

The final resolution that was passed was an amended version of the EB's resolution. It calls for ASHA to: (a) support the *concept* of doctoral degrees as the entry-level academic credentials for audiology; (b) support the development of the professional doctoral degree in audiology with Au.D. as an appropriate designator; (c) reaffirm its prior support for the development of the clinical doctoral program; (d) petition the Council on Post-Secondary Accreditation to expand ASHA's scope of accreditation authority to include clinical and professional doctoral programs; (e) urge the Standards Council to develop standards making the clinical or professional doctorate eligible for certification (a curious recommendation since the requirements for the Au.D. far exceed the new requirements for certification in audiology); and finally (f) report to the Legislative Council in 1993 with information about the feasibility and impact of the professional doctorate.

Following the 1992 convention, there was continuing controversy about the Au.D that reflected the view of many audiologists that the Executive Board, composed primarily of academicians and speech-language pathologists, had succeeded in thwarting the wishes of practicing audiologists to move their profession to a doctoral-level entry requirement in a timely way. Therefore, the original resolution (LC4A-92) was resubmitted to the Legislative Council at their meeting in Anaheim, California in November 1993. This time, the resolution (LC44-93) passed by a large margin. The 1993 resolution calls for ASHA to (a) support the *professional* doctorate as the entry-level credential for the practice of audiology; (b) support the Doctor of Audiology (Au.D.) as the preferred designation for the professional doctorate in audiology; (c) recommend that the Council on Professional Standards in Speech-Language Pathology and Audiology (Standards Council) change the degree requirement for the CCC in audiology from a master's degree to the professional doctorate; (d) recommend to the Standards Council that it develop standards for the CCC in audiology that reflect the academic and clinical training requirements necessary to earn a professional doctorate in audiology; and (e) recommend that the Standards Council disseminate the revised standards for peer review by January 1, 1997 with the year 2002 as the goal for implementation of the new standards.

It is now ASHA policy that a change in entry-level standards for the profession of audiology from the master's degree to the professional doctorate—designated by Doctor of Audiology (Au.D.)—should be in effect by the year 2002. The reports of the Feasibility and Impact Committees created by the Executive Council have not yet been released. Since passage of LC44-93, the Standards Council Committee on Audiology Standards Definition has been conducting a comprehensive review of the issues related to revising entry-level standards to incorporate the professional doctorate. The Standards Council is scheduled to begin consideration of this issue at its March 1994 meeting. Graduate program directors have continued to voice their opposition to the Au.D. For example, at its April 1993 meeting (Minutes and Proceedings of Council of Graduate programs in Communication Sciences and Disorders meeting, 1993), the Council voted 94 to 2 that the doctoral degree should be "one of," not "the only" entry-level degree in audiology. In other words, they voted to reject the vote of LC 1992 and in favor of the Executive Board's *original* resolution. The council also approved a resolution that the issue of the development of professional doctorates should be separated from the issue of minimal requirements for entry into the profession. Finally, the council voted against a resolution suggesting that it encourage academic programs to develop professional doctorates. It can be expected that some program directors will continue to oppose the implementation of LC44-93.

ASHA has received approval from COPA (Council on Professional Accreditation) to expand its accreditation function to graduate programs that provide entry-level education, whether the degree is the master's or a doctoral degree. Testimony was given to COPA by the Audiology Foundation of America (AFA) urg-

ing it to limit its approval to professional doctoral programs in order to maintain the integrity of the Ph.D. and halt the drift of Ph.D. programs into professional education and away from vigorous basic and applied research. The AFA testimony pointed out that both COPA and the Council of Graduate Programs had often noted the need to differentiate between academic doctorates and professional doctorates. In its official ruling, however, COPA did not require ASHA to differentiate between professional and academic doctorates.

PROFESSIONAL VERSUS CLINICAL DOCTORATES—THE FALLACY AND DANGER OF THE "ROBUST PH.D."

Throughout the years of debate about doctoral-level education, some members of our profession have continued to argue the concept that Ph.D. programs are "robust" and flexible enough to accommodate both our expanding professional and clinical training needs in Audiology and the rigors of preparing scientists and scholars. Others believe that the preparation of practitioners and the preparation of scholars/scientists are separate and distinct tasks and cannot be accomplished by the same degree structure. In fact, proponents of the latter view hold that attempting to combine the two tasks leads to inadequate preparation for either goal.

The Council of Graduate Schools (CGS) in the United States (1990) has defined the Doctor of Philosophy degree as "the highest academic degree granted by North American Universities. It is a research degree. . . [and] is designed to prepare a student to become a scholar" (p. 4). CGS defines the professional doctorate as "the highest university award given in a particular field in recognition of completion of academic preparation for professional practice" (p. 6). Aronson (1987) posed a new definition for a "clinical" Ph.D., as distinguished from a "research" Ph.D. He described it as a clinical track for those who wish to practice the profession as a direct service to the public. This definition was used by the ASHA Committee on Doctoral Education (ASHA, 1991b). Many, however, view this notion of a "clinical" Ph.D. as paradoxical. In fact, since the Ph.D. is defined as a research degree, it is redundant to say "research" Ph.D. Feldman (1989) stated that the Ph.D. is neither a clinical degree nor a professional degree—it is a graduate school academic degree dedicated to creating scholarship. Saxman (1989) asked how "robust" the Ph.D. can be before its essence is subverted. It is also reasonable to ask how one would differentiate between a research Ph.D. and a clinical Ph.D.? Would recipients of the research Ph.D. have to return to school for the clinical Ph.D. if their career goals changed from research to practice and vice versa?

Flower (1985) asserts that the erosion of scholarship in our Ph.D. programs can be attributed, at least in part, to efforts to use them for the preparation of clinicians. ASHA's Task Force on Science (1978) pointed out the dangers of diluting research training by including persons who really want a professional degree. Spriestersbach (1989) stated that "audiologists should be undeterred by the irrelevant discussion that has been swirling around clouding the issue. The bottom line is that traditional Ph.D. programs fail to graduate people with a high level of clinical competence; that the sanctity of the Ph.D. for research purposes must be preserved; that audiologists holding a professional doctorate will be better equipped to interact with other doctors" (p. 78).

Flower (1985) stated that "the assertion that the Ph.D. degree is robust enough to accommodate advanced preparation of service professionals would be regarded as oxymoronic in most of our nation's major universities" (p. 6). Oyer (1990) expressed concern about obscuring the boundaries between "graduate" and "professional" programs. He stated that making the difference more nebulous would compromise the development of both graduate and professional education and result in the inefficient use of available resources. Higher education accrediting bodies are concerned about the inappropriate use of the Ph.D. degree designation. The Western Association of Schools and Colleges, the accrediting body for universities in California, mandates that programs emphasizing research must offer the Ph.D., whereas those emphasizing professional objectives must offer the professional degree (Weiner, personal communication, December 1992). These standards are inconsistent with the notion that the Ph.D. can be redefined to accommodate professional education.

In addition to philosophical concerns about the purpose of the Ph.D., a number of other factors regarding Ph.D. education must be considered. Our educational institutions are currently producing fewer than one Ph.D. graduate per state per year. The shrinking numbers of Ph.D. candidates and the time required to complete a Ph.D. are both matters of concern, and do not augur well for the ability of Ph.D. programs to both meet the needs of the increasing population of consumers who need the audiologist's professional services and simultaneously produce adequate numbers of researchers, scholars, and teachers. Given that adequate preparation for the knowledge and skill needed to practice audiology requires at least 4 years post-BA, and given that adequate preparation for the scholarly pursuits represented by the Ph.D. requires at least 3 or 4 years (median figures are reported to be 7 to 12 years post-BA by Thurgood & Weinman, 1990) to complete, it is unreasonable to believe that Ph.D. programs in audiology could successfully produce individuals who are both scholars and skilled practitioners. Oyer (1990) stated that both the research doctorate (Ph.D.) and the professional doctorate (Au.D.) are extremely important, require rigorous training and significant achievement, and ultimately lead to services for society. Both have an equally important role to play in our professions, and one should not be compromised for the sake of the other.

THE PROFESSIONAL DOCTORATE (THE AU.D.)

Our current academic structure differentiates audiology from other traditional health care professions such as medicine, dentistry, and optometry in that professional education leads to a doctorate that is uniquely identified with the profession, for example, MD, DDS, and OD. Practitioners in other fields have long recognized the value of a professional doctorate and the unifying effect of a single degree designation. The Au.D. is a **48 month,** postbaccalaureate professional degree. Its primary objective is to produce audiologists who are competent to peform the wide array of diagnostic, remedial, and other services associated with the practice of audiology. The Au.D. places major emphasis on clinicial training.

In addition, student practitioners would be required to be familiar with the scientific and research literature that represents the foundation of audiology, and would be required to acquire the knowledge needed to interpret pertinent research and apply it to clinical practice. Au.D. prerequisites would include basic sciences (biology, chemistry, physics), mathematics, communication, statistics, English, psychology, humanities, social sciences, and foreign language. The initial 2 years of the program would be heavily weighted toward didactic instruction and laboratory classwork, while emphasis in the latter 2 years would be increasingly shifted to clinical learning experiences. The degree would require 2000 to 3000 hours of clinical experience.

Baylor College of Medicine, under the leadership of James Jerger, has announced the first Au.D. program and has begun accepting students in the spring semester of 1994. At the Spring, 1993, conference of the American Academy of Audiology, Baylor was given a $25,000 award by the Audiology Foundation of America as the first Au.D. program. A number of other institutions throughout the country are in various stages of development of Au.D. programs, but there is no doubt that the divisive actions of ASHA's leadership related to stopping the Au.D. have strengthened the resolve of those who do not desire change to occur.

RESISTANCE TO CHANGE

It is important to analyze the factors that create resistance to change in our educational and practicum standards in audiology when the need for change is so widely acknowledged. Support for the Au.D. has been expressed by virtually every related professional organization and in every survey conducted. In addition to support for requiring the Au.D. as the entry-level degree, there has been clear interest and support expressed by practicing audiologists in creative and innovative methods to allow practitioners who wish to upgrade their credentials to do so. Yet our universities, ASHA, and organizations such as the Council of Graduate Programs in Communication Sciences and Disorders continue to slow the pace of orderly and timely change.

Some of the resistance to change arising from academicians is based on the fear that their individual institutions would not or could not create or grant professional doctorates. Some express concern that, because of budgetary or other constraints, their programs would shut down if the professional doctorate was required. In the current economic climate in higher education, it is clearly not in the best interests of some programs to call attention to themselves by proposing a more rigorous degree program that would require additional expenditure by the university. A number of programs have already been jeopardized by budget analyses that could not support the expense of a graduate program that accommodates 5 or 6 students a year. In fact, the Au.D. discussions have highlighted a problem that has also been discussed for many years. We have over 160 ESB-accredited programs producing only about 700 master's level graduates per year—an extraordinarily inefficient system that greatly increases the cost of producing audiologists.

An additional source of resistance has to do with the feeling expressed by some academicians that the professional doctorate, especially if it does not require a research dissertation, is a "sham" degree. Susan Jerger (1989) states that the principles of science must be included in all doctoral programs and that we must mandate that maintaining standards of excellence can only be guaranteed if professional doctoral programs are in universities.

Others have been more forthright in stating that every doctoral degree should require a dissertation. It is interesting to note that schools of medicine, optometry, pharmacy, veterinary medicine have managed to maintain widely acknowledged standards of excellence in professional schools without requiring a dissertation. The real fear of some Ph.D. program administrators may have far less to do with the preservation of science and research than with the preservation of their programs. The fear is that, since some individuals who enter Ph.D. programs do so because they want advanced clinical training (not research), these individuals will choose Au.D. programs instead, thus decimating the already low enrollment of our Ph.D. programs.

Another argument often used by academicians is that ASHA as a professional organization cannot dictate the model of doctoral preparation to be used by universities. The minority report of the Ad Hoc Committee on Doctoral Preparation stated: "It is not within the purview of professional associations to determine academic institutions' curricula or degree requirements and titles." Of course, that is true—ASHA cannot tell university programs what degrees to offer. However, as an advocate for its audiology members, as an advocate for high standards of practice, and as an advocate for hearing impaired consumers, ASHA can choose to accredit **only** programs that offer the Au.D. Graduates of master's programs would not be eligible for certification. Some of these programs might be forced to close, however, because Au.D. programs would attract many students who would otherwise have gone to existing master's programs.

The assertion that ASHA cannot "force academia to offer a particular degree" is somewhat puzzling. It is clear that graduate audiology programs and their institutions of higher learning have accepted ASHA's degree, curricular, and practicum requirements in the past and have recently accepted ASHA's dictum that CCC and ESB accreditation go together. Why would such institutions be unwilling to accept and create Au.D. programs if such programs are financially viable, meet a defined need of the community, set standards higher than our existing master's programs, and produce excellent practitioners in the Audiology profession? Au.D. programs could be located in schools of health science or could be joint programs between health science and arts and sciences. Spriestersbach (1976) has suggested that, in an arts and science setting, the Au.D. could be overseen by a special council. The Au.D. model developed by the ADA conference is just that—a model that can be changed to create better fits to individual university structures. Baylor's model, for example, includes a research project and emphasis on medical audiology, in keeping with its location in a medical school.

It has also been difficult for some academicians to understand the importance of the unifying degree designation (Au.D.). Practicing audiologists in all settings are more acutely aware of the importance of recognizable designates in the practice arena. While the designate "Ph.D." is a unifying ticket in universities, the same letters, or the letters Ed.D., do not signify anything recognizable to consumers of the services of practicing audiologists. In fact, in the author's experience, patient's often ask: "Why is your degree in education if you are an audiologist?" or "What does the Doctor of Philosophy degree have to do with audiology?" ASHA's recent focus group studies of consumers on their familiarity with our profession and our services indicated how far we must go to improve our image with consumers. A recognizable and unifying degree designate will greatly assist in those marketing efforts.

THE FUTURE

What are the steps that must yet be taken to make the professional doctorate a reality for the audiologist of the 21st century? Audiologists must organize efforts to ensure timely implementation of LC 44-93. We must lobby for appointment of audiologists to the Standards Council who are supportive of the policy created by LC 44-93 and who will work to create the new standards needed for doctoral-level entry. In addition, audiologists must organize to inform our universities of the need for and success potential of Au.D. programs. Audiologists must actively pursue changes in ASHA's governance and board structure that will lead to separate decision-making and policy-making processes for audiologists and speech-language pathologists. Although we share many significant issues with our colleagues in speech-language pathology, matters relating to standards of education and practicum are not necessarily identical. Audiologists must decide these policy issues for themselves. In addition, audiologists must urge their state organizations to support their efforts toward the professional doctorate. Finally we must continue to build the strength of our newer professional organizations (AAA and ADA). It may be necessary to create our own accrediting bodies and perhaps our own institutions separate from speech-language pathology.

The chief deterrent to the creation of Au.D. programs appears to be the unwillingness of far too many of our academic colleagues to take positions of leadership in this arena. The movement for the Au.D. has been a practitioner-driven movement, and it has not yet been possible to convince many academians that the professional doctorate is the future of audiology. Audiologists must join in efforts on the state level to meet with university program administrators, deans, fiscal officers, and regents to encourage the development of Au.D. programs. Consumer-audiology coalitions could be formed to meet with university officials to stress the importance of the Au.D. to the hearing impaired consumer. Our future as a profession will be shaped by the efforts audiologists continue to make to set their course as an autonomous, doctoral-level profession.

SUMMARY

The professional doctorate is a controversial topic that has been discussed for many years and in many forums. The recent practitioner-driven movement for the Au.D., a professional doctorate in audiology, has brought this debate

to the forefront of professional issues in the American Speech-Language-Hearing Association. The Au.D. movement was precipitated by concerns about the rapid growth in scope of practice in audiology coupled with the widely acknowledged inadequacy of the master's degree model to accommodate necessary professional training and education. In addition, audiologists' ability to function autonomously in the current health care system, and in proposed reforms, is hampered by their entry-level preparation and by the absence of professional doctoral programs. The main opposition to the requirement of a professional doctorate for entry into the practice of audiology has come from academicians and the Executive Board of ASHA. Audiologists must continue to work toward the goal of timely progression to a professional doctorate as the entry level requirement for the practice of Audiology.

DISCUSSION

1. What are the differences between the requirements for the Au.D. and those for the master's degree?
2. What might some of the implications of doctoral-level entry requirements be for audiology and for consumers in the current health care reform environment?
3. How might a professional organization such as ASHA reorganize its governance structure to equitably reflect the needs of the two professions represented in its membership?

REFERENCES

Academy of Dispensing Audiologists. (1988, October). *Proceedings of conference on Professional Education.* Columbia, SC: Author.

American Speech-Language-Hearing Association. (1963). *Highland Park Conference: Graduate education in speech pathology and audiology.* Report of a National Conference. Washington, DC: Author.

American Speech-Language-Hearing Association. (1978). *Report of Task Force on Science.* Rockville, MD: Author.

American Speech-Language-Hearing Association. (1983). *Proceedings of the 1983 National Conference on*

Undergraduate, Graduate and Continuing Education. ASHA Reports 13. Rockville, MD: Author.

American Speech-Language-Hearing Association. (1987). *Evaluation of the requirements for the Certificates of Clinical Competence of ASHA.* Rockville, MD: Author.

American Speech-Language-Hearing Association. (1988). Report of the Task Force on Audiology II. *Asha, 30,* 41–45.

American Speech-Language-Hearing Association. (1990). Scope of practice, Speech-Language Pathology and Audiology. *Asha, 32*(Suppl. 2) 1–2.

American Speech-Language-Hearing Association. (1991a). Report on doctoral education. *Asha, 33*(Suppl. 3), 1–9.

American Speech-Language-Hearing Association. (1991b). Report on the survey of audiologists. Rockville, MD: Author.

American Speech-Language-Hearing Association. (1992a). Balance system assessment. *Asha, 34*(Suppl. 7), 13–16.

American Speech-Language-Hearing Association. (1992b). Electrical stimulation for cochlear implant selection and rehabilitation. *Asha, 34*(Suppl. 7), 17–21.

American Speech-Language-Hearing Association. (1992c). External auditory canal examination and cerumen management. *Asha, 34*(Suppl. 7), 22–24.

American Speech-Language-Hearing Association. (1992d). Neurophysiologic intraoperative monitoring. *Asha, 34*(Suppl. 7), 34–36.

American Speech-Language-Hearing Association. (1992e). Report of the Ad Hoc Committee on Professional Education. *Asha, 34*(Suppl. 7), 112–114.

American Speech-Language-Hearing Association. (1992f). Sedation and topical anesthetics in audiology and speech language pathology. *Asha, 34*(Suppl. 7), 41–46.

American Speech-Language-Hearing Association. (1993, August). [Mid-year demographic profile of the ASHA membership]. Unpublished raw data.

Aronson, A. (1987). The clinical PhD: Implications for the survival and liberation of communication disorders as a health care profession. *Asha, 29,* 35–39.

Beck, L. B. (1991, September). VA to endorse the professional doctorate. *Torchbearer* (Newsletter of the Audiology Foundation of America, West Lafayette, IN), 15–16.

Big Ten Conference. (1976, March). *The professional doctorate in speech pathology and audiology. A discussion of the issues.* Chicago, IL.

Blake, A. K. & Slater, S. C. (1993). Asha Data. How does ASHA compare, *Asha, 35,* 71.

Caccavo, M. T. (1992, Winter). Survey of audiologists. Feedback. *Academy of Dispensing Audiologists, 3,* 18.

Carhart, R. (1976). Introduction. *Amplification for the hearing impaired* (3rd ed.). New York: Grune & Stratton, Inc.

Council of Graduate Programs in Communication Sciences and Disorders. (April, 1993). *Proceedings.* Minneapolis, MN: Author.

Council of Graduate Schools in the United States. (1971). *The doctor's degree in professional fields. A statement by the Association of Graduate Schools in the Association of American Universities and the Council of Graduate Schools in the United States.* Washington, DC: Author.

Council of Graduate Schools in the United States. (1990). *The Doctor of Philosophy degree.* Washington, DC: Author.

Curtis, J. F. (1984). An emeritus looks at graduate education. *Proceedings of the Fifth Annual Conference on Graduate Education* (pp. 9–17). Minneapolis, MN: Council of Graduate Programs in Communication Sciences and Disorders.

Decker, T. N. (1990). Academic freedom. *Audiology Today, 2,* 8.

Educational Testing Service. (1991). *NTE programs: Interpreting NTE specialty area test scores, 1991–92.* Princeton, NJ: Author.

Ehrlich, C. H., Merton, K., Sweetman, R. H., & Arnold, C. (1983). Training issues—Graduate student externship. *Asha, 25–28.*

Engleman, L. (1992). Satisfaction, respect and income in audiology practice. *Audiology Today, 4,* 23–25.

Feldman, A. S. (1981). The challenge of autonomy [Presidential Address]. *Asha, 23,* 941-945.

Feldman, A. S. (1984). In support of the professional doctorate. *Asha 26,* 24–32.

Feldman, A. S. (1989). The professional doctorate: Wishing doesn't make it so. *Asha, 31,* 51–52.

Flower, R. (1985). ASHA standards: Where we've come from, where we're at, prospects for the future. In *Proceedings of the Sixth Annual Conference on Graduate Education* (pp. 1–9). Minneapolis: Council of Graduate Programs in Communication Sciences and Disorders.

Flower, R. (1987). The future of accreditation and ESB standards: Myth or reality? In *Proceedings of the Eighth Annual Conference on Graduate Education* (pp. 30–33). Minneapolis, MN: Council of Graduate Programs in Communication Sciences and Disorders.

Fowler, C. G., & Wilson, R. H. (1989). More degrees, but no more degrees. *Audiology Today, 1,* 22–23.

Goldstein, D. (1989). The AuD degree: The doctoring degree in audiology. *Asha, 31,* 33–35.

Jerger, S. (1989). Doctoring of the audiology degree. *Audiology Today, 1,* 20–21.

Lingwall, J. (1988a). Evaluation of the requirements for the certificate of clinical competence in speech-language pathology and audiology. *Asha, 30*, 75–78.

Lingwall, J. (1988b). *Professional domains, knowledges and skills in the practice of speech-language pathology and audiology.* Unpublished report. Rockville, MD: American Speech-Language-Hearing Association.

Loavenbruck, A. (1983). How may we better prepare clinicians for the reality of providing services to the communicatively disordered in a variety of settings? *ASHA Reports, 13*, 52–57.

Lovrinic, J. (1991). Focus. *Asha, 34*, 15.

Lynn, D., & Loavenbruck, A. (1991). Autonomy: The road directly to the public. *Asha, 33*, 41–43.

Miller, M., & Deutsch , L. (1983). Future directions in audiology. *Asha, 25*, 39–42.

Oyer, H. J. (1990). Professional/academic degree. *Audiology Today, 2*, 11–13.

Oyler, R. F., & Matkin, N. (1987). National Survey of Educational Preparation in Pediatric Audiology, *Asha, 29*, 27–31.

Saxman, J. H. (1989). A celebration of the tenth anniversary: Where have we been and where are we going? In *Proceedings of the Tenth Annual Conference on Graduate Education* (pp. 17–26). Minneapolis: Council of Graduate Programs in Communication Sciences and Disorders.

Speaks, C. (1989). *Standards Council notes, 10/23/89.* ASHA Council on Professional Standards.

Spriestersbach, D. C. (1976, April). *Doctoral programs: Patterns for change.* Paper presented at the Conference of the Big-Ten University Programs in Speech Pathology and Audiology, Chicago, IL.

Spriestersbach, D. C. (1989). Professional education and communication disorders. *Asha, 31*, 77–78.

Spriestersbach, D. C. (1991). The professional doctorate: Consensus and controversy. *Audiology Today, 3*, 24.

Thurgood, D. H., & Weinman, J. M. (1990). *Summary report 1989. Doctorate recipients from U.S. universities.* Washington, DC: National Academy Press, 15–17.

Van Vliet, D., Berkey, D., Marion, M., & Robinson, M. (1992). A survey of California audiologists' attitudes towards professional education in audiology. *Asha, 34*, 185.

■ INDEX ■